£2

THE TEMPLE OF PERFECTION

THE TEMPLE OF PERFECTION

A HISTORY OF THE GYM

ERIC CHALINE

REAKTION BOOKS

Published by Reaktion Books Ltd
33 Great Sutton Street
London EC1V 0DX, UK

www.reaktionbooks.co.uk

First published 2015

Printed and bound in Great Britain
by TJ International, Padstow, Cornwall

A catalogue record for this book is available from the British Library

ISBN 978 1 78023 449 6

CONTENTS

INTRODUCTION

The gymnasium's 2,800-year history places it among the oldest human institutions: it predates the foundation of the Christian church by eight centuries and of representative parliamentary democracy by 2,500 years. Its history, however, is not an unbroken one, and can be divided into four periods: its creation during classical antiquity; a long hiatus until the sixteenth century when, though it had not been forgotten, it had only an academic, medical and literary existence; its re-emergence as a place dedicated to exercise in early nineteenth-century Europe; and finally, its evolution into its modern form in twentieth-century America. For each of these phases, I shall provide a description of the gymnasium and of the activities performed there, but my principal concern in writing this book goes beyond descriptive history to finding the answers to two questions: why did the gym appear, disappear and then reappear at key moments in human history? And what motivated individuals to go to the gymnasium during each of its incarnations?

Embodying the Social and the Individual

The history of the gymnasium is also a history of the human body: its real and idealized forms, artistic representation, shaping, and public and private presentation. The body, despite its importance to all aspects of individual, social and cultural life, has long been a neglected topic in the social sciences. The study of its workings and mechanical uses has been entrusted to biology, medicine and sports science, and of its representation to the arts and art history. However, in the past decade more prominence has been given to the idea of 'embodiment', that is, the psychological, social, cultural and political significance of the body. The body, how it is interpreted, represented, used, shaped and presented in private and public, plays a central role in the transformation of abstract social discourses into lived actions and identities. How the body is interpreted and functions has changed with both historical period and culture. A simple but extreme example of different forms of embodiment is to contrast the representation of the naked human form in classical Greek art with the absolute prohibition of human representation in Islam. Between these two extremes of uncensored display and complete absence, there are many gradations of style and meaning. In addition, I would ask the reader to consider whether the statue of a naked fifth-century BCE Greek athlete in situ at Athens or Olympia conveyed the same social meaning as a first-century CE copy of the same work made to adorn a Roman palace, or a nineteenth-century plaster cast exhibited in a European or American museum. Although the statues are identical, their social contexts are completely different, as are the attitudes and backgrounds of those viewing them. An identical representation of the body can have completely different meanings depending on its historical and social context.

The body is the physical embodiment of an individual human being and the physical expression of identity. Although the basic blueprint of the body – height, skin tone, and eye and hair colour – is determined by an individual's genetic make-up, the actual expression of the genome as an individual's body shape, body composition, body-weight, muscularity, strength, health and overall physical fitness is a function of lifestyle and diet. These factors are themselves dependent on social factors such as status and occupation and other social constructs regulating appearance, grooming and physical fitness. During human prehistory, physical fitness and strength were necessary for survival; the body was shaped by the activities that it was expected to perform: hunting, gathering and travelling. With the advent of urban civilization, the shape of the body became a function of the job one did and one's position in society. Recent decades have seen the phasing out of most forms of heavy manual labour in the developed world, and social class rather than occupation has become the most likely determinant for physical appearance and physical fitness. In a reversal of what has happened for most of human history, when the poorer members of society were likely to be underweight and the wealthy to be overweight, in the developed world, it is now the economically most disadvantaged who are likely to be obese and the wealthy who are likely to be slim. Individual embodiment can be expressed in a number of impermanent and permanent ways. The former includes grooming, style of clothing and the wearing of jewellery and accessories, and the latter body decoration such as tattooing, scarification and piercing. While these methods affect the surface of the body, until the advent of advanced cosmetic surgery and the invention of surgical implants, physical exercise was the only proven method that could alter the shape of the human body.

Transformative Training

The gymnasium is the place where the body is transformed through physical practices, specifically different forms of exercise. For the purposes of this book I have divided gym-based exercise into four types of training: 'functional', 'therapeutic', 'aesthetic' and 'alternative'. To begin with the two types that are most familiar to the patrons of a contemporary gym, aesthetic training is designed to alter the shape of the body by increasing muscle mass and/or decreasing body fat. Traditionally this is achieved through a combination of weight training and cardiovascular exercise. Therapeutic training, while it might employ the same methods as aesthetic training, targets one or more aspects of the health of the individual, with the aesthetic effect as a by-product.

Functional training is specifically designed to develop skills for another field of physical activity, such as exercises designed for military training. Many athletic events were designed as forms of armed and unarmed combat training in the age before the dominance of gun-powder weapons on the battlefield. Functional training can also include what is known as 'assistance' or 'complementary' exercises for athletes – for example, weight training exercises that train muscle groups, skills or movements used in a specific sport. Functional training has also recently come into use to describe exercises performed in a gym that do not involve classical bodybuilding exercises with weights or cardiovascular training on aerobic exercisers, and which increase strength and stamina through the use of other types of equipment and bodyweight exercises and movements. This modern take on functional training goes beyond reshaping the surface of the body to developing new abilities and skills, bringing gym-based training back to its origins, when training for function was the primary motivation.

Alternative training describes those forms of exercise imported into the gym from other physical disciplines or non-Western fitness cultures, and either performed in their original forms or adapted to meet the fitness requirements of the modern exerciser. They are alternative because they might be designed to develop skills not associated with mainstream Western exercise that is usually practised in a gym. My definition includes non-Western exercise systems such as yoga and the martial arts, as well as disciplines such as classical dance, boxing and Pilates, which can be found on the group exercise-class schedules of most modern gyms.

Yoga and the East Asian martial arts are also alternative because they are based on theories of physical fitness that are completely different from those of science-based Western medicine. Although yoga brings students many physical benefits, especially in terms of flexibility, posture, balance and coordination, its claims to promote spiritual growth and well-being are a matter of faith, as they are based on the existence of subtle energies in the body for which there is no scientific evidence. There is naturally a considerable overlap in the four types of training outlined above. In a sense, all gym-based training is aesthetic, because it will change a person's appearance; therapeutic, because it is likely to have an effect on their state of health; functional, because improved strength and endurance can be applied in other areas of life; and even alternative, as it may develop skills that are not usually included in the conventional canon of Western fitness.

Converts and Entertainers

In the ancient world, gymnasia were often associated with sacred precincts dedicated to heroes, demigods and gods, and many of the practices connected with them played an important role in the religious life of the pagan *polis*, or city-state. At Olympia, the quadrennial men's games were held in honour of Zeus (Roman: Jupiter), and a separate women's competition in honour of his consort, the goddess Hera (Roman: Juno). The local festivals that were dedicated to the patron god or goddess of each polis also included athletic events for which men trained in the city's public gymnasia. In addition to these grand communal celebrations, there was a more individual association between religion, athletics and the gymnasium. In classical Greece, physical beauty had moral and spiritual dimensions: a beautiful man or woman was held to be morally superior and was compared to Apollo or Aphrodite (Roman: Venus), sharing in their divinity.

Readers might think that it would be stretching the argument a little too far to argue that in the modern period, in parts of the developed world where participation in organized religion has decreased, people go to the gym with the regularity and zeal they once reserved for attending religious services. But if we compare the practices of organized religion and the gym, we can identify many similarities: the faithful of both church and gym travel to a separate building, wear special clothes, eat special food and take part in shared rituals that are performed with complete absorption and dedication. For those for whom religion is no longer a marker of identity, and who do not take part in the social aspects of religious observance, going to the gym fulfils many of the same individual and social needs. The major difference is, of course, that churchgoers polish their eternal souls with a view to attaining happiness everlasting, while gym-goers train their bodies for rewards in the here and now.

Another important aspect of the gymnasium since its creation has been its close links to entertainment, either because it was a place where people came to watch athletes train and compete, or because the men and women who helped to create and define it had once been performers, or would use the physical attributes that they developed in the gym to become performers. In classical Greece, men went to the gymnasium to exercise, and also quite unashamedly to admire the bodies of other men and boys. This practice was carried over into the gymnasia of the nineteenth century, which were equipped with viewing galleries for spectators. This is not entirely surprising, because the first commercial gymnasium entrepreneurs were performers, a tradition that has continued into the modern period, when competitive bodybuilders have made the transition from the weights room to the big and small screens.

Fit for Purpose

Finally, any study of the gym must include a discussion of the meaning of fitness. Asked to define fitness, we might come up with a list of physical characteristics, capacities and abilities, but, in fact, there is no generally agreed definition of fitness. There are medically sanctioned physiological descriptions of the desirable functionality of our bodies' musculature, joints and cardiovascular systems at different life stages, as well as tables of ideal weight and height based on statistical averages, and formulae used to measure body composition that set the recommended ratio of lean muscle mass to body fat. In addition, there are definitions of fitness produced by public and private health management organizations (HMOs), by the fitness industry and sporting bodies, as well as definitions of dubious provenance crafted by health-and-fitness gurus to encourage you to buy their exercise books and DVDs. However, the truth is that given the genetic diversity of humans these can only ever be general guidelines rather than exact prescriptions. Two of the leading institutions advising the public on health and fitness and exercise in the U.S., the President's Council on Fitness, Sports and Nutrition and the American Council on Exercise, do not even attempt to provide simple definitions of fitness. The former, for example, lists twenty areas that it considers to be integral parts of physical fitness.[1] Until each of us gets a copy of our personal genome indicating our physical strengths and weaknesses, and highlighting specific health issues that we need to address through lifestyle choices, what we do to maintain our physical fitness is a matter of personal choice, and for many in the present day, that means going to the gym.

The original meaning of fitness, however, was 'fit for purpose'. Here we have the additional dimensions of for what and whose purpose? The ancient gymnasium was a state-sponsored institution with wide-ranging functions in addition to the physical training of its members. In this phase of its development the official purpose of the gymnasium was to create citizens and soldiers fit for the purposes of the *polis*. At the same time, because the government of the city-state was composed of its freeborn male citizens, the gymnasium was central to the pursuit and attainment of an individual's full physical, social, moral and intellectual potential, known to the ancient Greeks as *arete*. When we reach the genesis of the modern gymnasium in the institutions of the late eighteenth and early nineteenth centuries, the nation-state as the main sponsor implies that what was fit for purpose coincided more closely with the aims of the state rather than any individual motivation. It was only when the gymnasium became a commercial enterprise that was independent of the state that the relative importance of state and individual fitness for purpose became more balanced. However, even in the modern period, when the reader might think that going to the gym is entirely a personal choice, the state still retains considerable influence in defining why and how people choose to exercise.

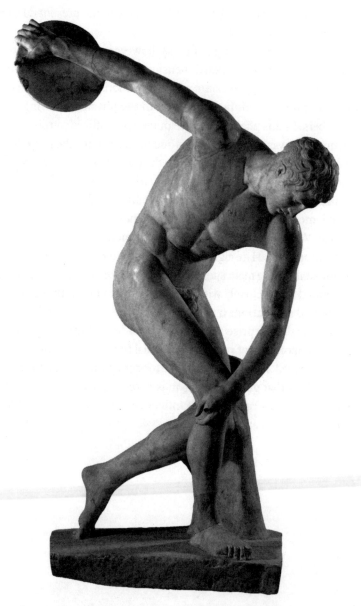

The 'Townley Discobolus' – discus thrower – embodies the classical Greek ideal of masculine beauty. The youthful athlete's lean, muscular physique has been honed in the gymnasium for the sporting arena and battlefield; it remains the basis of contemporary Western constructs of male fitness and attractiveness. Second-century Roman marble copy of a 5th-century BCE Greek bronze original by Myron (c. 480–440 BCE).

1

THE PURSUIT OF *ARETE*

You met my son coming from the bath after the gymnasium and you
neither spoke to him, nor kissed him, nor took him with you, nor ever
once felt his balls. Would anyone call you an old friend of mine?

Aristophanes, *The Birds*

Modernity's greatest debt to the ancient world is not to the Roman
Empire but to ancient Greece, and more specifically to the
polis (city-state) of Athens during its classical Golden Age, which
began at the end of the sixth century BCE with the emergence of the
city's democratic institutions and ended with the establishment of
Macedonian hegemony at the end of the fourth century BCE. Although
the Romans conquered and civilized regions of northern Europe
where few classical Greeks ever ventured, much of what was salvaged,
studied and admired from antiquity during the medieval and early
modern periods was Greek and not Roman, though a great deal of
it was transmitted through Latin sources. Our debt to the ancient Greeks
is so great in the fields of the arts, architecture, politics, philosophy,
mathematics, the applied sciences and, from the highly specialized
viewpoint of this book, of sporting and athletics cultures, that it would
be easy to imagine that they were not very different from contemporary
Westerners. This false sense of closeness has been fostered by decades
of sword-and-sandal epics, and by recent television and film portrayals
of ancient Greeks both historical and fictional, including Kevin
Sorbo's 'buff-bodybuilder' Herakles in *Hercules: The Legendary Journeys*
(1995–9); Brad Pitt's 'Californian-surfer-dude' Achilles in *Troy* (2004),
Hollywood's version of Homer's *Iliad* (mid-eighth century BCE); and

Gerard Butler's 'U.S.-marine-at-war-with-Iran' Leonidas (d. 480 BCE), king of Sparta, in 300 (2007) – three actors who have clearly spent time in the gym. However, the crucial fact that we must remember about the classical Greeks is that they are separated from us by a historical gulf of two and a half millennia.

A second possible cause of chronological confusion for the modern reader can be blamed on the classical Greeks themselves. They felt a direct kinship with the heroes in Homer's epic poems – Agamemnon, Paris, Achilles and Odysseus – whom they took to be historical figures. Modern scholarship, however, rejects the historicity of the characters and events described in the *Iliad* and *Odyssey* (both composed in the mid-eighth century BCE) and the Mycenaean Greeks, who are thought to be the 'Achaeans' who besieged and took Troy during the thirteenth century BCE, belonged to a different cultural tradition, spoke a different language and used a different alphabet from the classical Greeks, from whom they were separated by seven centuries. Ignoring this prolonged cultural break, the classical Greeks sought the origin of many of their institutions, including their gymnasia and sporting and athletics cultures, in the stories told in Homeric epics and in the myths and legends that underpinned their religious beliefs.

The Lands of Greater Greece

The classical Greeks were great explorers, navigators and merchants, but their journeys were confined to the Mediterranean and Black seas. Perennially short of land for their growing populations, the city-states of Greece founded colonies and trading posts east in Asia Minor (now Turkey) and on the coasts of the Black Sea, south in present-day Libya, and west in Sicily and southern Italy (known as *Megale Hellas* in Greek, *Magna Graecia* in Latin, meaning 'Greater Greece'), with outposts as far west as southern France and Spain. Wherever they settled, they brought their institutions and customs, including gymnasia and religious celebrations that featured athletic contests. Because they could trace their descent from the Hellenes of mainland Greece, these 'greater Greeks' were allowed to compete in all Pan-Hellenic competitions, and one of antiquity's greatest athletes, the wrestler Milo of Croton (*fl.* sixth century BCE), was a citizen of an Achaean colony in southern Italy.

Unlike the Macedonians and Romans who followed them, the classical Greeks were not conquerors and colonizers who established vast territorial empires. Even when they were the dominant power in the Mediterranean, their empires were commercial rather than territorial, and their 'leagues' – alliances of city-states – were short-lived. The most important thing to remember about the geopolitics of classical Greece is that its many polities only united when their survival was threatened by *barbaroi* (barbarians – in other words, all non-Hellenes), but their bitterest rivals and most vindictive adversaries were not the Persians, Macedonians or Romans, but fellow Greeks. The defining rivalry of the classical period was that between democratic Athens and oligarchic Sparta – a contest that was played out on the battlefield during the Peloponnesian War (431–404 BCE), and at great Pan-Hellenic sporting events such as the Olympic Games.

The disastrous war between Athens and Sparta allowed the Macedonians, a people from the northern fringes of the Greek world, whom many Greeks considered to be semi-barbarians, to conquer and unite the whole of Greece under Philip II (382–336 BCE). But it was his son, Alexander III (356–323 BCE), known to us simply as Alexander the Great, who conquered the Persian Empire, establishing the dominance of Hellenistic culture from the Mediterranean to the Indian subcontinent. As he travelled east, Alexander established permanent colonies of Macedonian and Greek veterans who intermarried with the local population. These foundations, which often bore his name, were modelled on Greek cities and were furnished with all the amenities that Greek citizens were accustomed to, including gymnasia.[1]

Gymnasion

The 1,170-year period covered by this chapter begins during Greece's archaic period (800–508 BCE). Although there is no archaeological evidence for gymnasia in the eighth century BCE, the year 776 BCE – the date I have chosen to start my history of the gymnasium – coincides with the first ancient Olympiad, held at the Pan-Hellenic sanctuary of Olympia in southern Greece. And while the programme of the first games featured only a single foot race, the occasion of such a major national contest implies the existence of some kind of training facilities – proto-gymnasia – however basic, where athletes could prepare for the competition in their home cities and in Olympia. We have some corroborating literary evidence for sporting competitions in the Iliad, which, though purporting to be an historical account of events that took place during the Greek Bronze Age (c. 1900–1100 BCE), is widely believed to describe much later athletics practices. In Book XXIII, Homer describes the funeral games held in honour of Patroklos (Patroclus), companion, and some say one-time lover, of Achilles, which included a very martial line-up of events, including foot and chariot races, the javelin and iron weight shot put, wrestling and boxing.[2] The martial nature of the events demonstrates that ancient Greek sporting competitions had their origin in functional military training. However, there is no mention in the Homeric epics of specific buildings set aside for exercise.

The first documentary evidence for gymnasia dates from the sixth century BCE, but the earliest surviving archaeological remains are from the late classical and Hellenistic periods, and the interpretation of the archaeology is further complicated by the many alterations and additions made during later periods. The Romans followed the Macedonians as the overlords of the Greek world, starting with their conquest of Megale Hellas in 275 BCE, and of Greece and the Aegean islands in 133 BCE. Although Greece and the Hellenistic kingdoms of Egypt and the Near East became Roman provinces, they never lost their Greek cultural identities. The Pan-Hellenic games and pagan festivals continued to be staged, albeit with new Roman imperial sponsors, and the gymnasia remained open.

What brought an end to the athletics culture of classical antiquity was not the coming of the Macedonians or Romans, but the decision of Constantine the Great (272–337 CE) to stop the persecution of Christianity in 313 CE. In 330 CE he founded a magnificent new capital in the east, Constantinople (formerly the Greek colony of Byzantium), which, though a majority Greek city, did not have public gymnasia. It was left to one of his successors, Emperor Theodosius I, the Great

(347–395 CE), to complete the Christianization of the empire when he closed all pagan temples and abolished the Olympic Games and all other festivals that featured athletics contests in the year 394 or 393 CE. The abolition of sporting competition made the infrastructure of gymnasia redundant, although a few survived as part of Roman bathhouses, until they, too, were closed, as remnants of a decadent pagan past out of tune with the new Christian morality.

Imagining the Ancient Gymnasium

Although every major classical Greek city had several gymnasia and *palaestrae* (Greek: *palaistrai*), we have no detailed description of their appearance, layout or facilities from the classical period. It is likely that gymnasia were so familiar that no chronicler of the time thought it necessary to describe them in detail. In reconstructing the appearance of ancient gymnasia, historians and archaeologists have used several sources. First, archaeological remains have been excavated across the Greek world, the majority of which date from the Hellenistic period, with Roman additions and restorations, giving us only partial or conjectural physical evidence for earlier classical gymnasia. Second, though we do not have descriptions of gymnasia from the classical period, we do have many references to them in period texts – poetry, prose and drama, such as the philosophical treatises and dialogues of Plato (424–348 BCE) and Xenophon (430–354 BCE), and the plays of Aristophanes (c. 446–386 BCE) and Euripides (480–406 BCE). We also have records of the regulations governing the management, staffing and funding of several ancient gymnasia. The best-known gymnasia of antiquity, for which we have many references in classical texts, are the three main public gymnasia of Athens: the Akademia (Academy), Lykeion (Lyceum) and Kinosarges (Cynosarges). The remains of both the Akademia and the Lykeion were discovered during construction work in Athens, confirming the existence of buildings at both sites. Unfortunately the available archaeological evidence does not allow us to reconstruct their exact appearance, layout or facilities during the classical period, as both sites were greatly altered during later periods.

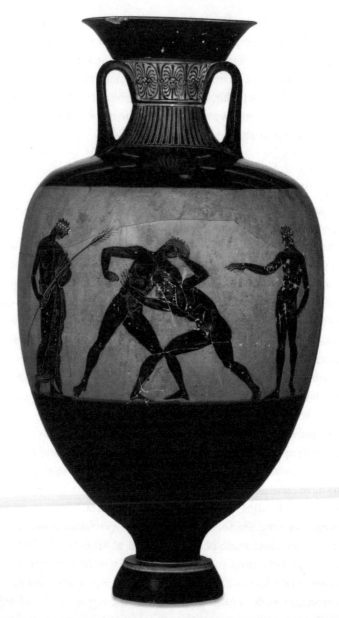

Sporting competition defined a Greek man's local, national and cultural identities. Though glory was the only prize awarded at the four Pan-Hellenic games, city competitions rewarded victorious athletes with valuable prizes, such as this Athenian Panathenaic prize amphora showing two wrestlers and a judge signed 'by Kittos', c. 367–6 BCE, which would have been filled with costly olive oil.

Third, Ancient Greek art is rich in depictions of athletic and sporting themes. Although many Greek statues, especially bronzes, have been lost, we have marble Roman copies of Greek originals. But perhaps the most numerous and revealing pictorial sources are the decorated ceramics of the classical period, which show scenes of sporting competition and training in the gymnasium. The conventions of Greek vase painting mean that the buildings are rarely represented, but we have visual clues and occasional textual references that give the context of the scenes depicted on ceramic objects. Fourth and finally, we have one complete description of a Greek gymnasium in *De Architectura* (c. 27 BCE) by the Roman architect and engineer Vitruvius (fl. first century BCE).[3] Archaeologists believe that he based his description on the Hellenistic gymnasium and *palaestra* at Olympia, whose ruins can be still be visited today.

As with the gyms of today, classical gymnasia did not follow a standardized plan. They shared a basic number of facilities, but their size and layout were affected by their date of construction, the wealth of the city, the geography of the site and the available space and proximity of nearby buildings. Examples of different configurations can be seen at two of the mainland Greek sites that hosted Pan-Hellenic contests: the city of Delphi, home of the Pythian Games, and the sanctuary of Olympia, the site of the ancient Olympic Games. During the classical period, Olympia was not a city but a sacred site with temples and shrines visited by pilgrims, and home of the stadium used for the quadrennial Olympic Games that were held to honour the father of the gods, Olympian Zeus, and of a separate women's games held in honour of his consort Hera. The sanctuary is built on a plain near a river with ample room for athletics facilities. In contrast, Delphi is built on the slopes of Mount Parnassus, which forced the city fathers to lay out the athletics and sporting facilities on several levels, with the stadium on a separate, spectacular mountaintop site. Delphi is believed to have the remains of the oldest surviving Greek gymnasium, with features dating from the late fourth century BCE, but here, too, there were many later additions and restorations.

The Origins of Ancient Greek Athletics

Although we do not have any documentary evidence for the existence of public and private gymnasia in Greece before the sixth century BCE, the existence of Pan-Hellenic contests from the eighth century onwards makes it likely that competitors would have had training facilities of some kind. This raises the question of whether classical Greek athletics culture and gymnasia had antecedents in the Aegean or elsewhere in the eastern Mediterranean.[4] The Aegean experienced a first flowering of urban civilization in the second millennium BCE in mainland Greece, the Aegean islands and Crete. The Mycenaean and Minoan elites lived in palace cities and left behind a rich artistic legacy, including many representations of an activity usually described as 'bull leaping', in which athletes are shown vaulting over charging bulls. Unfortunately, we do not know whether this practice was a religious ritual, a rite of passage or a spectator sport (or all three). But the practice is possibly linked to the Greek myth of the Minotaur, the monstrous half-man, half-bull, who fed on human flesh and died at the hands of the mythical hero and king of Athens, Theseus, who was honoured as one of the founders of the Olympic Games. The only documentary evidence for Mycenaean athletics culture is found in Homer. However, as Mark Golden and others have pointed out, the *Iliad*, while describing events that were supposed to have taken place during the Bronze Age, contains many anachronistic elements, and it is likely that the practices it describes are more representative of the eighth rather than the twelfth or thirteenth centuries BCE.

When we turn to examine the possible influence of neighbouring cultures in the eastern Mediterranean, Near East and Africa, we can discount the Hittites of Anatolia, whose culture vanished during a cataclysmic event known as the Bronze Age Collapse (c. 1250–1200 BCE), which took place several centuries before the archaic renaissance in Greece four centuries later. The only other civilization in the region with a well-developed athletics culture was ancient Egypt, whose tomb paintings depict riding, swimming, ball games, wrestling, stick fighting, archery and boxing. However, these were practised as leisure pursuits and for functional military training, and the Egyptians never valued or developed competitive sports in the same way as the classical Greeks. Sport, therefore, is a unique, significant and distinguishing characteristic of classical Greek culture that sets it apart from contemporary cultures in a way that neither religion nor warfare could do. If we follow Golden's argument to its logical conclusion, it is athletic competition and its related infrastructure of gymnasia that made Greek culture so distinctive.[5]

Although classical Greece produced the world's first historians, when they had little or no historical evidence to explain the origin of an event or institution, they fell back on mythological accounts. For example, one tradition ascribed the foundation of the Olympic Games to Herakles, another to King Theseus. Various ancient sources, including the Greek historian and travelogue writer Pausanias (fl. second century CE) and the Graeco-Roman physician Galen (129–c. 199 CE), cited differing explanations for the origins of gymnastics and gymnasia that combine historical fact with legend. The most trustworthy ancient sources suggested that gymnasia existed in many Greek cities during the lifetime of the Athenian statesman and lawmaker Solon (c. 638–558 BCE), as he referred to their management in his laws, and that they had become an established part of daily life by the time of the founder of Athenian democracy, Kleisthenes (b. c. 570 BCE).

Before Athens had gymnasia and other purpose-built athletics facilities, athletes trained in any available open space and competed in the Agora – the large open area that functioned as the city's main square and marketplace at the foot of the Acropolis, where the remains of a running track and starting blocks can still be seen. But as the city grew larger and its most important civic festival, the Panathenaia, which included a full programme of athletic events, became grander and more popular, it became necessary to provide both a stadium for the competition and training facilities for athletes. The tyrant Peisistratos (d. c. 527 BCE) set aside the sacred grove dedicated to the hero Akademos (or Hekademos), which became known as the Akademia, as the first public gymnasium for the freeborn male citizens of Athens, though at this date it was probably just an open-air training area without much in the way of buildings or facilities. His heirs and their democratic successors further developed the Akademia and founded the other two public gymnasia of the city.[6]

The Naked Greek

The ancient Greeks trained and competed naked (Greek: *gymnos*). Exercise and male nudity were so closely linked that the Greek verb 'to exercise', *gymnazein*, translates literally as 'to exercise naked', and the word *gymnasion*, from which we derive the words gymnasium and the abbreviation gym, as 'a place where athletic exercises are performed naked'. There are several stories, as well as several versions of the same story, that explain how the Greeks came to train and compete in the nude. According to Christopher Hallett, the earliest date given for an athlete competing naked is 720 BCE, when a Spartan runner called Akanthos, who was taking part in the fifteenth Olympiad, ran the foot race naked after his *perizoma* (loincloth) slipped off. Another contender for the title of the first naked competitor is Orsippos from the city of Megara.[7]

In both cases there is a debate as to what happened after the mishap: the athlete either won his race, demonstrating that an athlete unencumbered by a loincloth could run faster, leading other athletes to imitate his example; alternatively, he tripped, fell and died of his injuries, and thereafter athletes were allowed to compete naked to avoid future fatalities. The Greek historian Thucydides (c. 460–c. 395 BCE) is one of several ancient authorities who placed the origin of the custom much later, in the fifth century BCE. A Spartan connection does make a certain amount of sense, as in ancient times they were reputed for their physical fitness and toughness. Their offspring's rigorous training programme began at the age of seven, and they were also reputed to be the only Hellenic people who encouraged their daughters to train alongside their sons, though not naked but with their breasts exposed. Outside Sparta, women were banned from training in gymnasia and from competing alongside men at the Pan-Hellenic games or even watching male sporting competitions.

Although the patrons of gymnasia, like athletes, trained naked, they were not completely uncovered or unprotected. Before his training

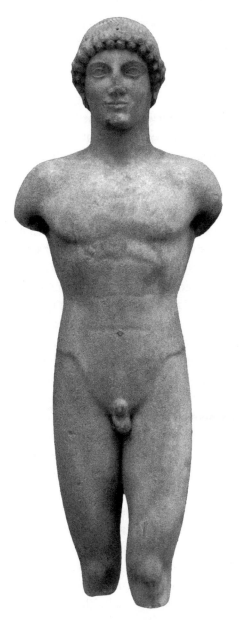

In classical Greece, male nudity was no mere sculptural convention, as it would be in later periods. Greek men and boys were expected to be naked when they trained at the gymnasium, as well as during religious festivals, social events and sporting competitions. The 'Strangford Apollo', Greek statue of a naked standing youth, *kouroi*, in Parian marble, *c*. 490 BCE.

session the naked athlete would be anointed with olive oil. According to Pliny the Elder (23–79 CE), 'Olive oil by nature makes the body warm and protects against the cold, and also cools the head when heated.'[8] He then moved to another room in the gymnasium where, according to Philostratos (c. 170–250 CE), he could choose between several kinds of dust that were supposed to have different physiological effects: clay disinfected and prevented excessive sweat; terracotta opened the pores, thereby promoting perspiration; and asphalt was heating.[9] In order to understand why the Greeks and Romans were so concerned with exactly the right amount of sweat during exercise, as well as with the 'heat' and 'coolness' of the body, we have to examine the basis of their medical system. In *The Greatest Benefit to Mankind* (1997), medical historian Dr Roy Porter explains that by the classical period, Greek doctors had abandoned the supernatural origin of disease caused by gods or demons. Hippocrates (c. 460–377 BCE) promoted a natural theory of disease, but ignorant of the micro-organisms that cause infectious diseases, he believed that ill health was caused by an imbalance of the four bodily fluids, or *chymoi*, the 'humours' of pre-modern Western medicine: blood, yellow bile, black bile and phlegm, associated with heat, dry, cold and wet, and with a specific temperament.[10] In order to treat disease, the doctors of the Hippocratic school prescribed dietary regulation and exercise, establishing a link between health and the gymnasium that has endured for more than two and a half millennia. The Roman physician Galen further refined the Hippocratic system, and his work remained a medical set text until the nineteenth century. Therefore, according to the medical knowledge of the day, the athlete, though naked, was not unprotected from the elements or disease through the application of a coating of olive oil and dust.

The finishing touch to the athlete's outfit before proceeding to the gymnasium, running track or stadium was the *kynodesme*, which translates literally as a 'dog lead'. The ancient Greek slang for a man's penis was his 'dog'. The *kynodesme* was a leather thong that was tied to the end of the foreskin and either secured to a waistband or tied to the base of the penis, curling the penis back on itself. Although this would prevent the male member from flopping around

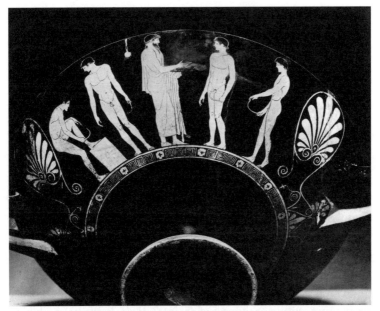

A group of young athletes use a metal *stlengis* (strigil) to scrape off the coating of oil, sweat and dirt that has accumulated on their bodies during exercise, prior to bathing. The scrapings were not discarded but were considered a valuable medical commodity. Attic cup, *c.* 460 BCE.

during training and competition, it left the scrotum unsecured and exposed. It could be that the *kynodesme* had more of an aesthetic than a practical function. The Greeks, unlike the moderns, though they greatly admired the naked male form, did not prize large, visibly displayed genitalia. As anyone visiting the Greek gallery of a museum can testify, the statues of naked athletes, heroes, demigods and gods, while they have very well-developed physiques, have comparatively small genitalia.

After exercising, the coating of dust, sweat and oil was scraped off the skin with a curved metal scraper known as a *stlengis* (the strigil of the Romans). The scrapings were not discarded, as they were believed to have therapeutic properties, and this unappetizing product was probably a profitable sideline for the employees of the gymnasia charged with cleaning and massaging exercisers after their workouts. Once scraped clean of oil, sweat and dust, the exerciser proceeded to the bath, which in the classical period would have consisted of cold water carried or piped into a stone basin, raised tub or small communal pool. It is only during the Roman period that furnaces to heat water and warm rooms would have been installed at Greek gymnasia.

Before we discuss why the ancient Greeks trained and competed naked, we have to be absolutely sure that this was the case. The male nude is a constant theme of ancient Greek art from the archaic period until late antiquity. Artistic representations, however, do not necessarily imply an accurate reflection of social practices. In the nineteenth century, for example, sculptors adorned Britain's buildings, monuments and public spaces with heroic marble and bronze nudes while concurrently even modest displays of bare flesh were hedged with complex moral, social and legal restrictions. Were future social scientists to base their interpretations of attitudes in our own time to male and female nudity on the advertisements for a range of consumer goods from underwear to car tyres, they might conclude that public nudity was a common and accepted feature of urban life in the early twenty-first century. In the case of ancient Greece, however, in addition to the many pictorial and sculptural representations of male nudity, we have written evidence from classical Greek, Hellenistic and Roman sources that confirms that the Greeks had very different attitudes to the practice and representation of public nudity from other ancient peoples. Greek men, and I must stress that our discussion deals almost exclusively with males (with the exception of Sparta), did not live their lives naked, but when it was deemed appropriate, they dispensed with clothing, and even when dressed did not seem overly concerned with preserving their modesty by making sure their genitalia remained covered at all times. Clothing in classical Greece was very basic. Men wore the *chiton* or *exomis*, two variations on the tunic, under the *chlamys* or *himation* – short and long cape- or shawl-like garments, which could also be worn without underclothing. Unlike peoples who use minimal clothing or dispense with it altogether because of climate, the Greeks did not go naked simply as a response to warm weather. Anyone who has been to Greece in the winter will know that cold weather and snow are not uncommon even in low-lying coastal regions. Men and boys chose or were expected to be naked under certain circumstances. In addition to when exercising and competing in athletics, they were naked during certain religious ceremonies, social events and public performances.

There is no evidence for this relaxed attitude to male nudity in the Bronze Age cultures of Mycenaean Greece and Minoan Crete. In the *Iliad*, when Achilles defeats and kills the Trojan Prince Hector in single combat, he dishonours the dead man by stripping his corpse and dragging it naked from his chariot around the walls of the besieged city. In other ancient cultures nakedness was usually associated with criminals, slaves and defeated enemies. In the bas-reliefs of Mesopotamia, Egypt and Assyria, nudity indicated a low or complete loss of social status. In contrast, clothing, accessories and headgear expressed royal and divine status. The Greeks were exceptional in representing their kings and gods as idealized naked humans. However, even in ancient Greece, convicted criminals were stripped before being punished or executed, and slaves serving at banquets were naked; hence athletic, heroic and divine nudity presents us with an interesting paradox that needs further explanation.

Although we can be pretty certain that Greek men and boys did exercise and compete naked, we have to explain their reasons for doing so. The answer to this question comes in two parts, and I shall give the first part here, and the second in the section dealing with personal motivations for attending a gymnasium. According to Hallett, the Greeks used athletic or heroic nudity to differentiate themselves from non-Greek barbarians, especially their main enemies during the classical period, the Persians, who attempted and failed to invade Greece twice (in 492–490 BCE and 480–479 BCE). He cites the example of several temple bas-reliefs where naked Greek warriors fight clothed barbarians.[11] In this case nudity does not imply submission or defeat but underlines the heroic element of the scene.

Hallett goes on to identify the mid-fifth century BCE as the period when images of male gods, demigods and heroes became younger and more idealized and were represented naked. The convention continued into the Hellenistic period, when, in imitation of the founder of the Macedonian Empire, Alexander the Great – who awarded himself divine status during his lifetime, claiming to be the son of Zeus – Greek rulers were depicted naked in the guise of Olympian gods and demigods. Hence, exercising and competing naked enabled Greek men to project their national and cultural identities, differentiating themselves from their barbarian neighbours and enemies. Additionally, heroic nude effigies of rulers projected their personal authority, their divine status and their political and military might.

Membership

Thanks to the efficient electronic record-keeping of our own time, we can be pretty certain of the percentage of the population of the developed world with an active gym membership. Unfortunately, we do not have the membership roll of a public gymnasium in the fifth century BCE, and it is unlikely that such a thing ever existed. The Greek world was divided into rival city-states of varying size and power, but they were small compared to modern nation-states, and the men and boys entitled to go to the gymnasium – freeborn male citizens and resident aliens – would have all known one another. Although we cannot give an exact number of members, for the best-known classical polis, Athens, capital of the province of Attica, we can estimate how many people were eligible to go to its public gymnasia. In the classical period Attica had a population of around 500,000, of which 130,000 were freeborn citizens and 70,000 were metoikoi (metics, or freeborn resident aliens) of both genders.[12] The remaining 300,000 were slaves.[13] As only freeborn male citizens and metics were entitled to use publicly funded gymnasia, around 100,000 men and boys, or 20 per cent of the total population, were eligible. Of course, this is a very rough-and-ready calculation, and we would have to exclude boys below the age of seven, who were too young to go to the gym, as well as those who would be unable to attend because of advanced age or physical disability.

Athletes

Unlike the majority of modern gym-goers who engage primarily in aesthetic or therapeutic training, the patrons of ancient Greek gymnasia had other well-defined motivations to exercise. Among the most important was to compete in local and Pan-Hellenic sporting contests. In his survey of ancient Greek sport, Mark Golden explains that competition was built into Greek society, between individuals and city-states. When domination by the Macedonians and Romans made war impossible, this competitive spirit was expressed entirely through athletic contests. During the early Roman period there were 206 city-sponsored sporting contests in addition to the four major Pan-Hellenic games held at Olympia, Delphi, Nemea and Corinth.[14] The Pan-Hellenic games featured both athletic and equestrian events, but the principal sports for which athletes would have trained at the gymnasium under the supervision of professional trainers were running, long jump, wrestling, discus, javelin and *pankration* (a no-holds-barred combination of wrestling and boxing). In addition to these sports, the patrons of gymnasia would have trained for local athletic events such as Athens' *Lampadephoria*, a night-time torch race run from the Akademia to the Acropolis, as well as for displays such as the Pyrrhic dance – a cross between dance and military drill performed by the *epheboi*, young cadets of eighteen to twenty doing their military service, performed naked but wearing items of armour and carrying shields.

To claim, however, that the Greeks engaged in athletics contests because they could no longer fight one another would be a gross over-simplification and incorrect for the archaic and classical periods when sacred truces in force during the Pan-Hellenic games interrupted their many internecine feuds and wars. Another reason the Greeks participated in sport was to differentiate themselves from non-Greeks. During the classical period, non-Greeks were excluded from the four main Pan-Hellenic contests, and in local festivals, such as the Pan-athenaic Games, participation in several events was restricted to men and boys born in the city. Sporting contests, therefore, were used to reinforce a man's local identity as a citizen of a specific city-state, as well as his national identity as a member of the Hellenic race.[15]

As individuals, athletes trained for personal fame, as well as the material rewards that victory in the Pan-Hellenic games would bring. It was not merely glory, laurel wreaths, statues and Pindaric odes that came with victory at the ancient Olympics.[16] Unlike local contests, such as the Panathenaic Games, where the winners won valuable prizes of olive oil in decorated amphorae, there were no prizes awarded at the Pan-Hellenic games; however, the victorious athlete was richly rewarded by his city. Fame and material rewards went hand in hand. Victory in competition brought the athlete an exalted position in his native city, one that elevated him well beyond the status of his fellow citizens and associated him with the gods themselves.[17] But the lifestyles of professional athletes who devoted themselves to training and victory at the Olympic and other Pan-Hellenic games were criticized during the classical period as being unhealthy and extreme, and lacking in the moderation and self-control that were considered part of the contemporary masculine ideal. In *Autolycus*, the Athenian dramatist Euripides has one of his characters say of them, 'Of every evil in the land of Greece there is no worse than the athletic tribe.'[18] However, just as today, the number of elite professional athletes training at gymnasia was small when compared with the total number of men and boys who attended on a regular basis. Hence, while sporting competition was an important motive for attendance, it alone cannot explain why gymnasia were so popular or well attended in the Greek world for more than a millennium.

Schoolboys, Cadets and Philosophers

In the absence of a school system run by the state or religious bodies, public gymnasia and private *palaestrae* provided for the formal education of freeborn boys from the age of seven to fourteen. The curriculum was divided into three parts: academic subjects, music and dance, and athletics. After the age of fourteen, boys dropped the first two to concentrate on athletics in preparation for their two-year military training as *epheboi*, which took place, in part, in the gymnasium.[19] The *epheboi* had their own room in the gymnasium, a cross between a lecture theatre, an indoor training area, a fraternity house and a mess hall. Classical Athens, like all other Greek city-states, was a warrior society, and while the slaves did all the hard labour and menial jobs in the city, mines and fields, freeborn citizens and metics were expected to fight in the city's armies and crew her war galleys. The athletic events for which men and boys trained at the gymnasium were also functional training for war, and there were festival events with an even more martial flavour, such as the mock cavalry battles, races run in the nude but carrying a shield and wearing greaves and helmet.[20]

Gymnasia also provided the closest thing to tertiary education in the ancient world. At first this was informal, with philosophers and sophists visiting the gymnasia to exercise themselves and to lecture to friends and pupils afterwards either in the shelter of the buildings of the gymnasium or under the trees in the parklands that surrounded them. But in the fourth century this became more formal with the establishment of 'schools' at Athens' three public gymnasia: Plato established his school at the Akademia in 386 BCE, forever associating the name 'Academy' with scholarly endeavours; one of Plato's star pupils and the most influential ancient Greek philosopher of the European Middle Ages, Aristotle (384–322 BCE), founded his school at the Lykeion in 355 BCE, whose name is linked to education in Francophone countries where a *lycée* is a secondary or high school; and another major Athenian philosophical school, the Cynics, owe their name to the city's third gymnasium, Kinosarges.[21]

Honouring the Gods

Sporting competition had an important religious function in classical Greek culture. The Pan-Hellenic games were dedicated to major Olympian gods, and local games were held as part of the festival in honour of the city's patron deity. The gymnasia themselves were often built within sacred precincts, as in Athens, Delphi and Olympia. Gymnasia were under the special patronage of the god Hermes (Roman: Mercury), and they had altars and shrines to other gods, demigods and heroes. Hence attendance at the gymnasium could also be interpreted as a religious obligation and observance. Unlike the hybrid animal-human deities of Egypt, the Olympian gods were human in appearance, and although immortal and much more powerful than humans, they were believed to feel the same emotions of love, hatred, lust, envy, joy, anger and jealousy, which motivated their actions, which could be just and fair, or petty and vindictive. Because the gods were so human, the

Greeks felt a direct kinship with them, and there were many myths of gods and goddesses taking mortal lovers and fathering demigods, such as the legendary Herakles, Theseus and Achilles. Through heroic deeds, humans could rival the gods, but this was dangerous, because the gods were vain and jealous, and they delighted in punishing human hubris.

Narcissists

In the preceding sections I examined the social motivations that drew men and boys to the gymnasium. However, while boys, younger men and professional athletes had formal reasons to go to the gymnasium, I also need to account for their continued attendance in later life. Among the more personal reasons why modern gym-goers train, we should not underestimate narcissism – another gift from the ancient Greeks through the myth of Narcissus, the youth who fell in love with his own reflection. The Greeks, who were great admirers of the male form, also trained at the gymnasium to attain an ideal physical appearance. However, this view is not one that is universally shared. In his study of the classical Greek embodiment, Robin Osborne, professor of ancient history at the University of Cambridge, warns us that we must not take for granted that the Greeks made the link between male beauty, a muscular physique and aesthetic training in the gymnasium. He dismisses the idea that the Greeks made a direct connection between exercise and muscularity, or that they saw the statues of athletes, heroes and gods as representations of gymnasium-trained bodies.

Osborne goes on to argue that Greek sculpture and painting do not depict musculature in the same way as Renaissance art, and that the Greeks themselves did not refer to muscularity as a desirable quality but contrasted a body's 'softness' and 'firmness' and stressed its 'articulation'.[22] I disagree with Osborne about the Greek indifference to muscularity. Although archaic nude *kouroi* and depictions of decorated ceramics are highly stylized and lack proper definition of the musculature, classical sculpture also shows several extraordinarily accurate studies of athletes and warriors in a variety of poses. In the case of athletes, they clearly have muscular bodies trained in the gymnasium. One ancient statue, known as the 'Farnese Hercules', discovered in Rome during the Renaissance, depicts the famous hero with an impressive musculature that would not look out of place in a modern bodybuilding competition.

What we can be sure of, from both artistic representations and documentary references, is that the ideal male body was not the same as it is today. In his comedy *The Clouds* (423 BCE), Aristophanes describes the ideal adolescent male body to be gained from regular attendance at the gym: 'A shining breast, a bright skin, big shoulders, a minute tongue, a big rump and a small ham (penis).' Unlike today, when large male genitalia seem to be highly prized, the most admired feature in a manly physique was well-developed buttocks. Regardless of exactly what characteristics they were admired for, Greek men valued physical beauty, and they took part in the equivalent of our own physique and bodybuilding competitions, known as *euandria*, in which they were judged on their physical fitness, strength, beauty and manliness.[23] These were not limited to younger men and boys, but also open to older men. The winners won places of honour in the processions of the festivals in honour of the city's patron deity. For the Greeks, physical beauty was always associated with moral virtue, summed up by the phrase *kalos kagathos* ('beautiful and good'). To quote the French classical historian Robert Flacelière, 'Physical beauty is the "flower of virtue" as though the soul always shaped the body, and a fine body could not be sorted with anything but a fine soul.'[24] Hence, if physical attractiveness was an important motivation for men of all ages to exercise, it is to the gymnasium that we should look, rather than to the stadium – that is, to regular attendance at the gymnasium rather than to sporting competition.[25]

The Love that Dare Speak its Name

The ancient gymnasium (with the exception of Sparta) was an all-male preserve, where men and boys socialized and trained naked, and where there were many opportunities for sexual encounters and more lasting relationships, both sexual and non-sexual. Same-sex relations were undoubtedly a powerful personal motivation for many men's regular attendance at the gymnasium, but it was not just the lure of sexual encounters that drew them there. Historically many cultures have proscribed and persecuted same-sex relations, others have declared them illegal but tolerated them, while a select few, including the elite cultures of medieval Japan, ancient China and ancient Greece, integrated them into their social and educational systems. In Greece they played an important role in the education and socialization of freeborn boys and adolescents, who were taken up by older patrons who were often their sexual partners. However, the nature of these relationships must be qualified. As Michel Foucault points out in The History of Sexuality, we cannot use modern labels and definitions to describe social and sexual practices that had a completely different social and ideological context. The homosexual as a 'separate sexual species', meaning a man who has an identity based on his sexual object choice, is a relatively recent invention, dating back to the late nineteenth century.[26]

Therefore, I have purposely avoided the terms 'gay' and 'homosexual' to describe same-sex relationships between males in ancient Greece because the two terms would be completely anachronistic. 'Homosexual' – itself a strange Greek-Latin hybrid – was coined in the 1860s as part of the medicalization of sexuality, while 'gay' is of even more recent vintage, coming into common use to refer to men whose sexual identity is based on the gender of their partners in the twentieth century. Several authors have used the term 'pederasty', which, though more accurate as same-sex relationships were usually between adult men and adolescents and boys, is tainted by its negative associations with modern-day paedophilia. If I had to use a modern term to describe Greek sexuality, I might opt for 'bisexuality', because though many Greek men had same-sex relationships, once they reached adulthood they were expected to marry and father children. All such terms are inaccurate, however, and their use saddles the ancient Greeks with modern sexual taboos, prejudices and values that they would not have understood. In volume two of The History of Sexuality, Foucault examines ancient Greek sexual practices in detail. The Greeks did not have a single term equivalent to 'sexuality', for which they used several words, including aphrodisia and eros (from the gods of love and sex Aphrodite and Eros).[27] According to Foucault, *aphrodisia* and *eros* were hedged with as many taboos, regulations, prohibitions, constraints and thorny moral questions as sexuality in any other culture, past or present.

This ambiguity has not prevented campaigners for homosexual rights to cite ancient Greece as a model of enlightened tolerance in all matters sexual, while more conservative admirers of the ancient Greeks have downplayed the sexual nature of relationships between men and boys by describing their relationships as 'platonic'. As is often the case, the truth probably lies somewhere in between the two extremes: Greek men were neither libertarian hedonists nor high-minded moral philosophers; they were men with sexual desires for which they found outlets, which included partners of both sexes. In contrast with the modern divide between homo- and heterosexuality, which defines straight and gay sexual identities according to the gender of partners, the most important criteria that determined the suitability of an individual as a potential partner was social status and age. The sons of well-to-do and aristocratic families remained with their mothers and sisters in the women's quarters until the age of seven, when they were sent to the gymnasium for their formal education until the age of eighteen, at which point they became *epheboi*. In *The Clouds*, Aristophanes paints a delightful, though probably idealized, picture of two boys going to the gymnasium together:

> You will go down to the Academy, and under the sacred olive-trees, wearing a chaplet of green reed, you will start a race together with a good decent companion of your own age, fragrant with green-brier and catkin-shedding poplar and freedom from cares, delighting in the season of spring, when the plane trees whispers to the elm.[28]

In practice, an older man, known as the *erastes*, would pursue a boy or adolescent aged between twelve and eighteen, known as the *eromenos*, courting him and offering to be his mentor in the ways of life and his political patron.[29] The relationship had clear advantages for the *eromenos*, especially if the *erastes* were a powerful man who could give him advancement in future life. There was no question of a same-sex relationship between two adult males, which would have struck the Greeks as bizarre in the extreme. Former *eromenos–erastes* pairings could and did establish lifelong friendships, modelled on the friendship between Achilles and Patroklos in the *Iliad*, but any sexual activity between two men was meant to end with the younger man's attainment of physical and civic maturity. In the *Erotic Essay*, Demosthenes (384–322 BCE) spoke of the 'razor severing the ties of love'.[30] The patrons of gymnasia were men and boys of the freeborn Athenian ruling class. The adults were the effective rulers of the city as members of the citizen assembly, the *Ekklesia*, and the boys would be their successors. Although the Greeks did not judge men by the gender of their partners, they did have very strong opinions about whether men should be sexually and morally active or passive. A boy could be the passive object of pursuit because he was not fully mature or male, but the opposite would have been unthinkable. However, even freeborn youths, because they would become adult citizens, could not be seen to give in too easily to their suitors, and should not submit passively to anal intercourse. Sex with a slave or prostitute of either gender was not subject to these rules, but as a social inferior, a male slave could never take the active role with a freeborn citizen.

In the many representations of same-sex activities on painted ceramics, the older man is usually portrayed reaching for the boy's genitals, suggesting that the *erastes* initiated the sexual act while the *eromenos* showed modest reticence. Although in classical Greece same-sex relations were not associated with effeminacy, as they were in the Western world in the nineteenth and twentieth centuries, same-sex passivity was seen as problematic for a freeborn youth.[31] Additionally, Foucault explains that Greek men were expected to show *sophrosyne* – moderation in their desires – if they wished to achieve full mastery of the self and true masculinity. This provides yet another link with the gymnasium, because the achievement of *sophrosyne* was often compared to winning an athletics contest. In *The Laws* Plato makes an even closer association, saying, 'A man will not be able to defeat his desires if he is *agymnastos* (untrained).'[32] The idealized relationship between *erastes* and *eromenos* was first one of mentor and pupil, then of friends, and lastly of sexual partners. However, we have to ask ourselves what the reality of same-sex relationships was in classical Greece. Unfortunately, we have no first-hand account of such a relationship written by an *erastes* or *eromenos*, which might show us what was really going on between men, adolescents and boys. We do, however, have rules and regulations governing admittance to and behaviour in gymnasia and *palaestrae*.

The Athenian lawgiver Solon, while not being against same-sex relationships, established rules about who should be admitted to gymnasia, as well as regulations to protect younger boys from the advances of adolescents and adults. As confirmation, we can cite the rules of the public gymnasium of the city of Beroea in northern Greece:

> With regard to the boys, let no one of the young men approach the boys, nor let any chat with them, but if he does, let the gymnasiarch punish him and let him keep the one doing it away from them.

The rules go on to state that the person in charge of the gymnasium, the *gymnasiarchos*, could be fined if he allowed persons 'without a share in the gymnasium' to strip off and train, meaning slaves, male prostitutes, drunks and artisans.[33] In *The Clouds*, one of Aristophanes' characters reminds his audience that boys should not sit naked on the ground in the gymnasium and leave the imprints of their genitals in the sand lest it overexcite their older admirers. The regulations cited above and Aristophanes' quip imply that sexual moderation and platonic love were ideals that were not always respected in day-to-day interaction in the gymnasium.

As we saw above, same-sex themes are common on decorated Greek ceramics, and the setting that is suggested by the inclusion of a piece of athletic equipment or a *stlengis* is often the gymnasium. According to Thomas K. Hubbard, one of the foremost authorities on same-sex relations in the ancient world, the heyday of same-sex relations was between the seventh and sixth centuries BCE. He explains that it was an aristocratic tradition, celebrated in homoerotic poetry and in stories such as that of the aristocratic pair of tyrannicides Harmodios and Aristogeiton (both d. 514 BCE).[34] However, he notes the beginning of a change of attitude in Athens after the establishment of democracy.[35] In *The Birds* (414 BCE), Aristophanes is able to poke fun at same-sex relations when he makes one of his characters complain to another,

> You met my son coming from the bath after the gymnasium and you neither spoke to him, nor kissed him, nor took him with you, nor ever once felt his balls. Would anyone call you an old friend of mine?[36]

Although they were much less important than in earlier centuries, age-graded, same-sex relations endured until late antiquity, when they became the target of moral censure by the early Christian Church.

Arete

One reason the classical Greeks strike us as being so familiar is the sense of individuality that seems absent from other ancient cultures. Even though the Greek worldview was very different from our own, when we watch the great tragedies of classical Athens we can identify with the plight of their tortured heroes and heroines – Electra, Orestes, Medea, Phaedra and Oedipus – as they struggle to overcome the obstacles put in their paths by the Fates and the capricious gods. Whereas the ancient Egyptians and Mesopotamians were the subjects of divine kings and, through them, servants of the gods, the Greeks of the classical period for the most part had dispensed with their kings (even Sparta, which had two hereditary kings, had a council of elders who oversaw the running of the state). When oligarchs or tyrants ruled city-states, they did so not by divine right but because they had seized power, which they kept with the support of the majority of the citizens or of powerful special-interest groups such as the landed aristocracy.

To be considered a success in life, ancient Greek men had to reach their full potential in all areas of life, private and public, physical and moral. Although the classical Greeks were profoundly self-identified as citizens of a particular city and as Hellenes, they have also been described as history's first self-conscious individualists. The ancient Greeks called a person's full potential his *arete*, a term for which there is no exact English equivalent. According to Stephen Miller, who edited a sourcebook on the concept, its definition includes but is not limited to 'virtue, skill, prowess, pride, excellence, valor, and nobility'.[37] In the section on athletic nudity above, I gave one reason why Greek men trained naked – to differentiate themselves from neighbouring barbarians. Athletic nudity also represented an individual's *arete*, which was revealed in his physical accomplishments, often compared in ancient texts to the *agones* ('labours') of Herakles or Theseus.[38] The nakedness of the exerciser also enabled him to demonstrate his complete self-control, especially when compared to clothed non-Hellenes. Hence, the pursuit of *arete* also involved the achievement of *sophrosyne* – mastery of the self and one's desire.

A Visit to the Classical Gymnasium

Unlike later Macedonian kings and Roman emperors, the ruling classes of classical Greek states did not build luxurious palaces and villas. In democratic Athens, the idea of such a conspicuous display of wealth by an individual – even the richest aristocratic landowner – would have struck citizens as unforgivably ostentatious and might have led to the person's banishment by the *Ekklesia*. Wealthy Greeks lived in larger homes, with better furnishings and decoration, but these were expanded versions of more humble dwellings. The Greeks reserved the most costly materials and elaborate designs for their public buildings, in particular their civic shrines and temples. In Athens, the main religious structures on the Acropolis – the Parthenon and Erechtheion – were built of marble and decorated with complex sculptural schemes by the leading artists of the day. Second to the temples and shrines came the stoa, a multi-purpose covered portico that could be plain and functional, such as the commercial stoas of the Emporion in Athens' port of Piraeus, or grand, faced with marble and decorated with bas-reliefs and statuary. In the Athenian Agora, for example, the richly decorated, marble Basileios Stoa (Royal Stoa), built in the fifth century BCE, was the repository of the city's laws.

Although public gymnasia were not as grand as temples, their entrances and main portico were built of stone and marble, decorated with inscriptions, bas-reliefs and statuary. Because they played their part in the religious life of the city, they contained shrines, altars and statues of gods, demigods and heroes, particularly those associated with athletics and sporting competition.

Gymnasium or *Palaestra*?

Before I use the available physical and documentary evidence to invite the reader to join me on a tour of an ancient Greek gymnasium, I shall attempt to clarify the difference between the terms gymnasium and *palaestra*. There are three major differences that can be inferred from the available documentary evidence: (1) gymnasia were public while *palaestrae* were private; (2) gymnasia were reserved for men and older boys while *palaestrae* were principally for the education of younger boys; and (3) although a *palaestra* could exist as an independent institution, a gymnasium had to include a *palaestra* as part of its facilities.[39] The major problem is that ancient sources do not make a clear distinction between the two institutions and their functions, and sometimes use the terms interchangeably. Vitruvius dispenses with the word gymnasium altogether and calls the entire complex that he describes a 'Greek *palaestra*'. A closer reading of period sources, however, reveals that although the large classical gymnasia were usually publicly funded, *palaestrae* could either be public or private. There is evidence of older men and adolescents attending *palaestrae*, and younger boys training in gymnasia, hence a neat age-based distinction is not possible. However, the third point, that a *palaestra* could exist independently of a gymnasium but that a gymnasium must have a *palaestra*, is essentially correct. For the purposes of this book, I shall use the term *palaestra* to refer to an open-air training area enclosed by porticos (either on its own or as part of a gymnasium), while I shall use the term gymnasium to refer to the entire athletics complex, which, in addition to the *palaestra* and running facilities, included separate bathing facilities and parklands. Although *palaestra* is often translated as 'wrestling school', as the word is derived from the Greek verb *palaiein* (to wrestle), its courtyard and porticoes were used for training in other forms of exercise and contained rooms with distinct functions.

Beyond Vitruvius

Although my aim is to describe a gymnasium of the classical period, I shall have to base my reconstruction on Vitruvius' much later description of a generic Greek *palaestra*, which includes Hellenistic and Roman elements. Therefore, I have supplemented his text with evidence from archaeological sites and other textual evidence from the classical period. There was no prescribed location for a gymnasium, although there were limiting factors to where they could be built. The facilities required of a gymnasium, as opposed to those of a smaller *palaestra*, which could be housed in the courtyard of a private dwelling, needed a large open area. Depending on the available space, gymnasia could be built within the city walls, as in Priene in Ionia (now southwestern Turkey), or outside the city walls, as was the case with the three public gymnasia of Athens. The gymnasium at Olympia presents a third type of location. During the classical period, Olympia was a religious sanctuary dedicated to the gods, with important temples and shrines and sporting facilities for the quadrennial Olympic Games, but it was not a residential town until much later. Olympia had ample space for the stadium to the east of the sanctuary, and for a large gymnasium to the west of the site on the banks of the Kladeos river. The three suburban Athenian gymnasia were also sited near rivers, which provided them with water for their baths and irrigation for their parklands.[40]

The Akademia of Athens was constructed outside the city walls within a pre-existing sacred precinct which contained shrines and the *moriai*, a grove of twelve olive trees sacred to Athena, patron deity of the city, whose crop was pressed to make the oil awarded as prizes presented in decorated amphorae to the victors of the Panathenaic Games. The Akademia would have had its own enclosure and entrance, but in a city gymnasium, such as the one in Priene, the entrance would have been directly into the main building of the complex, the *palaestra*, through a *pylon*, or monumental pillared entrance. The materials chosen for the construction and decoration of gymnasia are evidence of their importance to the communities that funded them. Rather than the functional wooden-framed wattle-and-daub construction of private dwellings, gymnasia had marble facades and colonnades ornamented with bas-relief decorations, statuary and inscriptions. Although they could not rival temples in terms of their sculptural decorations, they were as well built and finished as any other important civic building.

Once through the *pylon*, the visitor would find himself in an open courtyard, the *palaestra* proper (also simply called a *peristylos* or *peristoion* – peristyle), surrounded on all four sides by colonnaded porticos. As Greek cities became wealthier, their *palaestrae* and gymnasia became larger and more luxurious. The oldest remains of a *palaestra*, which date from the late classical period at Delphi, are also the smallest yet found, measuring 47½ ft. (14.5 m) square. The Hellenistic *palaestra* of the Priene gymnasium is approximately 115 ft (35 m) square, while the *palaestra* at Olympia, also from the Hellenistic period, is 216 ft (66 m) square. The largest Hellenistic *palaestra* was found at the site of Ai-Khanoum, Afghanistan, thought to be a foundation of Alexander the Great, Alexandria in Oxus, which measures 328 ft (100 m) square.[41] What the visitor would not see in the courtyard of the *palaestra* is any fixed athletics equipment, such as the free weights, benches, aerobic exercisers and weight-training machines that occupy most of the floor space in a modern gym, or the apparatus used for the sport of artistic gymnastics: parallel bars, balance beam, rings, vaulting horse and asymmetric and high bars. Instead of stone or wooden flooring, the courtyard was covered with a layer of fine sand, which was dug over every morning to loosen it to provide a softer surface for training. Ancient Greek exercisers did use equipment but none of it was particularly bulky, so it could be stored away when not in use.

The porticos could be little more than covered walkways about 15 ft (5 m) deep, which were used by spectators and exercisers socializing and resting. But one or two sides housed more substantial rooms. The most basic rooms contained seating (*exedrai*) and were used as schoolrooms and lecture halls. In *De Architectura*, Vitruvius lists ten different room types that were found in a Greek *palaestra*. As Stephen Miller and others have pointed out, the problem with Vitruvius' description is that he was writing in around 27 BCE, over a century after the

Romans had conquered Greece and several centuries after the end of the classical period. Therefore his *palaestra* is a hybrid complex with classical Greek, Hellenistic and Roman elements.[42] The Romans had a very different approach to athletics and sporting culture, and the buildings they described as gymnasia and *palaestrae* were often annexes to *thermae* (public baths), whose main functions were bathing and socializing and not exercise. During the Roman period, spa and bathing facilities were added to Greek gymnasia or sometimes superseded them completely. What Vitruvius is describing is a mixed Graeco-Roman building with facilities that would not have been present during the fifth century BCE, specifically the warm bath and sweating room.

From the available evidence, it is clear that classical gymnasia had much more basic facilities. The room closest to the entrance would have been the *apodyterion*, the undressing or changing room, which, strangely, Vitruvius leaves out of his otherwise fairly detailed description. We do not know how it would have been furnished, but one can imagine a fairly basic arrangement of benches, wall hooks and shelves to store the belongings of patrons under the watchful eye of a slave-attendant. Another important room was the *ephebeion*, the clubroom and mess for the *epheboi*, which was equipped with *exedrai*, and was large enough for the *epheboi* to exercise indoors during bad weather. In addition, Vitruvius also lists the *korykion* (punchbag room), *konisterion* (dusting room), *elaiothesion* or *aleipthrion* (oil storage and anointing room) and *loutron* (cold bath), which could be equipped with individual stone basins, raised tubs or a communal bath. Another room Vitruvius fails to mention is the *sphairisterion*, the room set aside for ball games. The dimensions of these different rooms would vary with the overall size of the *palaestra*. In Priene, for example, the ephebeion was approximately 31 ft × 24½ ft (9.5 m × 7.5 m), while in Delphi's *palaestra* they would have been considerably smaller.

Modern-day gyms are often plain, functional buildings with little or no decoration, but in addition to any sculptural elements and free-standing statuary, Greek gymnasia displayed trophies won in athletics contests, including decorative shields and torches. In terms of their equipment, the gymnasia would have provided balls of different sizes, hoops, punchbags for boxers, and *halteres*, small, handheld weights, hemispherical or shaped like modern dumb-bells, made of stone or metal, weighing between 4½ and 20 lb (2 and 9 kg), which were used both for light weight-training movements and to provide extra momentum in the long jump. Additionally, Waldo Sweet describes two 'lifting stones' at Olympia inscribed with the names of the athletes who had succeeded in lifting them. One stone, weighing 316 lb (143.5 kg), has a recessed handle indicating that it was designed to be lifted with one hand; the second weighed in at 1,056 lb (480 kg), which is almost 44 lb (20 kg) over the modern dead-lift record of 1,015 lb (460.4 kg), when the lifter had the benefit of a modern weightlifting bar and weights.[43] However, lifting stones have not been found in other gymnasia, and it is unlikely that they were a standard part of a gymnasium's equipment. They would have been used by professional athletes who required great muscular strength for their events, and also to perform crowd-pleasing feats of strength. While modern gym patrons develop their bodies following the principles of nineteenth-century progressive weight training and their cardiovascular fitness with equipment designed in the twentieth century, the patrons of Greek gymnasia exercised by practising one or more of the six Olympic sports. A training session would begin with *cheironomia* (warm-up exercises) and proceed to training in the different sports, which were performed to the musical accompaniment of the single or double *aulos* (flute).

Apart from a *palaestra*, at a minimum, a gymnasium was required to provide running facilities, because foot races were among the highlights of the Pan-Hellenic games, as well as featuring in the sporting competitions of local festivals. Suburban gyms such as the Akademia and Lykeion would have had room for several running tracks, both open-air and covered for training in bad weather. The tracks were approximately one *stadion* long with varying widths. There was no standard measurement for the *stadion*, which is usually given as averaging 600 ft (180 m). The covered running track, or *xystos*, Vitruvius comments, should be set below the level of the surrounding ground, so as not to disturb those walking along the tree-lined walkways of the gymnasium's park. In Delphi, because of the constraints of the site, there was only one *xystos*, but at Olympia a large quadrilateral of porticoes that served as covered training areas for athletes was erected just north of the *palaestra*. Finally, Vitruvius says that a gymnasium should have a stadium for competitions. However, this was rarely the case during the classical period. In both Delphi and Olympia, the stadiums used for the games were separate from the gymnasia. In Athens, the Panathenaic Stadium was located near the Kynosarges but was not part of the gymnasium complex proper.

Running an Ancient Gymnasium

The large public gymnasia were built and maintained by the city itself, or in the case of the Olympic facilities by donations from wealthy patrons and city-states from all over the Greek world that sent athletes to the games. The gymnasium was under the charge of a civic official known as the *gymnasiarchos* who, in Athens, was also responsible for the organization and funding of certain athletic events. The post, while conferring a great deal of honour, also incurred significant expense. It is not clear, however, how much he directed the day-to-day management of the gymnasium, and this may have varied from city to city and also from period to period. He was assisted by the *paidonomos*, who supervised the academic curriculum. The gymnasium employed coaches and athletics specialists – *paidotribes* and *gymnastes* – who supervised the training of men and boys, and also of professional athletes. Other important employees of the gymnasium were the *aleiptes*, who anointed and massaged the athletes and who were also the establishment's medical specialists, and, finally, the *auletes*, the musicians who played the flute during training. In addition to these, the gymnasium would have accommodated private tradesmen who catered to the needs of exercisers and visitors. During the classical period, admission to a public gymnasium was limited to male citizens. Women, girls (except in Sparta), slaves and foreigners were all excluded. Although the public gymnasia were notionally free of charge, in reality the wealthier patrons and the *gymnasiarchos* were expected to bear the cost of the training of poorer citizens and professional athletes, and to buy the most expensive commodity used in the gym, the olive oil used to anoint and massage exercisers both before and after training.

Temple of Hellenic Identity

During the classical period the gymnasium was the ancient Greek world's most important social institution, and one that was deeply embedded in all aspects of the lives of freeborn men and boys. It was the place where they were educated and trained for war and citizenship, and where they developed their sense of self. It was also the place where they experienced their first sexual relationships and forged their most enduring friendships. The ancient gymnasium was also the first human institution that actively promoted aesthetic training alongside functional and therapeutic training, underlining the importance of the naked male form and masculine embodiment in classical Greek culture. The nudity that was required of men and boys in the gymnasium and other social settings served a number of important functions in classical Greece: it was a marker of Hellenic identity, through which Greek men sought to differentiate themselves from their clothed barbarian enemies; and of regional identity, when naked athletes competed for their city-states in Pan-Hellenic contests; and it was a visible expression of an individual's *arete*, a man's mastery of his mind and body that allowed him to attain his full physical, moral, social and intellectual potential.

Although we use the abbreviation gym, derived from the Greek word *gymnasion*, the ancient institution was completely different physically and functionally from the contemporary gym. In terms of its appearance and layout, it was closer to a modern-day athletics field, with open-air and covered facilities used for the practice of the ancient Olympic sports and for the functional military training of the city-state's warrior cadets. Beyond physical training, which in ancient Greek thought was inseparable from moral, social and intellectual education, the gymnasium functioned as a schoolhouse for boys and adolescents aged from seven to eighteen, a dance studio, a soldier's mess, a men's club and a university, where lectures were given by the leading philosophers of the period. Equipped with altars and shrines, built within sacred precincts and making an important contribution to the religious life of the community, the ancient gymnasium functioned as a temple dedicated to the perfectibility of the human body, mind and spirit, in the service of the city-state, of the Hellenic race and of the Olympian gods.

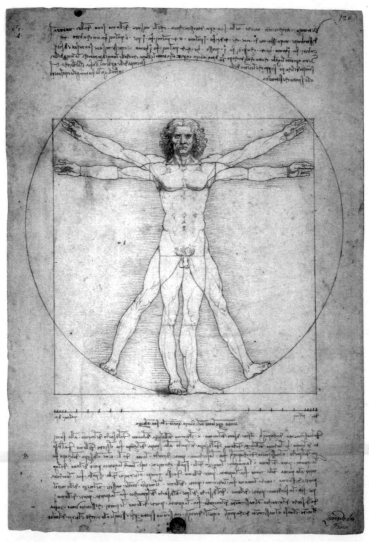

Vitruvian Man (c. 1487) by Leonardo da Vinci (1452–1519) expressed the new vision of humanity that was at the heart of the Renaissance project. Founded on the rediscovered texts and artworks of antiquity, yet informed by the preceding Christian centuries, humanism glorified the naked body, rehabilitating it as an artistic subject and at the same time re-creating it as an object of desire.

2

THE REBIRTH OF VITRUVIAN MAN

It remains for you, following the example of the ancients, to exercise
your own body so wisely that you do not only achieve the long life that
heaven promises you and your nature suggests, but also, if possible,
may extend it further.

Dedication of the first edition of *De Arte Gymnastica*
by Girolamo Mercuriale

The history of the collapse of Graeco-Roman civilization comes in
two versions: traditionalist and revisionist. *The History of the Decline
and Fall of the Roman Empire* (1776) by Edward Gibbon (1737–1794) presents readers with the most traditional view of the end of Roman rule
in the western provinces of the empire.[1] Gibbon highlights two major
factors that triggered the transition from late antiquity to the early
Middle Ages: the Norse-Germanic invasions of the Western Roman
Empire between the third and fifth centuries CE and the triumph of
Christianity at the end of the fourth century CE. The destruction of
classical Greece's public gymnasia, however, had begun centuries earlier, and had been initiated by Gibbons's heroes, the dour, upright
consuls and generals of the Roman Republic. In 86 BCE, when the
Greeks rebelled against Roman rule, Lucius Cornelius Sulla besieged
Athens. Recognizing the part that gymnasia played in the military
training of the citizenry, before taking and sacking the city Sulla laid
waste to the Akademia and Lykeion.

What the Romans had begun, the Norse-Germanic tribes continued
during their migrations into imperial territory. One of the most destruc-
tive raids into Greece took place in 267 CE, when the Germanic Heruli

sacked Delphi, the host city of the Pythian Games, and then destroyed Athens. The second cause that the Protestant Gibbon gives for the decline and fall of classical culture is the triumph of Roman Catholicism over paganism and its installation as the state religion of the empire by Emperor Constantine and his successors. However, though the Christian Church was fundamentally opposed to sporting competition because of its close associations with pagan festivals, and to gymnasia because of the culture of same-sex relations that they fostered, it nevertheless played a vital role in preserving knowledge of classical athletics by ensuring the survival of thousands of ancient manuscripts in its monastic libraries, where they would be rediscovered by scholars during the European Renaissance (fourteenth–seventeenth centuries).

Roman Questions

The Romans had an ambiguous relationship with the Greeks that can be compared to the uneasy friendship that often turned into open hostility between Great Britain and the United States of America during the course of the nineteenth century. Rome could not deny its enormous debt to Greece, but to offset its feelings of cultural inferiority, it stressed its moral superiority. In the previous chapter I quoted Pliny the Elder on the health benefits of anointing oneself with olive oil in the privacy of one's own home, but in the same entry in the *Natural History*, he berates the Greeks, calling them the 'progenitors of every vice', who have perverted olive oil 'to luxury by its public use in the gymnasia'. In the *Moralia*, compiled *c.* 100 CE, the Greek historian and philosopher Plutarch (*c.* 46–120 CE) summarizes the Roman suspicion of Greek athletics and gymnasium culture:

> For the Romans used to be very suspicious of rubbing down with oil, and even today they believe that nothing has been so much to blame for the enslavement and effeminacy of the Greeks as their gymnasia and wrestling schools, which engender much listless idleness and waste of time in their cities, as well as pederasty and the ruin of the bodies of the young men

with regulated sleeping, walking, rhythmical movements, and strict diet; by these practices they have unconsciously lapsed from the practice of arms, and have become content to be termed nimble athletes and handsome wrestlers rather than excellent men-at-arms and horsemen.[2]

Readers brought up on tales of insane, decadent Roman emperors who indulged themselves in every kind of vice and excess at orgies might be surprised at this prudishness, especially if they have seen in museums both Greek and Roman statues of naked gods, demigods, athletes, kings and emperors. However, the two cultures used the naked male form in markedly different ways. During the classical period, Greek men were expected to be nude on certain occasions and when performing certain activities, such as training in the gymnasium and competing in athletic events. The many representations of naked men and boys are not mere artistic convention but depictions of everyday reality. In contrast, the Romans were extremely prudish about public nudity, except in the semi-private setting of the public baths. Roman heroic nude sculpture was used to project a very different political and ideological message, which was similar in tone and function to the nude statuary of nineteenth-century Europe. If the Greeks had used heroic nudity to express their national, cultural and regional identities, in particular to differentiate themselves from their clothed barbarian neighbours and enemies, the Romans used it to project 'naked' military might.

The Romans disapproved of public displays of nudity, which they associated with barbarians, criminals and defeated soldiers. Many of the enemies of Rome, including the tattooed Picts, Gauls and Britons, fought naked. Reversing the earlier Greek tradition of heroic nudity that showed naked Greek warriors fighting clothed barbarians, the Romans saw nudity as a characteristic of their uncivilized and defeated foes. Condemned criminals and rebels, such as Jesus of Nazareth (c. 4 BCE–c. 30 CE), were stripped before being tortured and crucified. Vanquished soldiers were made to pass 'under the yoke' nudi (nude), though in reality, for Roman soldiers on the losing side of Rome's many civil wars, this probably meant stripped of their arms and armour in their undergarments rather than completely naked, which would have been a humiliation too far to inflict on fellow Roman citizens.[3]

The function of nudity in Roman art began to change with the advent of imperial rule in 27 BCE. During the republican period, Rome's consuls, senators and generals were represented realistically as old men in full senatorial garb, but a new idealized portrait of the ruler as a youthful god or demigod appeared during the reign of the first emperor, Augustus (63 BCE–14 CE). The concentration of power in the new office of *imperator* was expressed in the arts by borrowing and transforming earlier Greek royal and religious models. Heroic nude imperial portraits served to project the emperor's personal authority and divinity, as well as the military might of the imperial state.

After the conquest of Greece, several attempts were made to introduce Greek athletics to Rome. However, as is well known from recent film portrayals, such as *Gladiator* (2000), the Romans preferred far bloodier spectacles, such as gladiatorial contests to the death and the public execution of criminals in the arena. The Hellenizing Emperor Nero built gymnasia and instituted the Neronia, a Greek-style athletics contest, in 60 CE, but his freeborn Roman subjects refused to compete and preferred to watch the naked Greek athletes who had been brought to Rome for the occasion.[4] Athletics contests, nude or clothed, were never part of Roman religious observance, and writers such as Cicero (106–43 BCE), Seneca (54 BCE–c. 39 CE) and Tacitus (56–117 CE) considered them to be decadent, shameful and corrupting, describing them in terms reminiscent of a modern-day moral panic.[5]

Nude portraiture in Greek and Hellenistic art was used to represent idealized portraits of gods, demigods, heroes and kings, but there was also a tradition of portraiture representing the bodies of real people, including victorious Olympic athletes. Roman imperial nudes, however, were always idealized, and in Christopher Hallett's words, they 'transported the individual represented outside the realm of contemporary life, and into the world of myth, literature, and art' – a fact reflected in the name given to these images by the Romans themselves, *effigies Achilleae* (Achillean portraits).[6] The last nude imperial statues were those of Crispus (d. 326 CE) and his father, Constantine the Great, the first Christian emperor, whose statue in the guise of the naked sun god Apollo was placed on top of a column in his new capital, Constantinople, in about 324 CE.[7] In addition to the different conceptions and uses of nudity in Greece and Rome, the two cultures diverged considerably in their sexual mores. The aristocratic culture of same-sex relations that had played such an important role in the development of the classical Greek gymnasium was never adopted by Rome's senatorial elite. In Roman law, it was a criminal offence for an adult man to have same-sex relations with a freeborn youth. However, several emperors had male lovers, most famously Emperor Hadrian (76–138 CE), whose passionate but tragic affair with an adolescent boy is well documented. Antinöus (c. 111–130 CE), the object of Hadrian's obsessive attentions, was a Greek youth from the province of Bythnia in Asia Minor.[8]

Although the Christianization of the empire and the barbarian incursions did bring an end to the gymnasium, like many other classical Greek institutions, its decline had begun long before the fourth century CE. In the third volume of The History of Sexuality: The Care of the Self, which deals with the transition in attitudes to sexuality from ancient Greece to pagan Rome and then to the early Christian period, Michel Foucault documents the gradual changes in attitudes to same-sex relations.[9] The shift away from the cult of the body as an aspect of a man's moral and spiritual perfectibility was already present in ancient Greece in the concept of sophrosyne, the moderation of one's desires, which included controlling one's sexual desires for either gender. The Romans had an ever more highly developed sense of individual virtus, moral virtue and rigid self-control and self-restraint. What Christianity added was the concept of carnal sin, which defined the only legitimate sexual act as one with the aim of procreation between husband and wife. Same-sex relations, already suspect among pagan Romans, were destined to become 'sodomy', originally a much broader category than anal intercourse between two men, which included all sexual acts performed purely for pleasure between partners of the same or different genders.[10]

The shift in morality was expressed in artistic representations, especially of the deity. In late antiquity, the realistic, seductive, homoerotic bronzes and marbles of naked gods, demigods and divinized emperors disappeared and were replaced by highly stylized, austere images of Christ, the apostles, saints and fathers of the Church dressed in clothing more suited to the sixth-century Byzantine court than to first-century Judea. Late Roman iconography reflects the move away from the concept of the body as an aspect of divinity to be glorified and its transformation into an obstacle to salvation that needs to be hidden from view and mortified. A significant moment in Byzantine art history is the eighth-century movement known as iconoclasm, which proscribed any representations of God, Jesus and the saints as contrary to the Third Commandment.[11] Iconoclasm itself was heavily influenced by the Islamic ban on all human representation, and specifically of images of Allah and the Prophet Muhammad (c. 570–632).

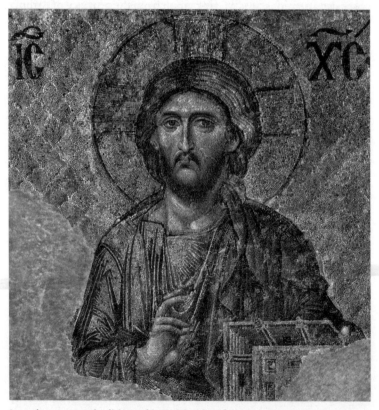

In stark contrast to the divine and imperial nudes of classical antiquity, late Roman and medieval art stressed Christianity's renunciation of the flesh by its depictions of the fully clothed Christ, apostles, saints and fathers of the Church. *Christ Pantocrator*, mosaic from Hagia Sofia, Istanbul, 13th century.

East versus West

The collapse of the Western, Latin-speaking half of the empire transformed the Eastern half, which gradually adopted Greek as its official language. The coronation of Charlemagne as Emperor of the Romans in 800 finally ended the fiction of a single undivided Roman world. At the same time, the Roman Catholic and Eastern Orthodox churches were diverging, and they would split permanently in the Great Schism of 1054. Henceforth, for Roman Catholic Western Europeans steeped in Latin culture, the Byzantine Empire was an alien, almost Asiatic entity, with a separate language and a heretical brand of Christianity. What united them in an uneasy alliance was their common fear of Islam, which continued to extend its borders and influence. Jerusalem fell to the Muslims in 637 and would remain under Muslim rule until the First Crusade (1096–9). The Crusades (eleventh–thirteenth centuries) saw a gradual reversal of the power balance in the Mediterranean. As the empire weakened, the power of Western Europe grew, until during the Fourth Crusade (1202–4), instead of attacking the Muslim forces in the Holy Land, a Venetian-led force captured and sacked Constantinople and established the Latin Empire of Constantinople, which lasted until 1261. Although Byzantine independence was restored, it faced a new and more dangerous threat in the rising power of the Ottoman Turks, who succeeded in taking the city in 1453. The fall of Constantinople – one of the dates used to mark the end of the Middle Ages – led to a migration to the West of Greek scholars who brought with them classical Greek manuscripts, many of which were translated into Latin for the first time. Western Europe, which had once been on the fringes of the civilized world, was now the seat of Christendom, the heir to the Roman Empire and the principal repository of Graeco-Roman learning.

Blues and Greens

Although much of the athletics culture of the ancient world disappeared in the fourth century with the proscription of paganism, sporting competition did not entirely vanish from the Byzantine Empire. Chariot racing remained Constantinople's most popular sporting pastime. Sponsored by emperors, it was the centrepiece of the spectacular games held at the city's great arena and race track, the Hippodrome, which was decorated with statues and architectural trophies brought from all over the Roman world. The games that took place in the Hippodrome were very different from the gladiatorial contests held in Rome's pagan Colosseum and were much closer in spirit to the equestrian events of the ancient Olympic Games. They continued to play an important role in the social and political life of the city throughout late antiquity. The demes – factions supporting different teams of charioteers, known by their colours as the Blues and Greens – were proto-political parties.[12] The Blues represented the interests of landowners, the Greens those of urban tradesmen, artisans and civil servants.[13]

The only other aspect of ancient athletics culture preserved during the Byzantine period was the therapeutic application of gymnastics described in the Greek and Roman texts preserved in the libraries of the Byzantine world. After the Arab conquest of Egypt and the Near East, this knowledge was transmitted to Islamic doctors, who further refined the ancient system of humorism outlined by Hippocrates and Galen. We do not know, however, to what extent exercise played a part in the treatments prescribed by Byzantine and Islamic physicians. Even if there was a limited survival and application of therapeutic exercise in medieval medical practice in the region, the gymnasium-based culture of aesthetic training would have been quite alien to Christian Byzantium and its Muslim neighbours, warrior societies whose exercise cultures and practices concentrated on functional military training. The Central Asian Ottoman Turks, for example, who moved westwards into Byzantine territory beginning in the thirteenth century, brought with them a style of wrestling that is still popular in present-day Turkey; however, this has no link to the sport practised in the gymnasia of the ancient world.

The Rediscovery of the Gymnasium

During the medieval period, the gymnasium as a physical space dedicated to the training of the body completely disappeared from the

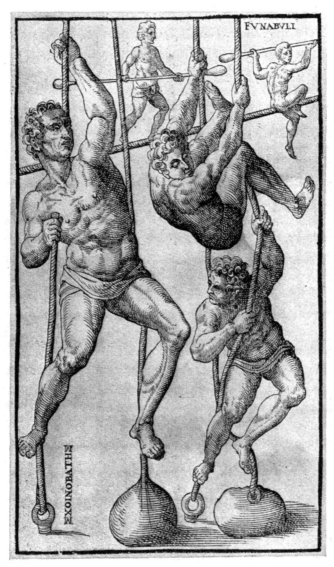

Illustration from Girolamo Mercuriale's *De Arte Gymnastica* (1569) purporting to show athletic training in an ancient gymnasium. Because Mercuriale had access to a limited number of classical texts and artworks on which to base the illustrations, his vision of ancient medical and gymnastic practices owes more to his imagination than to historical reality.

Byzantine Empire, from the former Roman provinces of the Near East and North Africa, now under Muslim rule, and from the successor states of the Western Roman Empire. However, descriptions of ancient gymnasia and athletics along with many other aspects of Graeco-Roman culture survived in the libraries of Western Europe, Constantinople and the Islamic world. The rediscovery of this cache of forgotten knowledge was known to later generations of scholars as the European Renaissance – an intellectual and artistic movement that began in Italy in the fourteenth century that would completely transform Western European society. Its most visible expression can be seen in the arts, in the emphasis placed on the naturalistic representation of the naked human form, as exemplified by Leonardo da Vinci's *Vitruvian Man* (c. 1487), which combined Vitruvius' ideal architectural proportions of the 'Golden Mean' with an anatomically correct representation of the body based on Leonardo's dissections of cadavers.

The fourteenth and fifteenth centuries witnessed the steady and irreversible decline of Byzantine power that could not resist the rise of the Ottoman Turks. Several Byzantine emperors attempted to end the schism between the Eastern Orthodox and Roman Catholic churches in order to obtain military support from the papacy and Western European states, but the violent opposition of their subjects to any reconciliation with Rome prevented any lasting rapprochement.[14] During several tours of Europe, Byzantine emperors took scholars with them to plead their cause. Among the most influential was the neo-Platonist philosopher George Gemistos Plethon (c. 1355–c. 1452), who, though considered a dangerous maverick in the empire for his open admiration of paganism, reintroduced the works of Plato to the West.[15] These were translated into Latin by scholars including the Florentine philosopher Marsilio Ficino (1433–1499), the founder of Florence's Platonic Academy. Unlike their ancient forebears, Ficino and his fellow academicians had little interest in athletics or gymnasia. They were the vanguard of the intellectual movement that oversaw the translation into Latin of ancient Greek manuscripts during the fifteenth and sixteenth centuries, making available for study many forgotten works of classical Greek philosophy, medicine, science, architecture and mathematics.

Among the rediscovered manuscripts were texts on ancient medicine, which included sections on exercise and gymnasia. In her study of Renaissance physicians, Eleanor English names a number of doctors who made extensive use of classical medical texts in their own works: Thomas Elyot (1490–1546), Girolamo Cardano (1501–1576) and Cristobal Méndez (c. 1500–c. 1553), the last of whom wrote a treatise entitled *Libro del Exercicio Corporal y de sus Provechos* (*The Book of Physical Exercise and its Benefits*) in 1553.[16] But by far the most famous and influential work on the subject written in the sixteenth century was *De Arte Gymnastica* by the Italian physician Girolamo Mercuriale (1530–1606), first published in 1569. Leafing through the pages of the only published facsimile, which has the Latin text facing the English translation, and reproductions of the original illustrations, the reader is struck by two things: the reverence in which all things ancient were held by scholars of the day, and the confusion about exercise that was caused by the lack of historical research, mistranslations and mistakes based on anachronistic interpretation of the material.

Mercuriale did not have access to the archaeological evidence that modern scholars have used to reconstruct ancient gymnasia and their facilities. He based his description of the Greek gymnasium entirely on Vitruvius' description, which mixed classical Greek with later Hellenistic and Roman features. As for his illustrations, they present his interpretation of textual references and possibly some very limited evidence available at the time from ancient sculpture and decorated ceramics; in other words, they are the result of his and his illustrator's fertile imaginations. Like many of his contemporaries, Mercuriale treats classical antiquity as a continuous, undifferentiated period, mixing Greek, Hellenistic and Roman athletic and therapeutic practices.

Although Méndez (who wrote in Spanish rather than in Latin, the universal language of the day) anticipated Mercuriale's book by three decades, his work remained undiscovered until the modern period. Mercuriale's book, by contrast, was circulated widely through the relatively new medium of the printing press.[17] Mercuriale and other Renaissance physicians did not set up gymnasia or try to re-establish ancient athletics contests, but they resurrected the notion of therapeutic training to promote good health and cure disease. The tone of the book, its constant reference to classical authorities, and the many repetitions in the text show exactly what Mercuriale was up against in trying to persuade Western Europeans of the virtues of exercise. Exercise in early modern Europe consisted of functional military training, hunting, dancing and racket games for the nobility, and manual labour, bare-knuckle fighting, wrestling, folk dancing and sundry savage team sports for the lower orders.

What Mercuriale stressed, as can be seen from the dedication of the first edition quoted on the opening page of this chapter, is first longevity, second improved health, both leading to 'the achievement of Human Happiness', and third, an improvement in military skill.[18] Like the health-and-fitness gurus of today, he understood the value of celebrity endorsement when he dedicated the edition of 1573 to the most powerful ruler of the day, the Holy Roman Emperor Maximilian I (1459–1519). De Arte begins with an examination of the origins of medicine, as it is therapeutic practices and not exercise that form the basis of the book. Like other Renaissance physicians who did not know about infectious diseases and degenerative conditions, he followed the ancients in ascribing the causes of illness to the imbalances of the humours, especially those caused by gluttony and drunkenness, the twin excesses to which his aristocratic patrons were particularly prone. His main classical source, Galen, features prominently throughout the text. He quotes Galen's Gymnastics, stating that exercise 'brings amazing benefits as regards averting future disease, protecting existing health and building strength in those recovering from illness'.[19] Mercuriale then gives an account of the gymnasia of antiquity based on references in Plato and Vitruvius' description, and covers the patrons of the gym, athletic nudity, equipment and anointing with oil. He also includes the ancient criticisms of the excesses of the 'athletic tribe' – the professional athletes who devoted their lives exclusively to exercise and competition.

His description of ancient life also includes a section on bathing, where his references are more to Roman than Greek practices, and also on the custom of reclining on couches to eat, which he does not recommend, citing the example of scripture (the Last Supper) to define sitting at table as a healthier and more modern way to eat. This is not the only biblical reference in the book, as – careful not to be accused of pagan sympathies or heresy – the Catholic Mercuriale includes many scriptural references to supplement and sanitize his classical sources. The next book defines different kinds of exercise, both ancient and modern, including the sports of the ancient Olympics, as well as running, which he calls 'supreme', walking, swimming, sailing, combat, hunting, riding, dancing, various games and, more bizarrely, holding one's breath, shouting, laughing and being carried in a litter.

The concluding books deal with who should and should not exercise; therapeutic exercises for different diseases; exercises for the elderly and those convalescing from illness; practical advice about where and when to exercise and how much exercise to do; and finally the effects of exercise on diseases and the body. Throughout the text Mercuriale shows himself to be a faithful disciple of Galen, who had a much more invasive approach to treatment, including bleeding and purging patients, than Hippocrates, who preferred to prescribe non-invasive treatments such as rest, dietary advice and exercise. Although Mercuriale describes and illustrates an ancient gymnasium, there is no evidence to suggest that he ever proposed building one, and it is unlikely that his aristocratic patients would have ever made use of it, preferring their traditional aristocratic pastimes. It is also unclear how much contemporary and later doctors took note of his recommendations for therapeutic exercise, as early modern medicine consisted of violent purges, cupping and bleeding, among several of the least pleasant treatments in vogue until the eighteenth century.

The Seductive Body Rediscovered

The Renaissance is seen primarily today as an artistic movement. Although the artistic conventions of Russia, Eastern Europe and the Balkans continued to follow Byzantine models even after the fall of Constantinople, in the West the rediscovery of ancient learning was paralleled by a reappraisal of ancient artistic models that were seen as the new models for both religious and lay art, in particular Graeco-Roman statuary. Eroticism and homoeroticism reappear in the works of such Renaissance masters as Donatello, Michelangelo and Leonardo da Vinci. Although the term 'gay' would be as anachronistic as the term 'homosexual' to refer to the sexual orientation of Leonardo and Michelangelo, they were known to have had same-sex relationships, only escaping the savage punishments meted out to sodomites because of their powerful patrons, who included popes, princes, kings and emperors. According to Hallett, there was greater concern about the correct anatomical representation of the musculature in Renaissance art than in its classical models. Leonardo, in particular, made careful anatomical studies, performing illegal dissections of cadavers to improve his understanding of musculoskeletal anatomy.

Along with Graeco-Roman manuscripts, several masterpieces of classical and Hellenistic art were rediscovered in the sixteenth century. In the 1540s, sections of two larger-than-life statues of Hercules standing 10 ft 33 in. (3.13 m) tall were unearthed in the ruins of the Baths of Caracalla in Rome. Now known as the 'Weary Hercules' or the 'Farnese Hercules', after Cardinal Alessandro Farnese (1520–1589), who acquired the statue to add to his collection of ancient art and who commissioned the sculptor Guglielmo della Porta to replace its missing lower half, the statue depicts the ancient hero as a hyper-muscular male who would not be out of place in a contemporary bodybuilding competition. The 'Farnese Hercules', a third-century CE Greek or Roman copy of a fourth-century BCE Greek original, would have been familiar to Mercuriale, who was the cardinal's personal physician, and would have influenced the engravings of heavily muscled gymnasts in De Arte Gymnastica.[20]

A renewed interest in the representation of the naked body did not imply a matching interest in gymnasia and physical exercise, however. Renaissance art dealt with the body as an abstract ideal that demonstrated the principles of the Vitruvian Golden Mean, rather than an actual flesh-and-blood body to be recreated through exercise in a gymnasium. Although Renaissance art restored the body as an aesthetic and erotic object, lived sexuality was hedged with Christian taboos, and same-sex relations were condemned as sodomy, which remained a capital offence. One of the most representative Renaissance works showing the new attitude to the body is Michelangelo's statue of David, sculpted for the city-state of Florence between 1501 and 1504.

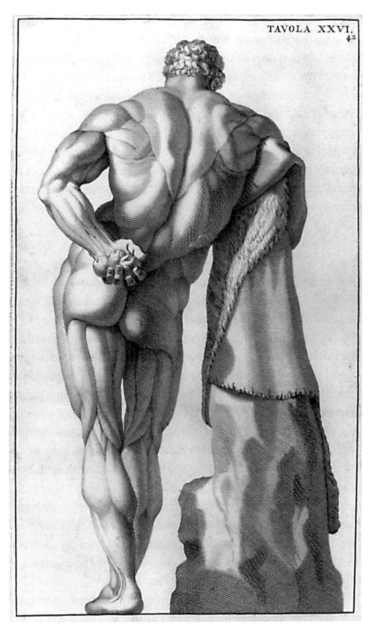

Unearthed in the ruins of the Baths of Caracalla in Rome, the 'Farnese Hercules' was one of the ancient statues that informed Renaissance artists and scholars about the physical appearance and muscularity of ancient athletes. Dutch artist Hendrik Goltzius (1558–1617) produced this engraving of the statue in 1591.

The subject combines the biblical hero David preparing for his encounter with Goliath, his sling trailing over one shoulder, with a classical pose borrowed from statues of ancient Greek athletes. The seductive David expresses the artist's sexual preferences for attractive, well-muscled young men, but much more significantly, it also carries a clear political message: David was the underdog who was supposed to lose to his giant opponent, just like the Republic of Florence that was surrounded by larger, more powerful enemies. The heroic, naked David projects Florence's political and military power and her vulnerability, as well as her claims to be the true heir of the culture and political institutions of classical antiquity.

Protestant Gymnasts

Philosophically, the Renaissance, in addition to rediscovering ancient learning and art, began the protracted and bloody process that would replace God with Man as the centre of the Universe. The name of the new academic curriculum, *studia humanitatis* (humanism), stressed the primacy of the human over the divine, triggering a profound challenge to the authority of the Roman Catholic Church. Recovered pagan philosophical and scientific texts encouraged scholars and the more radical clergy to question the dogmas of the Church, which were mired in corrupt practices, such as the selling of indulgences (pardons for sins) by official clergy and by freelance charlatans, such as the Pardoner in Geoffrey Chaucer's *Canterbury Tales* of the late fourteenth century. A century later, when Martin Luther nailed the *Ninety-five Theses* to the doors of All Saints' Church in Wittenberg, Germany, in 1517, he began what later became known as the Protestant Reformation, which plunged Europe into 124 years of bloody religious and civil wars (1524–1648), fought between Protestant and Catholic states and the followers of the two faiths within their own countries.

Education from primary school to university had been a monopoly of the Roman Catholic Church, which ensured that what was taught did not contradict Church teaching. However, the influx of classical learning disrupted the accord between scholars and clergy. Although many Italian scholars had initially tried to reconcile pagan philosophy with Catholic teaching because they did not want to run the risk of being excommunicated as heretics and imprisoned or executed by the Holy Inquisition, after the Protestant Reformation, when many churches broke away from Rome, there was greater freedom for scholars, as well as the ideological need to come up with rival scriptural interpretations. The Reformation broke the Church's monopoly on education.

Martin Luther was a strong supporter of education (at least for the aristocracy). He wrote: 'The best of schools should be instituted in all places for boys and girls . . . that men may be well able to rule land and people, and that women may know well how to rear children and to order house and servants.'[21] He also recommended adding mathematics and music to the traditional curriculum of Latin, Greek and Hebrew. His ideas were taken up in the independent Protestant Franco-German city of Strasbourg by the humanist educationalist Johann Sturm (1507–1589), who in 1538 founded the first institution to go by the name of a gymnasium since antiquity, the Gymnase Protestant de Strasbourg, taking over the buildings of a former Dominican priory. Sturm, a typical 'Renaissance man', was both a scholar and noted Ciceronian rhetorician and a man of action who worked as a spy for the Protestant queen of England, Elizabeth I (1533–1603). The Gymnase's curriculum was primarily academic, with little time for recreation or physical exercise. Pupils attended for eight years, studying Latin for the first three, after which Greek was added for a further three, with a final year devoted to Protestant theology.[22] However, in his essay 'For the Lauingen School', Sturm had the following to say about exercise or 'games' for his students:

> There are many things of this dangerous kind in fighting, swimming, fishing and hunting. It is, however, a characteristic of our schools to teach the Latin language in the games. So when the times of the games have been set, the moderator should be present, so that more suitable and more useful games are chosen, to set goals for the races, for running and jumping, also to pitch camp, to appoint leaders, centurions, decurions; to make the legions ready, and to separate them into cohorts.[23]

The quotation reveals that any games were to be subordinate to the academic curriculum, as the instructions were to be given in Latin, and the references to Roman military organization, ranks and practices also suggest that they were intended to be a history lesson with strong martial overtones. The Gymnase became a model for many other institutions across Europe, and in modern Germany and several other Central European countries, the term 'gymnasium' is still used to denote a secondary or high school.

Into the Wider World

The Macedonians and Greeks who conquered the Persian Empire with Alexander the Great and reached the Indian subcontinent were the first Europeans to encounter what Plutarch called 'gymnosophists', or naked philosophers. There is no general agreement as to who they were or what religion they followed. Sadhu, Hindu holy men, and Jain ascetics habitually are naked and share practices that include physical exercise. Several scholars have equated the gymnosophists with the ancestors of modern yogis, and claim that the exercises Alexander's soldiers saw them practise were archaic yoga asanas. Although asanas are undoubtedly extremely ancient and probably predate the fourth century BCE, their grouping into a formal exercise system dates to a much later period. The codification of hatha yoga is usually ascribed to the fifteenth-century Hindu sage Swatmarama, who composed the Hatha Yoga Pradipika.[24] It would be another four centuries before yoga was introduced to the West, and not until the last quarter of the twentieth century that it began to feature on the group exercise-class schedule of the contemporary gym.

The Hellenistic Greeks, like the other European explorers and conquerors who followed them, interpreted what they saw in terms of their own experience and beliefs. For them, naked holy men doing asana must be performing gymnastic exercises, and they must also be philosophers, because education and philosophical discourse were closely associated with gymnasia in the ancient Greek world. The Greeks trained for functional and aesthetic reasons, as the beauty of the body was equated with moral virtue. The yoga of posture, hatha

68

yoga (while it, too, has been turned in the West into a type of aesthetic training), is the physical component of a spiritual system intended to free the yogi from his attachment to the material world so that he can attain a state of transcendent enlightenment in which all physical desires are extinguished. Although it has been stripped of its philosophical and spiritual underpinnings, especially when it is taught as a group exercise class in a contemporary gym, yoga retains an aura of exoticism and Eastern mysticism that many teachers use to promote it as an alternative to conventional exercise to develop strength, stamina and flexibility, while at the same time claiming that it provides less tangible benefits such as an increased sense of physical and mental well-being.

The heirs of Alexander established Hellenistic kingdoms in Central Asia and northern India that endured until the first century CE, and built Greek cities with gymnasia, such as Ai-Khanoum in Afghanistan. Although these foundations did not survive the passing of the Indo-Greeks, they left an important artistic legacy, transmitting the classical Greek artistic canon to Central Asian Buddhist art, which in the following centuries would travel with Buddhist missionaries to East Asia, where its influence is clearly discernible in the Buddhist statuary of China, Korea and Japan of the early centuries CE. During his search for enlightenment, the historical Buddha, Siddhartha Gautama (c. 563–c. 483 BCE), followed the path of asceticism, which may well have included something resembling the physical practices of hatha yoga. However, when he devised the Eightfold Noble Path to enlightenment he did not include physical exercise.[25] Although there are statues showing the Buddha as a naked, emaciated ascetic, his most iconic representation is clothed and seated in a meditation posture. And while he is sometimes depicted bare-chested, his highly stylized features and body do not have the realism and homoerotic allure of Graeco-Roman depictions of gods and demigods. Representations of the body in Buddhism are not intended as projections of power or national identity but as expressions of spirituality.

Fighting Monks

Buddhist monks abandoned physical exercise as part of their quest for spiritual enlightenment in India and the countries most influenced by Indian Buddhism – Sri Lanka, Burma and Thailand – but according to traditional accounts, they were instrumental in the development of the second Asian exercise culture that has been imported into the modern gym for group exercise classes, the East Asian martial arts, known in Chinese as *wushu* or *gung fu*. Like hatha yoga, it is claimed that the Chinese martial arts have very ancient origins, dating back to the Han Dynasty (206 BCE–220 CE), when they were used as part of functional military training. In certain traditions, the invention of the first unarmed martial art is credited to the Indian Buddhist monk Bodhidarma (*fl.* sixth century CE), who created a style of *wushu* for the monks of the Shaolin Temple (Henan, China), in order to strengthen their meditation practice.[26] As with hatha yoga, however, the codification of different martial-arts styles is thought to have taken place much later, during the sixteenth and seventeenth centuries.[27] T'ai chi ch'uan (*tai-jiquan*), which is practised in the West primarily for its health benefits rather than as a fighting style, was codified in the seventeenth century, though its practitioners, too, claim that it has much more ancient origins in early Chinese therapeutic practices known as *qi gung* (energy work).[28] The codification of the Japanese martial arts of judo, jujitsu, karate and aikido is even later, dating to the nineteenth and twentieth centuries. Two things, however, link the exercise cultures of India and East Asia with that of ancient Greece: their role in the individual's moral and spiritual development and their therapeutic applications.

Asian religious philosophies, like Christianity, recognize that ultimately the body has to be transcended to achieve full spiritual enlightenment. But there is no Asian equivalent of the Christian dualism that opposes the divine essence of the soul to the corrupt baseness of the flesh. In Asian thought, the body may also be seen as a temporary vessel for an indestructible spirit – *Atman* or Buddha nature – but in order for individuals to attain liberation and enlightenment, they have to discipline and train their bodies, echoing Plato's previously quoted teaching that a man who is *agymnastos* – untrained – can never hope to attain full mastery over his own desires. In yoga and the martial art of t'ai chi, for example, it would be impossible to reach the first stages of spiritual awakening without the active training of the body.

Restoring Balance

Ancient China, India and Greece shared a belief in the therapeutic power of exercise, but they based it on completely different theories of how the body worked and how exercise affected it. Ancient Greek doctors developed the theory of the four *chymoi*, or humours; traditional Indian *Ayurveda* ('science of life') is based on a similar concept of three *doshas*, or elemental substances, that is combined in yogic practice with a belief in *prana*, the subtle energy that animates the body, flowing through a network of *nadis* (channels) and *chakras* (energy centres, or wheels); and Traditional Chinese Medicine (TCM) focuses on balancing the elemental forces of *yin* and *yang* in the body through the regulation of the subtle energy, *qi*, that flows through channels known as the meridians.[29] In the three systems health is seen as a balance and proper flow of different energies and elemental substances, and diseases as imbalances or blockages, many of which can be treated with therapeutic exercise. The main difference between *Ayurveda* and TCM and Western humorism can be seen in the different function of exercise in the three systems. For the early modern Western physician, exercise might assist in balancing the humours, but it was secondary to factors such as diet and climate, and treatments such as purging and bleeding. Traditional Indian and East Asian doctors, however, believe that practices such as hatha yoga and *qi gung* not only regulate and balance the subtle energies that animate the body but can be used to heal injuries and cure diseases.

Mesoamerican Ball Games

Yoga and the martial arts feature on the schedules of group exercises classes in most gyms, but in terms of layout, equipment and appearance, the yoga ashram and the martial arts *dojo* have not made a major contribution to contemporary gym design. However, there is one extremely important item of equipment now found in all contemporary gyms that we owe to a non-Western athletics culture: the rubber ball, which originated in pre-Columbian Mesoamerica. The Greeks trained in the *sphairisterion* with hard or soft leather balls of different weights and sizes, but these would have had absolutely no bounce, especially on the sandy floors of classical gymnasia. Soon after Christopher Columbus's discovery of the New World in four transatlantic journeys between 1492 and 1506, the Spanish conquered the Aztec and Maya civilizations of Mesoamerica. Among the many novelties that fascinated them were the rubber balls they saw bouncing off the hard stucco floors and sides of Mesoamerican ceremonial ball courts. Brought back to Europe as a curiosity, rubber was gradually adopted as the material of choice for sporting applications, especially for the balls used in team sports. Rubber balls and apparatus, such as fitness balls, exercise bands, medicine balls, rollers and BOSU balance exercisers (and not forgetting rubber mats, floor coverings and bench covers), are an integral part of gym equipment.

Dance Like a Butterfly, Sting Like a Bee

The rediscovery of ancient medical texts by Hippocrates and Galen caused a renewed interest in gymnastics and gymnasia, but had no impact on the sports and exercise cultures of the medieval and early modern periods. In *La gymnastique au XIXe siècle*, the historian of French physical education Gilbert Andrieu describes the athletic and sporting culture of Ancien Régime France.[30] As late as the closing decades of the eighteenth century, France's aristocrats exercised in the same way as their medieval forebears: they fenced, rode, hunted and danced. To this we can add sports such as the *jeu de paume*, a form of tennis played with the hand, which was popular with the French nobility. In England, Henry VIII (1491–1547), who must take his place among the kingdom's most sporting royals, favoured 'real' or 'royal' tennis (the ancestor of modern racket games), and he built a court that can still be visited at Hampton Court Palace in Richmond upon Thames, just west of London.

Kings, queens and courtiers danced in a style reminiscent of contemporary line dancing, with the genders segregated or just holding hands at a respectable distance from one another, lest too close physical contact inflame their carnal passions. Louis XIV of France (1638–1715), the self-proclaimed Roi-Soleil (Sun King), built the palace of Versailles near Paris as a backdrop for the elaborate court ceremonials and entertainments that glorified his own person and the absolute monarchy he had created. Reputed to be a talented dancer in his own right, Louis brought the Italian *balletto* to Versailles, and founded the world's first professional dance company, the Paris Opera Ballet, in 1672.[31] Professional dancers needed a place to practise their art, so the palace must have had a room set aside for rehearsal and training. It is unlikely that it was a custom-designed classical ballet studio with dance bars, mirrored walls and a sprung wooden floor, but however basic it was, for the first time since classical antiquity it would have reintroduced the idea of a space devoted entirely to physical exercise that had no link to functional military training.

Among the athletic pastimes of commoners, we can identify the origins of team sports such as football (soccer), which is attested to be the twelfth-century game of 'Shrovetide football', and cricket (the ancestor of all bat-and-ball games, including baseball), which may date as far back as the fourteenth century, but is known from the sixteenth century in something approaching its modern form. Other forms of exercise for commoners included wrestling and bare-knuckle fighting, though the early modern versions had no relationship with the classical Greek sports. In her cultural history of boxing, Kasia Boddy describes the development of boxing as a spectator sport from bare-knuckle fighting and prize fighting in sixteenth-century England.[32] As with dance, with the passing of several centuries a pastime for amateurs slowly became professionalized: bare-knuckle fighters turned into professional prizefighters and boxers – athletes who needed equipment and places to train. It would be several centuries before specialized boxing gyms emerged in Europe and North America, but, as with the proto-dance studio in seventeenth-century France, early training facilities for boxers re-established a space for functional training for athletic competition.

The Death and Rebirth of an Idea

To draw the rather disparate historical and geographic threads of this chapter together, though the 2,000-year period we have covered witnessed the disappearance of the classical gymnasium, it also saw a number of key social, religious, political, intellectual and artistic developments in the Western world that would lead to the re-emergence of the gymnasium as a place dedicated to physical exercise in the early nineteenth century. The decline of the ancient Greek gymnasium began long before the Christianization of the Roman Empire in the fourth century and the collapse of the Western Roman Empire in the fifth century. As the Greek city-states lost their autonomy first to the Macedonians and then to the Romans, gymnasia were deprived of several of their core functions. They were no longer the institutions where freeborn men and boys were educated, socialized and trained as citizens and soldiers. Instead they became facilities specializing in functional training for athletic competition and in aesthetic training. As a result, the gymnasia of the Hellenistic and Roman periods were viewed as decadent institutions that bred only indolence and vice. The Romans themselves hastened the process of decline by turning Greek gymnasia into annexes of their much larger and more luxurious public bathhouses.

Although it was a Christian emperor who effectively put an end to classical gymnasium culture by abolishing all pagan festivals and the Pan-Hellenic athletics contests, the destruction of many gymnasia during barbarian incursions and the Church's reconfiguration of the body as sinful and same-sex relations as sodomy completed the process. By the fifth century CE there was no social, moral or intellectual space left for an institution dedicated to the care and glorification of the naked male form. With the end of Pax Romana in Western Europe, imperial provinces became independent kingdoms ruled by Germanic and Norse migrants who had their own martial exercise cultures. Paradoxically, their attitudes to public and heroic nudity were more similar to those of the classical Greeks than to those of the prudish Romans. Like other warrior societies, the Germans and Norse valued manliness, strength and martial skill, and for many tribal peoples, barbarian machismo meant going into battle lightly clad or naked. Across much of Western Europe, a new civilization emerged from the collision between Graeco-Roman and Norse-Germanic cultures. The medieval knight is a Christian hybrid of the naked barbarian warrior and the armoured Roman cataphract. For the remainder of the medieval and early modern periods, exercise culture would be dominated by the functional military training of Europe's military elite, the mounted and armoured warrior.

In the Renaissance, the rediscovery of Graeco-Roman texts sparked a new appreciation of the therapeutic value of exercise but did not lead to the opening of gymnasia on the classical model. During the Protestant Reformation, the term gymnasium was revived to denote an establishment devoted to academic and religious education but which paid little or no attention to the development of the body. However, the period witnessed a series of events in Western Europe and the wider world that would play a significant role in the development of the contemporary gym. In the medieval and early modern periods, alternative exercise systems were codified in India and East Asia, and in Europe, the appearance of a new class of professional dancer and prizefighter created the need for places for them to train: the embryonic dance studio and boxing gym.

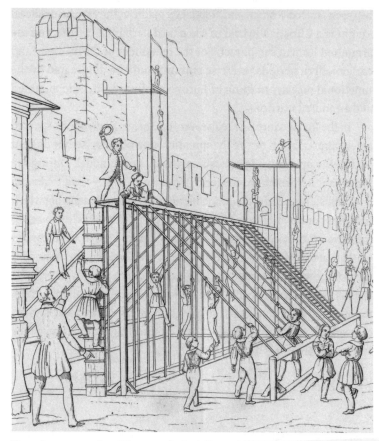

The 19th-century version of the gymnasium was the outdoor *Turnplatz*, or gymnastics field. With its parallel bars, vaulting horses, climbing frames, masts and towers, it was the preferred training ground for schoolchildren, amateur athletes and conscripts throughout the century. This engraving shows a school *Turnplatz* in Basel, Switzerland, in 1847.

3
THE HEALTH OF NATIONS

Military exercises are well calculated to animate the courage of youth,
to fortify their naturally bold, enterprising spirit, and to harden them
against bodily pain, which the effeminacy of our common mode of
living renders highly necessary.

Gymnastics for Youth by Johann Guts Muths (1800)

The many wars that opposed shifting alliances of Western European
powers between 1792 and 1945 could be thought of as a single
153-year conflict, interspersed with interludes of peace of varying
duration. Before 1792, Europe had also constantly been at war, but
for the most part these were dynastic squabbles fought over land and
inheritance rights by rival royal houses that shared the same ideology
of monarchical absolutism. The French Revolution, which attempted
but failed to establish a constitutional monarchy on the British model
in 1789, and resulted instead in the creation of the First French Republic
in 1792, transformed the social and political landscape of Europe,
creating a new kind of conflict underpinned by profound ideological
differences between the combatants. Once the French had guillotined
their last absolute monarch, Louis XVI (1754–1793), successive coalitions
of European monarchies, including Prussia, Austria, Russia and the
United Kingdom, who feared for their own crowned heads, attempted
to restore France's Bourbon Ancien Régime.

In 1793, after many of France's aristocratic generals and officer
corps had defected to the enemy, and with Austrian and Prussian armies
poised to invade and royalist rebellions breaking out all over the
country, the new republic resorted to a *levée en masse* (mass mobilization)

of 300,000 of the motherland's able-bodied male citizens, forever transforming European warfare and tactics, just as the Revolution had overturned European politics. After initial successes against the poorly equipped French citizen armies, the royalist coalitions met constant defeat at the hands of France's generals, the most brilliant of whom was Napoleon Bonaparte (1769–1821). Despite some early setbacks, most notably in his planned invasion of Egypt and Syria (1798–1801), Napoleon so decisively defeated the coalitions whose aims were to crush the Revolution and restore the Bourbon monarchy that he himself decided to overthrow the republic and establish a monarchy of his own. The First French Empire lasted from 1804 to 1814 (with a further hundred-day interlude in 1815), but its effect on Europe was much further-reaching and longer-lasting.

Napoleon's crushing defeat of Frederick William III of Prussia at the Battle of Jena-Auerstedt in 1806 was the opening salvo of a conflict that would not be settled until the mid-twentieth century. Its high, or low, points, depending on your nationality, continued with the Franco–Prussian War (1870–71), fought between Napoleon III's Second Empire (1852–70) and Otto von Bismarck's Prussia, which led to the creation of the Second German Reich (1871–1918). France's desire for revenge was a major factor in the outbreak of the First World War, and similarly, French *revanchisme* after Germany's defeat facilitated Adolf Hitler's rise to power as the Führer of the Third Reich (1933–45), which triggered the final act of this European tragedy with the outbreak of the Second World War.

Each of these conflicts took warfare further away from the formal battlefields of the eighteenth century, in which soldiers in brightly coloured uniforms formed into lines and squares like so many pawns on a chessboard. In the wake of the Revolutionary and Napoleonic Wars, large conscript armies replaced much smaller professional armed forces, while at the same time advances in military technology made set-piece battles redundant. Where pre-Revolutionary armies had required 'a few good men', those of the new 'total war' required large numbers as cannon and later machine-gun fodder. The problem was that, even though the new citizen soldiers did not need the same amount of training as their professional forebears, they still needed a basic level of physical fitness to get to the front to be slaughtered. In other words, they had to be 'fit for purpose', the purpose in this case being military and dictated by the nation-state. For a group of educational pioneers in Germany, Scandinavia and France, the solution was to raise the level of fitness of the general population by developing national physical-education programmes and providing places dedicated to exercise. Initially, these new gymnasia were intended for men of fighting age, but during the course of the nineteenth century it became obvious that the most sensible approach would be to start young and improve the health and fitness of the children who were destined to become the nation-state's future conscripts.

Progress in improving the physical condition of the populations of the industrialized nations of Europe and North America, however, remained painfully slow, and the governments of the major world powers became concerned that their citizens were woefully unfit and incapable of defending the father- or motherland against their near neighbours, who were held up as exemplars of rude health and aggressive vitality. Hence the French Republic terrorized its citizens with tales of German *Übermenschen* (supermen); the Second Reich bemoaned the effeminacy of the Teutonic race when compared to the empire-building Britons; and members of the British establishment, whose own privileged upbringings had been spent 'on the playing fields of Eton' (from the Duke of Wellington's famous quotation about the Allied victory at Waterloo in 1815), bemoaned the puny, consumptive physiques of Albion's lower orders, of whom between one-third and half failed the medicals for admission into the British armed forces during the nineteenth and early twentieth centuries.

'Neither Holy, nor Roman, nor an Empire'

The ancient Greeks invented the gymnasium, and the sixteenth-century Italian scholar and physician Girolamo Mercuriale revived the notion of therapeutic exercise, using ancient sources to give a description of a generic Graeco-Roman gymnasium. However, the first institution devoted to the training of the body since antiquity did not emerge in Greece or Italy, nor from within a province of the Western Roman

Empire, but in suburban Berlin, the capital of the kingdom of Prussia – a region far removed from ancient Rome's easternmost frontiers. There were two Roman provinces, known as Germania Inferior and Germania Superior, whose borders followed the course of the Rhine from the North Sea to Lake Geneva, with an eastward salient between the Main and the Danube, but whose territories excluded most of historical Germany that stretched far to the east into what is now Poland, the Baltic States and European Russia.

During the fifth century, instead of the empire Latinizing the Germanic and Norse tribes, it was the Goths, Franks, Angles, Saxons, Jutes and Vandals who Germanized the Western provinces of the empire. In the year 800, it was their heir, Charlemagne, king of the Franks, who was crowned the first Emperor of the Romans in the West since 476 CE, absolute ruler of a realm that encompassed France, Belgium, the Netherlands, Luxemburg, Germany, Austria, Catalonia, the Czech Republic, Switzerland and Italy. The division of the empire in 843 after the death of Charlemagne's son Louis the Pious marked the creation of the two kingdoms that centuries later would become present-day France and Germany. Although during the following millennium France coalesced into a centralized monarchy, Germany moved in the opposite direction, becoming a federation of autonomous kingdoms, principalities, dukedoms, bishoprics and free cities loosely united within the Holy Roman Empire, an unwieldy political institution that the French philosopher Voltaire described in 1756: 'This body which was called and which still calls itself the Holy Roman Empire was neither holy, nor Roman, nor an empire.'[1]

In 962, the pope crowned Otto the Great the first Holy Roman Emperor, a title that would endure until 1806, when the last incumbent, Francis II, abdicated after being defeated by the first French emperor since Charlemagne, Napoleon Bonaparte. The propagandists of the day attempted to cast the event as a French descendant of Charlemagne reclaiming his rightful throne, but the truth was that Charlemagne could have been claimed by either the Germans or the French, as his empire had united the territories of both countries, and his favourite residence was the Rhineland town of Aachen on the borders of Germany, Belgium and the Netherlands – a town periodically claimed by the French, to whom it is known as Aix-la-Chapelle.[2] There are interesting parallels between classical Greece and the German heartland of the Holy Roman Empire in the late eighteenth and early nineteenth centuries. Like the ancient Greek world, Germany was divided into rival polities, with different forms of government, ideologies and religious affiliations (within the empire, Catholic and Protestant), but a common linguistic and cultural identity. Like Greece's ancient rulers, the German kings and princes patronized a small group of philosophers, political and social reformers, economists and scientists, who together promoted a reform movement known as the Enlightenment, which consciously looked back to ancient precedents by comparing the *philosophes* of eighteenth-century Paris with the sages of classical Athens. In 1995 one of the leading scholars on the eighteenth century, Peter Gay, defined the Enlightenment project as

A vastly ambitious program, a program of secularism, humanity, cosmopolitanism, and above all freedom, freedom in its many forms – freedom from arbitrary power, freedom of speech, freedom of trade, freedom to realize one's talents, freedom of aesthetic response, freedom, in a word, of moral man to make his own way in the world.[3]

For all their influence on the modern world, the *philosophes* were few in number, and they disagreed violently among themselves. In addition, their proposals were not always very practical: they presented utopian solutions to the problems of their age without providing any clear guidance about how to achieve them. The German Enlightenment philosopher Immanuel Kant (1724–1804) encouraged his readers to *sapere aude* (dare to know), but when he asked himself the question, 'Are we living in an enlightened age?' he was forced to admit: 'No. We are living in an Age of Enlightenment.'[4] Although the Enlightenment's political and social reforms were well intentioned, they were beset by internal contradictions. The main tenets of the Enlightenment were secularism, cosmopolitanism and individual freedom, but the reforms were imposed from above by absolute princes who ruled by divine right over subjects who remained steeped in religious bigotry and xenophobia and were opposed by reactionary vested interests among feudal landowners and the clergy. Taken to their logical conclusion, the reforms would have meant the complete overhaul of the established power structure, which would happen during the two Enlightenment-inspired revolutions: the American Revolution and War of Independence (1776–83) and the French Revolution and First Republic (1789–1804). One of the key areas identified by the reformers was education. But here, too, despite the support of absolute rulers, reform was stymied because education was in the hands of the institutions most likely to support the status quo, the Christian churches.

'Everything According to Nature'

After the fall of the Western Roman Empire, the Roman Church preserved what survived of Graeco-Roman learning in Western Europe. As new Christian kingdoms emerged from the wreck of empire, the Church became an indispensable adjunct of the state, lending it its administrative and judicial know-how, and providing education, social care and healthcare to the general population. The Renaissance and the emergence of embryonic nation-states during the early modern period weakened the power of the universal Church of Rome. After the Reformation there were at least two versions of religious truth in Western Europe – Catholic and Protestant – and with the Age of Enlightenment came a third truth based on observation of the world, scientific experimentation and the application of human reason. The Enlightenment reformers understood that education was the key to transforming the social, economic and political institutions of Europe, but education at every level, from elementary schools for commoners to the elite gymnasia (high schools) and universities, was in the charge of the churches. The Catholic Church had long capitalized on the enormous power of education, which the founder of the Jesuit order, Francis Xavier (1506–1552), summarized thus: 'Give me the children until the age of seven, and anyone may have them afterwards.' For the churches, however, the body remained suspect and sinful, and they concerned themselves with the education of the mind as a means to achieve the salvation of the spirit.

Two of the leading figures of the Enlightenment, John Locke (1632–1704) and Jean-Jacques Rousseau (1712–1778), wrote influential books about educational reform. To the modern reader, many of the ideas put forward in Locke's *Some Thoughts Concerning Education* (1693) and Rousseau's *Emile; or, On Education* (1762) not only are eminently sensible but seem to be stating the obvious: boys and girls, rich and poor, should be educated together; education should be child-centred; learning should be enjoyable and encourage pupils to develop their critical faculties through observation of and interaction with the world, and not be limited to rote-learning imposed by harsh physical punishment; and the school curriculum should provide for the development of the body and of manual skills. Locke opens *Some Thoughts* with his take on the famous Latin saying *Mens sana in corpore sano*: 'A sound mind in a sound body, is a short but full description of a happy state in this world.' Although he does not mention physical education specifically, he lauds the value of play, dancing, fencing, riding and wrestling.[5]

Rousseau's injunction to do 'everything according to Nature' and not to start the child's instruction until the age of twelve is much less practical, but in its main outline his programme follows Locke and other contemporary educational reformers.[6] In *Emile*, he agrees with the French essayist Michel de Montaigne (1533–1592), who wrote that for education to 'strengthen the mind you must harden the muscles'. Rousseau underlined the value of play and of practical subjects that brought children into contact with the real world, rather than the traditional curriculum of grammar, rhetoric and theology taught in Latin and Greek. While recognizing the importance of developing the body, Locke and Rousseau did not recommend the teaching of physical education beyond the existing exercise practices of their day and allowing children to follow their natural inclination to play. How children's bodies should be trained through more formal physical education was left to the next generation of educationalists, who tried to turn Rousseau's and Locke's abstract theories into practical reforms.

Before the Revolution of 1789, it was not in France's royal court at Versailles that the Enlightenment received its most enthusiastic reception but in the palaces and chancelleries of the loose confederation of self-governing German states notionally ruled by the Holy Roman emperor. Duke Leopold III, absolute ruler of the small principality of Anhalt-Dessau (now in the German Land of Saxony-Anhalt), was a fervent supporter of the Enlightenment. He invited the educational reformer Johann Basedow (1724–1790) to open a new school in his capital of Dessau in 1774. In the curriculum of the Philanthropinum (derived from the Greek word philanthropia, meaning humanity, benevolence and love of mankind), Basedow attempted to put into practice Locke's and Rousseau's theories. Although the school remained open for less than twenty years, it became a model for other establishments throughout Europe, including the Salzmannschule (the Schnepfenthal Institution) in Schnepfenthal, near Gotha (now in the German Land of Thuringia), founded by Christian Salzmann in 1784.

Salzmann employed Johann Guts Muths (1759–1839), initially as a teacher of academic subjects, but Guts Muths went on to devote much of his 50-year career at the school to the theory and practice of teaching physical education. Now recognized as one of the pioneers of the modern sport of gymnastics, he revived ancient Greek training methods and also devised exercises and equipment of his own.[7] In 1793 he published the first manual of physical education for schoolchildren, Gymnastik für die Jugend, translated into English as Gymnastics for Youth, and published in London in 1800 and in Philadelphia in 1802. In it, Guts Muths made frequent references to the ancient Greeks, making no secret of his admiration for their achievements and lifestyles:

> It is universally acknowledged, that the Greeks were eminent for beauty, and symmetry of form. In my opinion, this is ascribable to their happy climate, excellent works of art, dress, and way of life; though their gymnastic exercises had a particular influence on it. The limbs were as far from being deformed, and the physiognomy disfigured by oppressive labour, and those from being relaxed, by soft and effeminate people.[8]

Guts Muths's exercises included leaping (the high and long jump, and pole vaulting); running; throwing (including the javelin and discus);

wrestling; climbing (ropes, masts and ladders); balancing (on beams and poles); lifting weights (with the description of a primitive adjustable barbell); skipping (with a rope and metal hoops); walking and drilling; games; and swimming. However, he did not see the need for 'spacious edifices' or the 'superb gymnastic structures of the ancients', stating that, 'Our *gymnasium* is, as far as is practicable, *the open air*' (author's italics). He described his ideal spot for exercise as a field covered with dry turf with trees for shade, a little handy hill and a brook or river.[9] According to Guts Muths, regular gymnastic exercises not only ensured the proper physical development of the child and prevented disease and deformity, but saved the individual from succumbing to the greatest danger of civilized life: 'effeminacy'. His definition of the word, which he uses throughout the book, does not carry the sexual implications of later periods but refers to a lack of physical strength and moral fibre. Like many Enlightenment thinkers, he believed that 'civilized' men and women, when compared to the ancient Greeks and Germans who lived more in accordance with the precepts of 'Nature', had become weak and soft from too much luxurious living.

Another early northern European pioneer of physical education influenced by the Enlightenment and by Guts Muths's writings was the Dane Franz Nachtegall (1777–1847). He opened a private outdoor gymnasium in Copenhagen in 1799 and later obtained the support and patronage of Frederick VI of Denmark (1768–1839) who, deeply imbued with Enlightenment ideas, set out to reform his realm. In 1804 Frederick established the Military Gymnastic Institute to provide a systematic programme of physical education for the Danish armed forces, appointing Nachtegall as its first director.[10] The equivalence between soft living and moral decay, contrasted with the social and moral benefits of physical education, will be a leitmotiv for the remainder of the chapter. For the ancient Greeks, physical exercise was part of their moral and intellectual training to achieve their full individual potential, or *arete*, which also included the service of their native city-state; but in the writings of Guts Muths and his disciples in late eighteenth-century Western Europe, there was an inversion in the nature and function of physical education. As the century progressed it would be the nation-state that increasingly defined and controlled what exercise was, and imposed it on the children in its care to mould them into the kind of citizen it required. Physical fitness, or fitness for purpose, was not an individual attainment freely offered to the state by the citizen, but a social obligation demanded by the state of its citizens.

When Guts Muths published *Gymnastics for Youth*, the French had already guillotined their last absolute ruler and established the First French Republic, signalling for some the final wreck of the Enlightenment, and for others its fullest expression. The pace of reform sped up all over Europe, but not through the peaceful efforts of reformers basing their theories on the writings of philosophers and supported by enlightened despots, but disseminated across the continent by wars and revolutions. Having disposed of their absolute monarchy, aristocratic privilege and religious conformity, the French were keen to export their brand of revolution to the rest of Europe, producing a kind of eighteenth-century domino effect that saw radicals among France's neighbours deposing their rulers and setting up republics on the French model. When Napoleon overthrew the Directoire, the final incarnation of France's First Republic, to award himself the ancient Roman title of First Consul in 1799, it was merely a prelude to his restoration of the monarchy with himself as emperor. Self-crowned as the new Caesar or Charlemagne in Paris, with the pope sidelined as a mere spectator, and in Milan, as king of Italy, Napoleon set about subjugating the rest of Europe. After his crushing defeat of imperial Russia and Austria at the Battle of Austerlitz in 1805, he brought an end to the 898-year-old Holy Roman Empire, uniting its western territories into the pro-French Confederation of the Rhine (1806–13), whose 35 members were meant to keep the power of Austria and Prussia in check. When Prussia rebelled, Napoleon destroyed her armies in a single campaign, occupied Berlin and confiscated much of her territory, distributing it among his new German allies in the west and Poland in the east.

Turning the Napoleonic Tide

Napoleon's defeat of Prussia was as shocking to Europeans as the Hitlerian *Blitzkrieg* that overran France in 1940. It inspired one of Guts Muths's disciples, Friedrich Jahn (1778–1852), who taught physical education at several secondary schools in Berlin, to redefine exercise as a mass movement of national salvation for Prussia, in the broader framework of a Pan-German revival to counter growing French influence in the former states of the now defunct Holy Roman Empire. Instead of concentrating his efforts on schoolchildren, Jahn targeted men of fighting age, who, he hoped, would succeed where Prussia's professional army had failed in defeating the seemingly invincible French. Like Guts Muths, Jahn favoured training in the open air, but unlike his mentor, he would go much further than 'a field of dry turf with a few trees and a little handy hill' when he established the first *Turnplatz* at Hasenheide on the outskirts of Berlin in 1811. Jahn explained why he had decided to call his system of exercise *Turnen* and not *Gymnastik*: 'It is an undisputed right to give a German thing or activity a name from the German language. Why go begging words from foreign languages when we have a better and more appropriate word in the mother tongue?'[11] In any case, he could not use the word gymnasium as it had been used to denote secondary schools in Germany since the sixteenth century; hence the first institution dedicated to physical exercise since antiquity was called a *Turnplatz* (*Turnen* field or place).

As with the ancient Greek gymnasium, a modern visitor transported to Hasenheide in 1811 would be hard pressed to identify a *Turnplatz* as a gym. A *Treatise on Gymnasticks* (1828) contained plans for different *Turnplätze*, with detailed descriptions of the layout and equipment required for establishments of between 80 and 400 'turners' (gymnasts). The book was intended as a manual for schools, but the descriptions are probably representative of the 150 *Turnplätze* that Jahn claimed existed in Germany by 1815. He recommended that a *Turnplatz* should be one or two miles (2 or 3 km) outside the city in the open country, providing a healthy walk for younger turners of eight or nine years of age, while the adults came on horseback or by horse-drawn transport.

He specified a 'level but high situation', where the air was healthier, with firm soil and where wet and damp would not interrupt the exercises too frequently. In ancient times, slaves or the junior members of a gymnasium dug and turned the sandy surface of the palaestra in preparation for the day's exercises, but for the Turnplatz Jahn favoured turf, conceding that if the soil were not firm enough for running or jumping, it should be covered with clay, stamped down and strewn with sand.

A Turnplatz suitable for 400 turners should occupy a large rectangular field about 465 × 260 ft (140 × 80 m) with a fixed boundary – a fence or ditch – with the very practical aim of keeping animals out, but also bordered with trees to increase its 'pleasantness', and with one or more entrances for turners and spectators, allowing free access to the field for pedestrians and vehicles without the need to cross any of the exercise grounds. Trees, in particular lindens (limes), could also be used to demarcate the different areas, provide shade and support climbing apparatus. If the field were to be used for more than three hours at a time, it would require a regular water supply, but this seemed to be intended for drinking, as there is no mention in the book of facilities for washing or bathing after a training session. The only building on the site was a large barn-like structure in the centre of the field that would be used to store the moveable apparatus daily, and the larger equipment when not in use in the winter. The building could also be used as a place to hang clothing, and as a rest area with benches and a blackboard for notices.

One of the major differences between the modern gym and the classical gymnasium was the lack of permanent equipment on display, as most training was done either without equipment or with small, portable pieces such as the discus, javelin and halteres. Jahn's list of apparatus to be stored in the barn daily shows the wide range of activities practised in the Turnplatz: ropes and yokes for pulling and drawing; ropes for skipping; strings, pegs and poles for vaulting; lances and balls for throwing; saddle cushions; and weights and dumb-bells for lifting. The Turnplatz had a running track, 300–400 ft long × 24–30 ft wide (90–120 × 7–9 m), with further grounds of various sizes for running in circles, leaping, throwing, skipping, wrestling, warm-up exercises and gymnastic games, all marked out with trees or furrows. The main difference between the Turnplatz and the Greek gymnasium, as well as the modern gym, was the type of fixed equipment on which the turners exercised. Several items would be familiar to someone who has seen or practised the modern sport of gymnastics – the long and short vaulting horses, single bar, balancing beam and parallel bars – and several more would be familiar from an athletics field, such as the pole-vaulting and high-jump stands, but towering over the field were apparatus that today, for reasons of safety alone, you would be unlikely to find anywhere apart from military assault courses and the more dangerous kind of adventure playground: climbing frames with poles, ropes, ladders and one, two or four masts, measuring 30 ft (10 m) or more in height, without the provision of any safety harnesses.[12]

Men in ancient Greece visited the gymnasium daily from childhood, and trained all year round, but Jahn recommended that turners train two afternoons a week; and because of the lack of covered facilities, and the harshness of the Prussian winter, training was only possible during the drier and warmer months of the year. Climate and morality also dictated the proper dress for a turner. Although Neoclassicism was in full swing and heroic nude statues in the Graeco-Roman style adorned public squares and buildings, there was no question of men and boys stripping off for exercise, even to a modest baggy undershirt and shorts. Jahn advised that clothes should be 'durable, cheap, and fit for all movements. Linen, not yet bleached, is the best material; a jacket, or roundabout, and pantaloons, the best form.'[13] However, he did specify in the Turnplatz rules that 'Every gymnick shall exercise only with coat, hat, and neckcloth laid aside', adding that cravats and neck cloths would be inconvenient or injurious, as well as braces with crosspieces in the traditional German style, because they would constrict breathing and free movement.[14] On his feet, the turner should wear boots that were neither too high nor too heavy. To translate this into modern terms: the turner trained wearing a linen shirt, long trousers held up by braces, a short fitted jacket and leather shoes.

Jahn did not go into detail about the financial management of the Turnvereine (Turnen clubs) that opened all over Germany in the 1810s and '20s, but as there was little in the way of buildings or investment needed for the equipment and apparatus, they were probably community enterprises paid for by small government subsidies, and modest subscriptions or fees for use, with the turners themselves providing the labour to build and maintain the Turnplatz, as well as any coaching necessary. In their first incarnation, the Turnvereine were open to all regardless of age, ability or gender, though early nineteenth-century prints show men and boys disporting themselves on the apparatus with women and girls looking on. Jahn was adamant that spectators should be welcome so that everyone gained 'a correct idea of the character and value of gymnastick exercises'. And, as a bonus, the presence of the public also ensured that proper moral conduct would be maintained.[15]

In one respect, the Turnplatz was quite close to its ancient predecessor: it was also a place primarily intended for functional military training. Jahn saw it as a means of revitalizing and uniting the German race, and allowing it to throw off the yoke of the hated French oppressor. Although there is some mention of the therapeutic value of exercise in his work, his initial aim is always to prepare men and boys to be soldiers, and many of the exercises are martial in nature. The whole concept of the Turnplatz is as a place for group and not individual exercise, and unlike the single-exerciser versions of today, the smaller apparatus, such as the vaulting horses, balance beams and parallel bars, were designed to be used by between eight and twelve turners at a time. In an age when the civic amenities – public or private – that we take for granted did not exist, and theatres and concert halls were reserved for the rich, a Turnplatz open to all would have been revolutionary in itself. The radical nature of the idea, and of the Pan-German ideology that underpinned it, while it had suited the governments of Austria, Prussia and the German states during the Napoleonic Wars, was considered dangerous once France had been defeated and as much of the pre-Revolution status quo as could be salvaged had been restored. In 1819, under pressure from Austria's ultra-conservative government, states across Germany banned the Turnvereine, and Jahn was imprisoned until 1825. He was released after agreeing not to teach or take part in Turnen. Although gymnastics continued under other names and guises in Germany during this period, the ban on the turners would not be lifted until 1842.[16]

Turners and the State

Apart from a brief period between 1811 and 1815, when *Turnvereine* were subsidized by the governments of the German states, they remained independent of state control and funding. They were civic enterprises more akin to modern municipal sports centres than private commercial gymnasia, but they were not sanctioned or controlled by the authorities, and therefore, potentially, could become breeding grounds for revolutionaries and radicals. It is a bit difficult for the modern reader to understand what the conservative regimes of early nineteenth-century Germany were so worried about. After all, exercising on the parallel bars is not the same as erecting barricades or cutting off the heads of aristocrats, but what they were really worried about was the ideology associated with the turners, many of whom were radical, egalitarian democrats who wanted to see an end to the many feudal regimes that prevented the unification and modernization of Germany.

We could compare the fears inspired by the *Turnen* movement in the 1820s to present-day concerns about what is being taught in Islamic schools, mosques and madrasas. Despite the ban in its homeland, Jahn's *Turnen* was influential all over the Western world. Two former Hasenheide turners, Charles Follen (1796–1840) and Charles Beck (1798–1866), emigrated to the U.S. in 1824 to escape persecution in Germany. Each established *Turnplätze*: Follen in Boston and Beck at Round Hill School in Northampton, Massachusetts. In 1826 they worked together to establish the first collegiate gymnasium in the U.S., at Harvard University in Cambridge, Massachusetts. The introduction of *Turnen* was only partially successful, and the Harvard gymnasium was not popular with the student body and was forced to close. A second wave of radical turners emigrated to the U.S. in the wake of the failed liberal revolutions of 1848. At the outbreak of the American Civil War (1861–5) there were 150 *Turnvereine* in the U.S. with an estimated 10,000 members.[17] The turners continued to thrive in America through the two world wars, despite their associations with Germany and German nationalism.[18]

Ironically, it was in Germany that the Turnen movement faced its greatest challenge in the first half of the twentieth century. Although Hitler made use of German nationalism for his own twisted ends, and supported physical education to breed stronger, fitter citizens and soldiers for his 1,000-year Reich, he could not tolerate the competition from the independent Turnvereine, which he banned after he came to power in 1933. Having taken over organized gymnastics, the Nazi propaganda machine used it to promote its corporatist, racist ideology at displays and rallies across the Reich and the occupied territories. The ultimate expression of gymnastics subverted to the ends of the state in the twentieth century are recorded in Leni Riefenstahl's film of the Berlin summer Olympics of 1936, when in the 'Pageant of Youth', held on the evening of the opening ceremony on 1 August, 10,000 carefully chosen Aryan youths of both sexes performed synchronized gymnastics movements wearing a modern interpretation of ancient Greek dress.[19] Although the Nazis made use of Graeco-Roman imagery in their pageants and propaganda, inventing the Olympic torch ceremony at Olympia and the torch relay, they did not build an infrastructure of Nazi gymnasia, nor develop physical education programmes of their own. They merely appropriated and perverted Jahn's Turnen for their own militaristic and nationalistic ends.

European Rivals and Collaborators

By the first decades of the nineteenth century, the idea of universal public education had come of age. France's First Republic had laicized public education in the 1790s, extending primary schooling to all children and establishing the modern lycée system of high schools. The reform had become so entrenched that it survived the restoration of the Bourbon monarchy in 1815. What its curriculum did not provide, however, was a coherent or sustained programme of physical education, precisely at a time when this was becoming more necessary. Industrialization and urbanization were transforming the Western world from a landscape of agrarian communities and market towns linked by roads into one of industrial cities linked by railways. Factories and offices were creating an ever-growing demand for skilled workers and clerks; and the new conscript armies needed not only educated soldiers who could operate the increasingly sophisticated military technology, but able-bodied men who could survive the rigours of army life without an extended period of preparatory training. Unfortunately, at the same time, the lack of public provision of sanitation, housing or healthcare, and long hours and poor working conditions combined with low wages, meant that working-class boys and men were becoming unhealthier and physically smaller and weaker.

It was a problem that would plague the industrializing nations of Europe and North America for the rest of the century. Between 1864 and 1867, the British army rejected 380 out of every 1,000 volunteers, and as the century wore on, the situation worsened.[20] At the turn of the twentieth century, the rejection rate had risen to 50 per cent.[21] Tackling the problem was complex because it required major reform in a number of areas, including public sanitation, housing and healthcare; labour legislation to outlaw child labour and control working hours and increase wages; and the provision of physical education classes for schoolchildren and conscripts. Ultimately the problem of the health and fitness of the citizens of the Western world would not be addressed until the middle of the twentieth century, but following in Jahn's footsteps, physical-education pioneers in Europe and North America canvassed governments, cities and universities to establish physical fitness programmes and public gymnasia. The first countries that took their lead from Germany to provide state physical education were Denmark, Sweden and France.

The Free Scandinavian Exercises

Denmark was among the first states to develop a systematic approach to the teaching of physical education, beginning with the Military Gymnastic Institute in 1804, and the provision of physical education in secondary schools in 1809 and in elementary schools from 1814, after which Frederick VI appointed Franz Nachtegall director of gymnastics for the entire country.[22] Unfortunately, after the end of the Napoleonic Wars, during which Denmark had been allied with France, the union between the crowns of Norway and Denmark was dissolved, and Denmark was effectively bankrupted, slowing the pace of educational reform. Nevertheless, by the year 1829, when France had only fourteen military and school gymnasia, Denmark had around 4,000.[23]

Nachtegall's work was taken forward by one of his Swedish students, Pehr Henrik Ling (1776–1839), who studied intermittently in Copenhagen from 1800 to 1805 while taking part in military actions against the British alongside the Danes, as well as travelling all over Europe until he was forced to return to Scandinavia because of financial difficulties and ill health. Having obtained a teaching post in Sweden, he took up fencing as a hobby, which restored his health, convincing him of the therapeutic benefits of exercise.[24] According to V. K. Rao, 'Ling's greatest contribution is that he strove to make physical education a science.' He studied anatomy and physiology in order to understand the effects of exercise on the human body, dividing gymnastics into three fields: 'educational', 'military' and 'medical'.[25] In 1815, he founded the Royal Gymnastic Institute in Stockholm to train teachers of physical education for Sweden's schools and armed forces.

Ling's gymnastics do not play a direct role in the development of the gymnasium. Unlike Nachtegall and Jahn, who established outdoor gymnasia with training apparatus, Ling based his system on free movements of the body that could be practised without equipment in any open space. He rejected the use of equipment because it might overtax the body, and also of music, as it could be a dangerous distraction.[26] His system stressed the importance of foot placement in each exercise and the synchronized performance of the exercises by all students, who trained like soldiers performing drills on the parade ground.[27] Because the system did not require any major outlay for apparatus or buildings, it was widely adopted by schools across the world. In 1881, when the London School Board decided to introduce physical education in all elementary schools in the British capital, it opted for Ling's gymnastics because the system could be used to teach both boys and girls at minimal expense.[28]

In *Here Comes the Sun*, Ken Worpole describes the continuing popularity of the synchronized free exercises in Europe during the interwar years. But rather than being performed in an indoor setting, they were part of an outdoor health-and-fitness culture that included sports and naturism, practised in a new type of resort setting specifically aimed at the more affluent and leisured members of the working class – the seaside holiday camp. Men and women were encouraged to socialize in swimwear, and were able to show off their bodies and see those of others in ways unthinkable to previous generations.[29] In the context of the modern gym, Ling's gymnastics is the origin of callisthenics, which are used as warm-up exercises for sports and weight training, as well as of the basic movements used in many group exercise classes.

Le Gymnase à la Française

Despite the influence of the Enlightenment philosophers on the teaching of physical education, compared to the Germans and Scandinavians the French were relative latecomers to the creation of purpose-built gymnasia. Before the French Revolution, schools were reserved for the elites – the aristocracy and those among the bourgeoisie who were rich enough to emulate their social superiors. Their sons (women's education did not exist) engaged in the physical pursuits suited to their class: riding, hunting, fencing and training at arms, and dancing.[30]

During the revolutionary and Napoleonic periods, though there were sweeping reforms to public education, in the field of physical education there was no mass civic movement such as the turners, nor a state-led initiative such as Ling's Royal Gymnastic Institute. Since the establishment of the absolute monarchy in the late seventeenth century, the philosophy and practice of government in France had been leading to an inexorable centralization of power, talent and resources in the capital. This trend only strengthened during the First Republic and Empire, when reforms were imposed from the centre on the provinces. In this climate, it was not surprising that any educational reforms should be pursued by the central government in the capital rather than by any grassroots movement, as was possible in the relatively decentralized German and Anglo-Saxon settings.

France's first physical-education reformer was not a Frenchman but a Spaniard, Don Francisco Amoros y Ondeano, Marquis of Sotelo

(1770–1848), who based his ideas on the work of the Swiss educational reformer Johann Heinrich Pestalozzi (1746–1827). Like Rousseau, Pestalozzi promoted a child-centred method that placed greater emphasis on physical education than the conventional schooling of the day, though, also like Rousseau, he did not make any specific recommendations beyond the creation of an 'ABC of practical power'.[31] An army colonel, Amoros was appointed preceptor to King Charles IV (1748–1819) of Spain's youngest son, and obtained funds from the king to establish a military gymnasium in Madrid. When Napoleon invaded Spain in 1807, and placed his brother Joseph (1768–1844) on the Spanish throne, Amoros collaborated with the new regime, and when the French were expelled from Spain in 1813, Amoros followed them across the Pyrenees, becoming a naturalized French citizen in 1816. Perhaps because he was of Spanish origin and thus not involved in the preceding quarter century of political turmoil, he survived the transition from the First Empire to the Bourbon Restoration with the accession to the throne of Louis XVIII in 1814.

Using his royal Spanish credentials rather than his now tarnished Napoleonic connections, Amoros established a small open-air gymnasium with a Greek-style covered portico at the Institution Durdan, a private boarding school in Paris' fifth arrondissement. He used this as a model to propose to Louis XVIII's government a plan for a much grander national institution, the Gymnase Normal, Militaire et Civil, to be established on a 47,500-square-metre (12-acre) site at the Parc de Grenelle on the south bank of the Seine, an area now dominated by the Eiffel Tower, to cater for students of France's elite lycées, renamed collèges royaux (royal colleges) during the Restoration, and for the French armed forces, which had several barracks and training establishments in the neighbourhood.[32]

Although there were similarities between the proposed gymnase and Jahn's Turnplatz, what Amoros envisaged was on a much grander scale. In volume one of his Manuel de l'éducation physique, gymnastique et morale (1830), Amoros described the extraordinary plans that he had for the gymnase, which were only partially realized, because to complete the whole scheme would have probably bankrupted an already strained French exchequer. Visitors arriving by carriage would drive through a

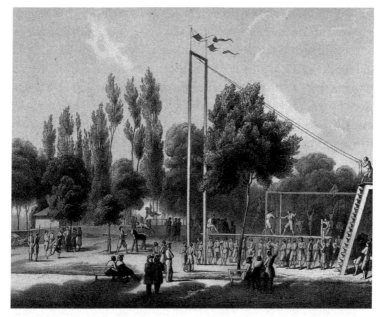

Outdoor gymnasia with their fixed equipment required little financial outlay to set up and had minimal running costs. Originally established by political and social reformers, they were gradually taken over by nation-states to serve their own ends. Pictured here is the outdoor gymnasium of the Colonie de Mettray, in central France, an institution for young offenders opened in 1839.

grand Neoclassical stone gateway and alight in a covered reception area. The proposed buildings around the entrance included an amphitheatre for classes in physiology and singing, demonstrations and lectures; the residences of the *directeur gymnasiarque*, that is, Amoros himself, consciously identified with the official in charge of an ancient Greek gymnasium, and of the teaching staff; and other sundry classrooms and storerooms.

Moving on to the facilities themselves, Amoros enumerated a changing room; a fencing school; a large gymnastic hall with apparatus for training in winter; a long portico open to a park, which he associated with an ancient running track, or *xystos*, for training under cover; a riding school, hippodrome for horse and chariot races, and stable block with its subsidiary buildings; two swimming pools, one heated for winter use, two further pools for marine exercises, one with a bridge for jumping into the water, and ships' masts with full rigging for naval training; 22 courts for *jeux de balle au mur* and a large court for ball games. The military theme of the facilities was underlined by the names he gave them, such as the *Montagne de la Gloire* (Mount Glory) – an artificial hill 100 ft (30 m) high, with one side completely vertical, and with a tower, a well or mine, and fortifications. The park would also house several porticos between 7 and 16 ft high (2–5 m) with climbing apparatus; two ditches for leaping on foot and horseback; masts ranging in height from 20 to 50 ft (6–15 m); wooden ladders from 9 to 15 ft (2.7–4.5 m), ropes and rope ladders; several sets of parallel bars; two *octogones* – a 30-ft (10-m) eight-sided climbing tower built around a mast of Amoros's own design; rifle and pistol ranges; archery and javelin fields; fortifications for mock assaults; an area for warm-up exercises and games; and finally an area set aside for the 'agreeable exercise of parents'.[33]

Apart from any qualifications he had in the teaching of physical education, Amoros was a gifted PR man and self-publicist. In 1820 he obtained the backing of the French minister of the interior, Count Siméon, who wrote to him, clearly intending the letter to be seen by a wider readership. The goals that the director of the Gymnase Civil Normal must set himself, Siméon wrote, must be: 'To strengthen the health of children, improve their manners, and develop their moral, intellectual, and physical qualities; to train virtuous French citizens and loyal subjects of the king.'[34] While Amoros made allusion to the therapeutic value of exercise in his writings, the aims of his system and of the Gymnase were made clear in the title of his two-volume *Manuel de l'éducation physique, gymnastique et morale* ('Manual of Physical, Gymnastic and Moral Education'), which became the standard text for schools and the military for the next two decades. Gymnastics, the author argued – and the king and his government no doubt fervently hoped – would breed a new kind of fitter and more disciplined French citizen, who would be less inclined to overthrow their government.

The Gymnase Normal, Militaire et Civil opened in 1820, and within a year, with little of the buildings and equipment in place, Amoros published a second book, entitled *Gymnase normal, militaire et civil*, which, along with a brief description of the state of the *gymnase* at the beginning of 1821, consists almost entirely of testimonials from the great and the good – ministers, military men, aristocrats and doctors – endorsing the aims of the institution and extolling the abilities of its first *directeur gymnasiarque*. On the frontispiece, Amoros is styled rather grandly as 'Former colonel, Director of the Pestalozzi Institute in Madrid, Counsellor and Secretary to Charles IV, Preceptor to the Infante Don Francisco de Paula, and Member of several learned societies'. Amoros succeeded in opening his Gymnase, but period illustrations show something much more akin to a *Turnplatz* than the athletics-military Disneyland he had originally envisaged.

In 1830 the restored Bourbon monarchy made way for France's second constitutional monarchical experiment, when Louis-Philippe I of the Orléans branch of the French ruling house replaced the un-popular Charles X. Amoros managed to keep his post under the new regime, but he lost the funding for the civilian section of the Gymnase, which was forced to close in 1833, and then for the military section, leading to its closure in 1837.[35] Amoros's dream of two national centres of excellence – a civilian *gymnase* that would accommodate all the students of Paris' elite *lycées* and train teachers for the nation's schools, and a sister institution for the military – met internal opposition from school principals, who thought that to send their pupils to a central location would be too disruptive, and politicians, who were not entirely convinced of the value of physical education or who baulked at the enormous cost of the project. Although France's first experiment in state-funded physical education had lasted only seventeen years, it had set the pattern for future school and military gymnasia, many run by men trained by Amoros. With his books, Amoros had established a style of gymnastics, gymnasia and gymnastic apparatus that, though they owed a great deal to Jahn and the *Turnplatz*, and were devised by a man of Spanish origins, were nevertheless recognized as quintessentially French.

It would take several further failed attempts at reform during the next three decades before every *lycée* in the country had its own in-door gymnasium. A photograph taken in about 1875 of the indoor gymnasium of the Lycée de Louis-le-Grand in Paris shows a large, high-ceilinged hall with benches on three sides and a raised stage on the fourth side, showing that the room could also be used for school

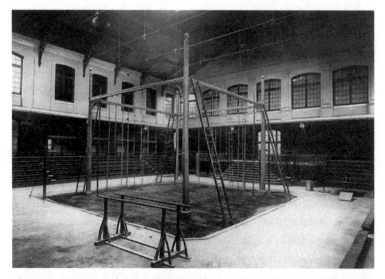

The successor to the outdoor *Turnplatz*, the late 19th-century indoor school gymnasium is still not recognizable as a contemporary gym but more like a hall for artistic gymnastics. The *gymnase* of the Lycée Louis-le-Grand in Paris, photographed in 1875, remained the model for French school gymnasia well into the 20th century.

assemblies, plays, concerts and prize-giving ceremonies. A large oblong cast-iron frame occupies the centre of the hall, built over what appears to be a sandpit or an area of loose soil. A wooden ladder in each corner gives access to the upper transverse beams. Hanging from the upper members of two sides are a selection of ropes, rope ladders and poles, some with footholds, for students to climb, and a set of gymnastics rings. In the foreground a set of parallel bars is visible, and running the length of one side of the frame is what looks like a single horizontal bar, and at the back, a lower balance beam. As only two sides of the hall are visible in the lithograph, it is likely that other pieces of apparatus, such as a vaulting horse, are present but out of shot. The caption accompanying the image explains that this indoor gymnasium was complemented by an outdoor one, with apparatus shaded by a stand of trees.[36]

There were two main reasons why the Amoros formula of a large, central open-air gymnasium did not succeed. For one, the climate in the Paris region, though milder than the Prussian climate, is no more suited to outdoor training in the colder and wetter months. Hence, for students to have their weekly training sessions, a covered space was essential. In terms of the disruption to the school day and the travel time for thousands of pupils across Paris, it also made much more sense to bring the gymnasium to the students rather than the other way around. During the course of the nineteenth century, the French system was adopted all over Europe, leading to the provision of physical education (PE) for all school students in purpose-built indoor gymnasia.

The type of PE on offer in French schools remained unchanged well into the twentieth century. As the son of French parents who settled in London when I was a child, I completed my education from elementary through to high school (primary and secondary education in the UK) at the Lycée Français de Londres (opened in 1915, and later renamed the Lycée Français Charles de Gaulle for the leader of the Free French during the Second World War, later the first president of the Fifth Republic from 1959 to 1969). The Lycée is part of a worldwide network of schools operated by the French state with the dual aims of educating its expatriate sons and daughters and promoting French culture across an increasingly English-speaking world. London's Lycée was a particularly significant foundation because it had been established in the capital of France's principal European enemy and rival from the Middle Ages to the signing of the *Entente Cordiale* (Friendship Accord) between the two countries in 1904.

Adhering to the national curriculum set centrally by the French Ministry of Education in all subjects, the Lycée provided one hour a week of state-sanctioned *education physique* (gym class in the U.S. and PE in the UK) or *gymnastique* in a purpose-built *salle de gymnastique* (gymnasium), in addition to one afternoon a week set aside for team sports. The *salle* was a large, high-ceilinged hall with a wooden floor; it doubled as a gymnasium where students did their weekly gym class and an indoor sports court with handball goals and basketball hoops at either end. One wall was fitted with ladders and ropes, and various pieces of antique gymnastic equipment lined the back and sides of the hall, including a vaulting horse, a set of parallel bars, floor mats and different-sized leather balls, while other sundry athletics equipment was packed away in large wicker baskets and cupboards. What was noticeably absent was any of the equipment that you would expect to find in a contemporary gym: free weights and benches, weight-training machines and cardio equipment such as stationary cycles and treadmills. What I did not realize at the time was that the *salle de gymnastique* was the product of a European health-and-fitness culture whose origin could be traced back to the first quarter of the nineteenth century and the outdoor gymnasia designed by Amoros and his disciples.

The other health-related practice common to the Lycée and all other French state-run schools was the yearly *visite médicale*, or medical examination, performed by a French doctor who was summoned from France to perform the task. From my hazy memories as a pupil, the examination consisted of being weighed and measured, being given a fairly cursory medical with a stethoscope, and being tapped on the back to check for signs of pulmonary disease or tuberculosis – one of the medical scourges of nineteenth-century Europe against which French children have been routinely vaccinated since before the Second World War. The next stage of the examination was devoted entirely to postural problems, and there was not one among my fellow students who was not diagnosed with either *scoliose* (scoliosis) or *lordose* (lordosis) – two deformities of the spine whose most serious manifestations would require surgical intervention. Like most school pupils of our age, we slouched and were round-shouldered from poorly designed school furniture combined with the preferred pose of the teenager, but to diagnose serious spinal defects was an act of medical terrorism that can be understood only in light of the concerns of nineteenth- and twentieth-century nation-states obsessed with the physical condition of future citizen-conscripts.

Although by the 1890s training in France's schools had moved indoors, the transformation of the nation's health remained a slow and ongoing process.[37] On the eve of the Great War, Georges Hébert (1875–1957), who pioneered the 'Natural Method' of physical education and is credited with the invention of the obstacle course for functional military training, complained of the low levels of physical fitness of French men and boys when compared to the Germans, British, Americans and Japanese. In *La culture virile et les devoirs physiques de l'officier combatant* ('The Virile Culture and Physical Duties of the Serving Officer',

1913), he claimed that up to 65 per cent of schoolchildren suffered from serious spinal defects, and shocked his readers when he revealed that in 1908, of the 318,000 conscript intake, 30,000 had been rejected on health grounds, while a further 22,000 had been invalided out of the army during their first two years of service.[38]

The Anglo-Saxon Contribution

Britain is known as a country with a sporting tradition that dates back to the medieval period. The English invented many of the world's most popular team sports, including football (soccer), rugby, rounders (softball) and cricket, as well as the main racquet sports such as tennis, badminton and squash, while the Scots gave the world the noble art of golf. It is also to England that we owe the transformation of bareknuckle fighting into the sport of boxing.[39] In terms of the teaching of physical education, however, Great Britain lagged far behind Continental Europe. There was no British Jahn, Ling or Amoros. When the British army was casting around for someone to devise a programme of physical education for its recruits in the early nineteenth century, it turned to an American-born, naturalized Swiss citizen with the splendid Graeco-Germanic name of Phokion Heinrich Clias (1782–1854), whose system was largely based on Jahn's *Turnen*.

There are several reasons why the British did not follow the French or Scandinavian models. For one, Britain is far larger and more regionally diverse than the Scandinavian countries and much less centralized than France. Britain had always had (and retains) a mixed educational system of church, state, charity and elite private (known as 'public') schools, each accorded a high degree of autonomy in the choice of curriculum and teaching methods. In his writings and speeches, Pierre de Coubertin (1863–1937), the founder of the modern Olympic movement, contrasted the freedom of the Anglo-Saxon games-based method of physical education with the rigid discipline of German gymnastics, arguing for a mixed system that would combine the best of both.

When it came to teaching physical education, the British had an advantage over the Germans in that there were no radical political associations with *Turnen*-gymnastics, and over the French, because they were not limited by having to get approval and funding for their experiments from the central government in the capital. In his career, Archibald MacLaren (1820–1884) combined government service, devising a system of physical education for the British armed forces in 1860, with his own personal experiments in the teaching of physical education.[40] In his case, however, the funding came not from a wealthy aristocratic patron or the Crown, but from the independent and very wealthy University of Oxford. While the French Ministry of Education was still discussing whether indoor or outdoor gymnasia would be best suited to France's *lycées*, MacLaren argued successfully that exercise should take place indoors, to preserve the health of students and the condition of the apparatus, and in a building that was not only soundly constructed, well lit and well ventilated but also heated in cold weather.[41]

The result was a two-storey, purpose-designed gymnasium in the centre of Oxford with a central dome topped with an octagonal lantern and with windows providing light and ventilation, and, a luxury at the time, a central-heating system. MacLaren's Oxford Gymnasium opened in 1858, and received glowing reviews from the publications of the day, including the *London Illustrated News*. The lower floor housed

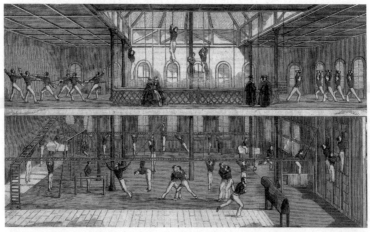

The move to indoor gymnasia attached to school premises, colleges and barracks served both practical and political ends: it enabled training to continue throughout the year and gave the authorities greater control over what was taught and by whom. Interior of the Oxford Gymnasium, from the *Illustrated London News*, 5 November 1859.

gymnastic fittings and apparatus familiar from the French *gymnase* and the German *Turnplatz*; the second floor was set aside for fencing, free exercises and training with dumb-bells and barbells that were performed not individually, but as a type of early group exercise class. In the centre of the gymnasium, and running through the two floors up into the central lantern, was a 60-ft (18-m) mast – the trunk of a Norwegian spruce – which, along with ropes and ladders, was used for climbing exercises.[42]

In the mid-nineteenth century, Britain was the world's undisputed military superpower, far outstripping its rivals technologically, industrially and commercially, controlling many of the world's natural resources through a vast colonial empire on which the sun proverbially never set. But Britain, like its European and American rivals, was not immune from fears that its population was becoming morally and physically degenerate – fears that might not be unfounded if one examines the living conditions of the working class of Victorian England that can be glimpsed in the novels of Charles Dickens, including *Oliver Twist* (1838), *Hard Times* (1854) and *Little Dorrit* (1856). The British response, however, was not a grand civic or state-funded project like Jahn's *Turnen* or Amoros' Gymnase Normal, but more individual efforts, such as MacLaren's Oxford Gymnasium described above, which he hoped would become a model for all British universities, military academies and public schools.

Nevertheless, according to Michael Budd's *The Sculpture Machine*, physical education in Britain served the needs of the imperial nation-state just as it did in France and Germany, but in more subtle ways, through charitable organizations such as the YMCA (Young Men's Christian Association), founded in 1844 by George Williams (1821–1905) to promote the physical health and moral welfare of men in London's drapery trade. By the 1860s the YMCA had become established as a worldwide movement promoting the values of 'Muscular Christianity'.[43] The irony of the association between Christian morality, manliness and self-discipline akin to ancient Greek *arete* and training at the YMCA will not be lost on readers who are familiar with the Village People's chart-topping gay anthem of 1979, 'Y.M.C.A.' But like Jahn and Amoros, the advocates of Muscular Christianity made a direct link between physical and moral health, and by extension between church attendance, good works and going to the gym.

The Triumph of the Nation-state

Although there had been academic and medical interest in classical gymnastics and gymnasia since the sixteenth century, there were no practical moves to teach physical education or recreate ancient gymnasia until the end of the eighteenth century, when reformers began to experiment with the provision of physical training as part of a more rounded, child-centred education. In the first instance, however, the real impetus leading to the rebirth of the gymnasium as an institution dedicated to physical education was not peaceful reform but war and revolution. France's overwhelming victories in the first decade of the nineteenth century led to the establishment of the first open-air gymnasia in Prussia.

From their foundation, gymnasia were institutions with radical social and political agendas that made them both suspect and attractive to Europe's emerging nation-states. In divided, ultra-conservative Germany, they were seen as dangerous, and efforts were made to control or suppress them; in more liberal France and Scandinavia, they were co-opted by the state to produce citizen conscripts and workers who would be fit for the nation-state's purposes. The one exception to state control was the Anglo-Saxon world, which had a mixed educational system and a physical-education culture based on team sports outside the gymnasium. In this more tolerant environment, reformers were able to experiment with the teaching of different styles of European gymnastics.

At the beginning of the nineteenth century, a gymnasium was an open-air training ground where children and adults were drilled in groups in free exercises or in the use of fixed gymnastics apparatus. The training was functional in nature, with a clear military purpose. Gymnasts were training to be better, fitter soldiers. A gymnasium could be built almost anywhere, on a suitable piece of open ground, and at relatively little expense. For the more authoritarian European states, this presented too many risks. The move to indoor purpose-built gymnasia was not only dictated by practical reasons, such as the need to be able to train in bad weather and in winter, but also by political motives: moving the gymnasium into the school or barracks meant that the state exercised complete control over what was taught and by whom.

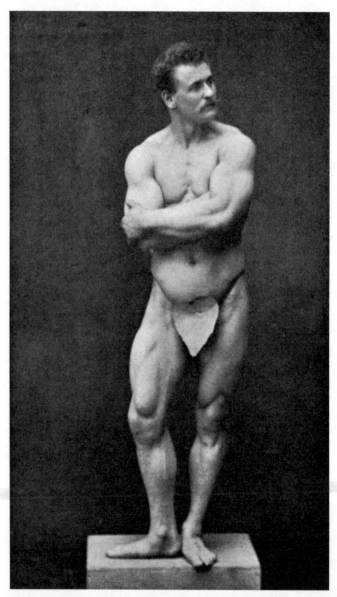

Vaudeville strongman turned fitness entrepreneur Eugen Sandow (1867–1925) made skilful use of his own image to promote both his stage career and his business interests. He marketed erotic photosets of himself, giving them a veneer of respectability as reproductions of famous Graeco-Roman artworks, to attract both male and female admirers to his stage shows, and to recruit members for his gymnasia and customers for his home exercise equipment and exercise manuals.

4
THE WORLD'S STRONGEST MAN

No Other Man Looked Like Sandow

Up Jumped Sandow like a Hercules,
Lifting up the iron bars
And breaking them with ease.
Sampson looked astonished and said it wasn't fair.
But everyone knows Sandow was the winner there.

The century from 1714 to 1814 was marked by a succession of bloody wars and revolutions, but the following century was one of relative peace and stability in Europe. Of course there were wars and revolutions, but nothing on the scale of what had come before or of what was to come in the twentieth century. The victors of the Seventh Coalition against Napoleon – Britain, Prussia, Russia and Austria – met with France at the Congress of Vienna (1814–15) to resolve the many issues arising from the previous quarter century of revolution and war.[1] The Bourbon claimant, Louis XVIII, was restored to the throne on the condition that France became a constitutional monarchy on the British model.[2] Of the three major wars fought between the European powers between 1814 and 1914, the first – the Crimean War (1853–6), which pitched Britain in an alliance with France against Russia – was fought in faraway Crimea; the Prussian-Austrian War of 1866, also known as the Seven Weeks War, was a short inter-German wrangle to settle which of the two countries would go on to unite Germany; and the Franco-Prussian War (1870–71), which could have easily turned into a protracted, bloody stalemate involving all the European powers like the First World War, lasted less than a year. Ideologically, however, there was no shift from militarism to pacifism of the kind that would mark the post-Second World War settlement. Each time a European power fought a war, and regardless of whether it was on the winning or losing side, politicians, educators and doctors voiced anxieties about the physical fitness of volunteers and conscripts and made damning comparisons with the fighting men of their allies and enemies.

The Birth of the Modern World

The relative calm on the military and political fronts was more than counterbalanced by radical social transformations wrought by advances in science and technology. Industrialization and globalization promoted by the expansion of European colonial empires provided both the raw materials for European industry and the markets for its manufactured goods. The First Industrial Revolution had initiated the transformation of Europe's agrarian-mercantile economies, with the majority of the population living in small towns and villages, into industrial-mercantile economies in which the population became ever more concentrated in new manufacturing and urban centres, linked by a network of railways. The Second Industrial Revolution (1860–1914) created the global economic system and the conveniences and inconveniences of modern life: the car, aircraft, telephone, gramophone, camera, cinema, telegraph, radio, electric motor, light bulb, linotype machine and typewriter.[3]

For the purposes of this study, the most important invention of the nineteenth century was the photographic camera, which transformed how people perceived their own bodies. Although cumbersome and requiring long exposures of one minute or more, the daguerreotype, developed in the late 1830s, was the first practical photographic medium, revolutionizing portraiture, which had hitherto been the province of the fine arts. As the century progressed, taking and developing photographs became much easier, faster and cheaper, until George Eastman produced the first mass-market camera using paper film, the Kodak 'Brownie', in 1900.[4] With improvements in printing, too, photographic images became commonplace, replacing idealized artistic representations with photographs of real people and real bodies. Looking at the enduring power of the still image in our own age, we cannot dismiss the enormous transformative power of photography when, for the first time, people were able to see themselves as they appeared to others.

The economic and technological transformation of society, however, came at a very high cost for many working men and women who had been uprooted from the countryside by agrarian reform, or drawn to the new cities by the promise of better paid factory jobs and higher living standards. Pre-industrial communities had provided a measure of community support and a welfare net, however inadequate, but with industrialization and urbanization, these networks disappeared. With poor working conditions and low wages, and without basic health-and-safety and labour legislation, or public sanitation and healthcare, life for the working population of the new industrial towns was grim and squalid, especially during the regular downturns of the economic cycle. Our impression of living and working conditions during the nineteenth century is still based on the novels of writers and social reformers such as Charles Dickens. To this day, the adjective 'Dickensian' stands for extreme squalor, social exclusion and exploitation. The population statistics for the period, however, tell a different story. For the century from 1800 to 1900, the population of the UK registered a more than threefold increase, from 10.5 to 38 million, while during the same period, the population of the U.S. saw an even more impressive rise from 5.7 to 77 million, during a period that witnessed the American Civil War (1861–5), the costliest war in U.S. history in terms of lives lost.

For many workers and their families, existence was a bitter struggle to survive, but for a significant number, conditions steadily improved over the century. Although wages registered only a modest rise during the nineteenth century, prices fell, creating the impression that the vast wealth accumulated by the great industrialists was trickling down to the most disadvantaged levels of society. However, very real and steady improvements in sanitation and healthcare reduced child mortality, allowing parents to limit the size of their families. Gradual reform of labour laws meant that workers had better living and working conditions, which together with advances in science and technology led to the appearance of new types of employee: skilled blue-collar and white-collar workers, with something that earlier generations of working men and women had not had: disposable income and leisure time in which to spend it.

In the previous chapter I examined the rebirth of the gymnasium as a state institution that focused on providing physical education for school pupils and conscripts with the aim of making them fit for the state's purposes. Even Jahn's *Turnvereine*, although they later became private members' gymnastics clubs, began life as state-backed civic enterprises with very similar functions and aims to the state-backed gymnasia set up in other European countries during the nineteenth century. This chapter, though its time frame falls within that covered by the previous chapter, deals with a radical transformation of the gymnasium from a public institution into a purely commercial enterprise, run by businessmen, built and equipped with funds raised from private investors, its day-to-day running paid for by membership fees.

In order for such an institution to appear at all, there had to be several existing socio-economic factors: at the very least, a large urban population with sufficient leisure time and disposable income to support this type of commercial enterprise. The first commercial gymnasia appeared in Brussels and Paris in the middle of the nineteenth century. Even in pre-Revolutionary days, these two cities had large populations of well-to-do citizens, and they were much larger than classical Athens, a city that supported three major public gymnasia and many private *palaestrae*. But as the French historian of physical education Gilbert Andrieu points out in the opening chapter of *La gymnastique au xixe siècle*, the Ancien Régime aristocrats and the wealthy among the *haute bourgeoisie* who imitated them had their own health-and-fitness pursuits.[5] They would have had no interest in going to a *Turnplatz* or *gymnase*, as they would have regarded the type of physical training practised there as being too close to manual labour, which they abhorred, and they would have been appalled by the democratic mixing of different social classes that they encouraged.

With the large urban population with sufficient leisure time and disposable income came two new types of individual: the fitness entrepreneur, who created commercial gymnasia and who was quite different from the educational reformers and *gymnasiarques* featured in the previous chapter; and the commercial gymnasium member whose main motivation in joining a gym and exercising was not for the common good or imposed by the state but to improve their own physical appearance and health – aesthetic and therapeutic training – both of which were trumpeted by the gymnasia's promotional literature. To claim, however, that these were the sole or even the principal motivations of this new breed of gym member is not entirely satisfactory.

Even in the days before Botox and cosmetic surgery, men and women with money had access to sufficient artifice to appear more attractive, slimmer, fitter and younger than they really were. And if they did want to exercise, the traditional aristocratic pursuits of riding, hunting, fencing and dancing were still available, as were other rowdier pastimes, such as prizefighting and wrestling, which also attracted the participation of the Parisian beau monde. Andrieu reveals that France's nineteenth-century aristocrats and wealthy bourgeois were to be seen performing in Paris's permanent circuses doing stunts on horseback and on the high-flying trapeze.[6] Therefore, something far more subtle, and at the same time, much more profound, was taking place in the elegant *salons* of mid-nineteenth-century Paris that concerned not only the appearance of the body, *l'art de paraître* in Andrieu's terms, but its physical fitness and abilities, which one could define as *l'art de pouvoir*, to borrow from Foucault.

The Pursuit of Happiness

There is a vast gulf to bridge between the grand religious, philosophical, artistic and scientific movements of early modernity – the Renaissance, Protestant Reformation and Enlightenment – that are seen as the basis for the development of Western individualism, and the very private, personal decisions of European citizens to spend a significant part of their disposable income and leisure time in going to a commercial gymnasium. I know of no grand statements of civil rights penned in the seventeenth and eighteenth centuries that guaranteed citizens the right to work out 'according to the laws of Nature', but clearly, an interest in one's physical embodiment was one of the unintended consequences of the social and political reforms of the late eighteenth and early nineteenth centuries. Individualism emerged during the

Renaissance and the Protestant Reformation, which liberated the Western mind from the absolute obedience expected by the medieval Church. The individual was placed in a direct relationship with the deity, without the mediation of the priestly hierarchy through the rituals of confession and absolution.

Greater freedom of conscience in turn weakened the Christian vilification of the flesh and the characterization of non-procreative sexual acts as sinful and sodomitic. For the first time since antiquity, artists glorified and idealized the human body, while scholars and physicians began to explore the therapeutic value of classical gymnastics. During the Enlightenment, educational reformers put earlier abstract theories of physical education into practice, which further stimulated the change of the individual's relationship to his or her body. This transformation was given a social dimension as the Age of Enlightenment turned into the Age of Revolutions: the old order based on birth into a particular class or caste was replaced by a democratic meritocracy based on personal qualities, which included appearance. And though I do not wish to establish an over-simplistic link between the early stages of Western individualism and a narcissistic interest in personal appearance and physical fitness, it is clear that the new conception of the rights and value of the individual promoted by the Enlightenment was mirrored by a growing concern with embodiment.

The second major stage in the development of modern individualism is expressed in the high-minded political declarations of the Age of Revolutions: the English Bill of Rights of 1689, the Constitution of the United States of 1787 and the two French Declarations of the Rights of Man and the Citizen of 1789 and 1793, which limited the power of the state and guaranteed the citizen's basic civil rights – at least if he were male, over 25, sane and a householder.[7] While these documents celebrated the birth of a truly liberated, modern individual, they dealt in lofty abstractions, such as the French Revolution's Liberté, égalité, fraternité, and Locke's doctrine of Natural Rights. There is one document, however, that succeeds in marrying the political with the personal in a remarkably modern national mission statement: the United States Declaration of Independence, ratified by the Continental Congress on 4 July 1776, whose preamble reads: 'We hold these truths to be self-evident, that all men are created equal, that they are endowed by their Creator with certain unalienable Rights, that among these are Life, Liberty and the pursuit of Happiness.' What the Founding Fathers meant by the pursuit of Happiness was probably very different from the modern interpretation of the phrase, and probably had a great deal to do with the untrammelled enjoyment of property, the ownership of slaves and freedom of religious belief, without royal interference and taxation without representation, but nevertheless, the term introduces a sense of intimacy and individuality that is lacking in the other grand political declarations of the period.

If the Enlightenment created the intellectual space for individuals to seek new ways of achieving personal fulfilment, the pursuit of Happiness found its fullest expression in the work of the English Utilitarians Jeremy Bentham (1748–1832) and John Stuart Mill (1808–1873), who held that happiness was the highest goal to be pursued by both individuals and society, through the application of the 'Principle of Utility' or the 'Greatest Happiness Principle'.[8] Neither man has much to say about physical exercise, but Bentham, in his review of 'The Pleasures', does list: '8. The pleasure of health, or, the internal pleasurable feeling or flow of spirits which accompanies a state of full health and vigour; especially at times of moderate bodily exertion.'[9] In *On Liberty* (1859), Mill championed the cause of the individual to pursue 'our own good in our own way', against the rights of society to interfere, and one whole chapter of the essay equates individuality with well-being.[10] Mill's work was the fullest statement of Enlightenment rationalism and became the basis for the small-c conservative liberal democracy of late nineteenth- and early twentieth-century Britain and America. As the individual took centre stage in the socio-political debate, we can infer that embodiment – the social and personal significance of the body to the individual – also became much more important. The body's health and appearance were now an indissoluble part of the individual's pursuit of his or her own self-actualization.

Turning from the public and political to the private and personal, the second half of the nineteenth century witnessed the 'invention' of a very important component of modern life: sexuality. Clearly, people had been having sexual intercourse before 1850, otherwise the human species would have died out long ago, but as Michel Foucault and Jeffrey Weeks point out, it is to this period that we owe the definition and classification of the paraphilias, which the more politically correct now call 'alternative sexualities'.[11] From the definition of what was considered perverse and abnormal, psychology and sexology gave the first definitions of what was sexually 'normal'. Heterosexual normality could come into being only once sexual abnormality had been defined.

During the medieval and early modern periods, sex was seen as consisting of discrete acts, some of which were sanctioned by the State and Church, while others were condemned as sinful and illegal. In the late nineteenth century, the forensic psychologist and sexologist Richard von Krafft-Ebing (1840–1902), who wrote the encyclopaedic *Psychopathia Sexualis* (1886), recast sexual sins and criminal acts as psychological conditions that needed to be treated and, if possible, cured. Paradoxically, the medicalization of alternative sexual practices became the basis for modern sexual identities. The twentieth century's out-and-proud gay man could not have existed without the invention of the nineteenth-century homosexual. Krafft-Ebing's book, which contained descriptions and case histories of homosexuals, fetishists, lesbians and sadomasochists, became an instant best-seller, avidly read by the public but more as a prurient guide to the forbidden pleasures of the flesh than as a serious work of forensic psychiatry. This was not the kind of freedom of choice and pursuit of Happiness that the Enlightenment philosophers and Utilitarians had intended, but it was definitely one that North Americans and Europeans were beginning to explore in growing numbers.

The Disempowered

Just as John Stuart Mill sought to convince his readers that they controlled their own destinies through the free application of rational choice, new ideas were emerging that put into question the fundamental premises of the Enlightenment. In the same year as Mill published *On Liberty*, Charles Darwin (1809–1882) published *On the Origin of Species*, which recast humanity from the favoured creation of the deity into the product of millions of years of unplanned, accidental evolution –

a process blind to the welfare of the individual, who is usually sacrificed for the survival of the species. Less than a decade later, Karl Marx (1818–1883) began to publish the monumental *Das Kapital* (1867–94), in which he argued that humans were impotent actors driven by social and economic forces and subject to historical imperatives that they could never hope to influence; and Sigmund Freud (1856–1939), in a series of essays and books, explained that humans, far from being rational beings in charge of their own destinies, were at the mercy of biology, primal drives and unconscious desires.

In the second decade of the twentieth century, humans discovered that they had little or no control over the future shape of society, or even over their own bodies and lives – a fact tragically confirmed by the First World War, during which a generation of young men was sacrificed in a conflict whose ideological justification is still extremely troubling, and whose conduct and tactics demonstrated a breathtaking lack of care on the part of the state for the individuals they were sending to their deaths for a few hundred metres of muddy ground in northern France and Flanders.[12] In contradiction to the greater control and freedom of choice to improve their own lives that individuals had gained at the beginning of the nineteenth century, and that is one possible explanation of why the care of the body became important enough to allow for the creation of commercial gymnasia, by the beginning of the twentieth century, the only thing that individuals could hope to discipline and master were their own bodies.

Les Hommes Phénomènes

The remainder of this chapter will focus on the careers of two nineteenth-century fitness entrepreneurs: the man who is credited with opening the first commercial gymnasia in Brussels and Paris, Hippolyte Triat (1813–1881), and Eugen Sandow (1867–1925), who, among his many accomplishments, could claim to have created the first modern health club in London's fashionable West End. Although they were born half a century apart, and active in different countries – Triat in Belgium and France and Sandow in the UK and U.S. – in terms of their backgrounds, personal lives and modus operandi these two men had a great deal in common, starting with how they began their careers as entertainers, or what Andrieu called *hommes phénomènes*.[13] The literal English translation of the phrase should be the rather flattering 'human phenomena', but the real meaning is closer to sideshow freaks.

What Andrieu described, and the French chronicler of strength athletes Edmond Desbonnet (1868–1953) lovingly listed in *Les rois de la force* ('The Kings of Strength', 1911), were circus, fairground and Vaudeville strongmen (and strongwomen) who, from the early modern period, made a precarious living, exhibiting their bodies, wrestling and performing feats of strength alongside other travelling entertainers, such as jugglers, trapeze artists and tightrope walkers. Unlike the professional athletes of classical antiquity, who won fame, wealth and honour, the *hommes phénomènes* had a very low social status with earnings to match, though they were sometimes hired to appear at princely courts to amuse the bored rich and powerful. The social, political and intellectual changes of the post-revolutionary period gave the ablest of these men opportunities that previous generations of strongmen could not have dreamed of. With the advent of photography, they became the first male pinups, sometimes photographed baring almost all – a freedom that clashes with our view of an age that placed so many taboos on public displays of nudity and had deep anxieties about sexuality and sexual impropriety, especially in connection with homosexuality.[14]

In every sense of the term, Triat and Sandow were self-made men. They began by transforming their bodies, although each clearly benefited from some genetic advantage in terms of their strength and muscularity. Neither of them had ever been a sickly or underweight child, and from their photographs it is likely that each had a natural aptitude for building lean muscle mass. In that they were not unique, as Desbonnet included dozens of contemporary strongmen with stage names such as 'le Briseur de chaînes' ('Chain breaker') and 'la Poitrine d'acier' ('Chest of steel'), which referred to their stage specialities. But where Triat and Sandow excelled was in converting their fame as performers – often achieved through daring acts of self-promotion, as well as quite a lot of stage artistry (or trickery) – into a kind of respectable celebrity that gave them access to the higher echelons of society, which in mid-nineteenth-century Paris and late nineteenth-century London were far more open than they

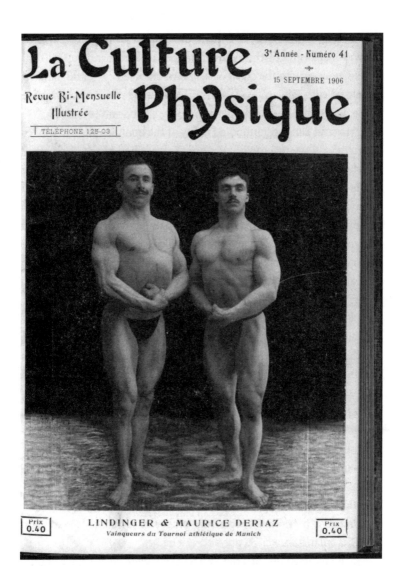

La Culture Physique

Revue Bi-Mensuelle
Illustrée

TÉLÉPHONE 125-03

3ᵉ Année - Numéro 41

15 SEPTEMBRE 1906

Physique

Prix
0.40

Prix
0.40

LINDINGER & MAURICE DERIAZ
Vainqueurs du Tournoi athlétique de Munich

Advances in printing and photography in the second half of the 19th century made possible the mass-production of cheap books, periodicals and magazines, such as Desbonnet's *La Culture Physique* and Sandow's *Physical Culture*, that promoted weight training and body-building. Cover of *La Culture Physique* (September 1906) showing two strength athletes, victors of a bodybuilding competition in Munich.

had been in earlier periods. During their careers, both men counted crowned heads among their acquaintances, admirers and pupils. Triat was a favourite with the court of Emperor Napoleon III, and Sandow socialized with Edward VII (1841–1910) when he was the incorrigible Bertie, living the life of a dissolute playboy in Paris and London.

Triat and Sandow embodied many of the qualities and paradoxes of the new Western individual whom I described above. They were men of humble origins, without status, connections or wealth, driven by the ambition to succeed in any way they could, who cashed in on the advantages they had been given over their fellow men – their looks and physiques. They were among the small band of strongmen who realized that there was a market for their skills beyond the stage, as the personal trainers of men and women who, while they might have been born rich and powerful, did not have the physique that had become a highly desirable personal attribute.

Like the fitness gurus of today, they made full use of the photographic and publishing technology of their day to promote themselves and their exercise systems and gymnasia. Sandow, in particular, was a prolific author, publishing half a dozen books that married health-and-fitness advice with colourful episodes from his own life as a wandering strongman. But as Sandow's biographer, David Chapman, points out, in Strength and How to Obtain It (1897) Sandow manufactured an autobiography that not only made him sound more respectable and interesting to his middle- and upper-class readers, but made his physical achievements seem much more attainable by the ordinary man. For example, he claimed to have been a sickly and delicate child who through his own efforts had achieved his spectacular muscular physique, a statement that Chapman says was an out-and-out lie.[15]

If the biographies of Triat and Sandow were suspect, we should also be wary of their stated motives for starting their businesses. Of the two, Triat had the greater intellectual pretensions. He founded the 'Societé Milonienne', named after the six-time ancient Olympic champion Milo of Croton, a Greek wrestler and strength athlete of the sixth century BCE, whose aims were nothing short of the 'physical regeneration of man'.[16] The society's prospectus boasted: 'The majority of M. Triat's students become models of physical perfection, which would stand comparison to most beautiful models of antiquity.'[17] Triat married the appeal of aesthetic training with the value to the state of therapeutic training, and hoped to build on Francisco Amoros's partial success in persuading Napoleon III's government to back his plan for a grand Gymnase Civil Normal – a national centre in Paris that would teach his style of gymnastics and train a corps of instructors who would disseminate it throughout France. Sandow, too, had national ambitions: he approached the British army, proposing his exercise system to train volunteers whose poor level of physical fitness had been demonstrated during the South African Boer Wars (1880–81 and 1899–1902), when many potential army recruits had been rejected on grounds of health and fitness.[18]

In the end neither man realized his grand ambitions, but, looking at their careers and undoubted self-promotion and marketing skill, I imagine that these schemes were part of the PR and advertising hype surrounding their core gymnasium businesses. Like many businessmen past and present, they were primarily interested in making their fortunes and achieving a position in society that they had been denied by their humble origins. In 1870 Triat became embroiled in the political upheaval associated with the fall of the Second French Empire and the founding of the short-lived Paris Commune (March–May 1871). After the fall of the Commune, his gymnasium was closed, and he died disgraced and impoverished. Sandow, though more successful, died in obscure but comfortable retirement. For all their vaunted strength and the health-giving powers of their exercise systems, neither man lived to a great age: Sandow died at the age of 58; Triat lived to be 68.

In their respective gymnasia, Triat and Sandow had quite different approaches to exercise. Triat, while he is credited with opening the first commercial gymnasium and devising the first sets of graduated metal dumb-bells and barbells, concentrated on what we would now call group exercise classes in his *gymnastique de plancher* (floor gymnastics). Sandow also used free weights in his English health clubs, and his approach was much closer to what we would find in a modern gym: individual stations with racks of dumb-bells and barbells supervised by gymnasium staff that doubled as personal trainers. What both men shared from their time on the stage was a certain theatrical flair. Triat in particular married the two worlds of exercise and performance in his extraordinary Grand Gymnase, over whose entrance was inscribed the Société Milonienne's stirring motto: La régénération de l'homme (the regeneration of man).[19]

Theatre of Strength

Hippolyte Triat's biography reads like something dreamed up by his great literary contemporary Alexandre Dumas. According to Desbonnet's hero-worshipping biography of Triat, little orphan Hippolyte was kidnapped by Roma travellers at the age of six and given or sold to an Italian circus troupe, who dressed him up as a girl and made him perform a rope-skipping routine under the name of Iselda for the next seven years.[20] When the troupe broke up, the thirteen-year-old Hippolyte took up with a Spanish strongman called Consuelo and his sons to be part of their poses plastiques stage routine, in which a lightly clad but clearly well-developed Hippolyte performed feats of strength and reproduced famous classical statues for the delectation of paying audiences.

Triat remained with Consuelo until 1828, when he was injured while rescuing a wealthy lady from a runaway carriage in Burgos, Spain. Out of gratitude, the distressed damsel gave the young man a home and paid for his education at the local Jesuit college. He remained in Burgos until he turned 21, when he went back to the stage with a solo strongman act. He toured Europe, finally settling in Brussels, where he opened his first commercial gymnasium in 1840. He remained in the Belgian capital until 1849, but having conquered the pinnacles of Belgian society and failed to persuade the Belgian government to back his scheme for a national gymnastics school, he moved to Paris, where he opened the first commercial, purpose-built gymnasium – not in an outlying district, like Amoros's Gymnase Civil et Militaire, but in the fashionable centre of the capital, on the Avenue Montaigne, just off the Champs-Elysées.

So much for the official biography. But with 165 years' hindsight, the modern reader should be able to fill in the obvious blanks in Desbonnet's romanticized and sanitized version of Triat's life story with the episodes of slavery, people-trafficking, and physical and possibly sexual abuse and exploitation that he must have experienced as a child and adolescent. It is a testament to his sheer strength of character, ambition and determination, combined with his intelligence and physical attractiveness, that he managed to get himself educated and then that he succeeded in the career path that he had chosen for himself as the personal trainer to the imperial court and the beau monde of the Second Empire.

The first of Triat's two Paris gymnasia, on the Avenue Montaigne, anticipating later developments in French school gymnasia, and unlike Jahn's Turnplatz or Amoros's *gymnase*, was an entirely covered space in a purpose-designed building. Constructed in the fashionable cast iron and glass architecture of the day that we now associate with railway stations, exhibition halls and greenhouses, the Gymnase Triat, or Grand Gymnase, was a vast cathedral-like structure dedicated to physical culture, measuring 131 ft (40 m) long, 69 ft (21 m) wide and 33 ft (10 m) high, with three spectator galleries running around the whole interior. It was hung with a network of ropes and ladders from the roof supports, which seem, however, to have been mostly decorative as Triat's system, unlike earlier French gymnastics, was focused on synchronized movements on the ground, using portable equipment including dumb-bells, Indian clubs and barbells. The huge floor space was largely unencumbered, again allowing spectators to observe the action without hindrance.

What Desbonnet describes in detail is a group exercise class for adult men in the Gymnase, which was led by Triat himself dressed in a uniform reminiscent of a circus ringmaster, carrying a long silver filigree cane and with the accompaniment of a drummer dressed as Francis I (1494–1547). The students were dressed in red tights and stripped to the waist, which might explain why the classes were so popular with Parisian ladies, who were depicted as appreciative spectators in the advertising material for the Grand Gymnase. Following Triat's booming commands that no doubt echoed and reverberated in the cavernous space, the 50 students, standing in two lines facing one another, went through a complicated routine of exercises of Triat's *gymnastique de plancher*, which included synchronized bodyweight movements, jumping and running on the spot, wrestling and exercises with light and heavy dumb-bells, barbells and Indian clubs that, like a modern circuit class, were designed to work the whole body and build up a considerable sweat.[21] The session ended with a cold shower and a vigorous rubdown given by the master himself. The *gymnase* offered sessions for gentlemen, boys and small boys, and ladies, girls and small girls, though for the women and girls' classes, Triat employed female trainers to teach and perform the vigorous after-workout rubdowns.

Among the financial innovations that we owe to Triat is that he financed the building of his Paris gymnasia by setting up a limited stock company which raised money from small investors. In order to cover his considerable running costs, he offered different kinds of membership, with rates for three or six sessions a week, and monthly, six-monthly and yearly terms, with discounted rates for the longer memberships. Unlike a modern gym-goer, a member of the gymnase could not turn up to train on his or her own, as Triat offered only group classes. Although his classes were popular, boasting large numbers of students and spectators, and he was the toast of Parisian society until the fall of the Second Empire, he only managed to pay his considerable overheads and staff costs, and when the Gymnase was closed he did not have any savings or other income to fall back on. Although he himself was destined to fail, Triat founded the Paris fitness industry. In 1845, the Paris Chamber of Commerce's directory listed no commercial gymnasia in the city, but by 1860 there were twenty, including several women-only establishments.[22]

Success and How to Obtain It

Our second fitness entrepreneur, Eugen Sandow, was born Friedrich Wilhelm Müller, a subject of the militaristic, authoritarian kingdom of Prussia four years before it created the Second German Reich in 1871. David Chapman's biography of Sandow has uncovered his real life story, while Sandow's *Strength and How to Obtain It* featured Sandow's embellished version. As a young man he joined his local Turnverein in Königsberg (Russian Kaliningrad since the end of the Second World War), where he developed the defined but relatively slender physique of a turner. At the age of eighteen, to escape the draft, he left Germany and joined a touring circus as an acrobat and stunt jockey. In 1886 or

1887, when the circus reached Brussels, it went out of business, leaving the nineteen-year-old Sandow stranded, friendless and penniless. It would not be the first or last time that Sandow would find himself alone and friendless in a foreign country, and it would also not be the first time that a chance meeting set his life on a new completely new course. In the autumn or winter of 1887 he met Louis Durlacher (b. 1844), a former Vaudeville strongman who had adopted the stage name Attila and granted himself the bogus title of 'Professeur', and who ran a gymnasium in Brussels. Professor Attila immediately recognized Sandow's potential as a strongman and stage performer, and trained him using what we would now consider to be standard progressive weight-training exercises, then considered a radical and dangerous innovation that went against the medical orthodoxy of the day, which claimed that it would lead to gradual paralysis through 'muscle binding'.[23]

Sandow and Attila soon parted company, however, and Sandow continued his adventures across Europe, performing as a strongman and accepting challenges as a wrestler. When he visited Italy he claimed to have met the German Crown Prince, the future Kaiser Wilhelm II, although this is probably one of Sandow's many self-aggrandizing inventions. When he was in Venice he struck up a friendship with the American painter E. Aubrey Hunt (1855–1922), who painted the young Sandow as a Roman gladiator, and who was quite possibly his lover.[24] In his autobiography, Sandow claimed that it was Hunt who told him of a duo of Vaudeville strongmen in London who were offering the then considerable sum of £500 to anyone who could match or better their feats of strength.[25] In Desbonnet's version, it was Attila who saw in the challenge the ideal opportunity to launch his protégé's career in London, and earn lucrative fees as his agent and manager. In 1889 the two men travelled to London, where they carefully prepared their challenge of the man who styled himself 'The World's Strongest Man', Charles A. Sampson (b. 1859), known simply as Sampson, and of his sidekick, the giant Polish wrestler and strongman Franz Bienkowski (b. 1862), who went under the stage name of Cyclops.

The story of the encounter is a classic of the genre, with the impetuous young challenger stepping on to the stage in foppish evening dress,

Life of the Author as told in Photographs.

Series of Photos

showing the Author at different periods of his varied career. These are presented here for the encouragement of the youth of the nation, and to show what can be accomplished by anyone who patiently and conscientiously follows out the methods described in this book.

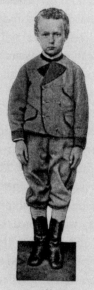

(1)

The Author at the age of 10. Delicate as a boy; he became enthused with a fervour for physical development, after seeing the statues and pictures of ancient and classical heroes in the art galleries of Europe, and lived afterwards with one ambition only, to become as well-developed and strong as they were.

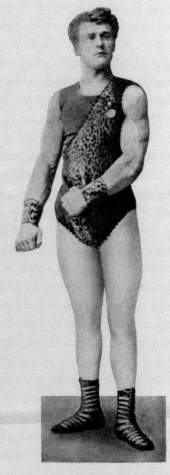

II

Photo taken at the age of 18, showing the remarkable increase of development in the intervening eight years.

482

Sandow was a master of self-promotion, using photography and the print media to promote his fitness businesses. However, he often embroidered or made up the colourful anecdotes that illustrated and enlivened his training manuals. In this illustrated biographical sketch included in *Strength and How to Obtain It*, Sandow made the false claim that he was 'delicate as a boy'.

complete with a monocle, cane and top hat, initially to the derision and catcalls of the audience. But when Sandow stripped off to reveal his muscular physique, Sampson knew that he had finally met a dangerous adversary. Rather than depending on brute strength alone, Sampson used stage trickery to achieve his stunts, which also ensured that no one could successfully challenge him and win the £500 prize. But Sandow and Attila had come forewarned, and Sandow easily defeated first Cyclops and then Sampson, instantly establishing his reputation on the London stage.

Success in London was followed by acclaim in the U.S., where Sandow teamed up with the impresario and creator of the *Follies*, Florenz Ziegfeld, Jr (1867–1932), who hired him to be the headline act at the Ziegfeld Theater at the Chicago World's Fair of 1893. On his subsequent tour of the U.S., Sandow made full use of the medium of photography to promote his stage act. He was photographed by several leading American society photographers, including Napoleon Sarony (1821–1896), sometimes dressed in Victorian versions of antique costumes, or with his modesty preserved by a large artificial fig leaf that must have riveted the many young blushing American and European admirers. Aware of the promotional possibilities of the new visual media that were appearing at the time, Sandow also agreed to perform for Thomas Edison's Kinetoscope, an early precursor of the cinema, becoming the first bodybuilder to be filmed.[26]

In 1897, back in London and now married, Sandow decided to convert his considerable fame as a performer into the world's first health-and-fitness business empire. He opened his first gymnasium, which he called the Institute of Physical Culture, at 32A St James's Street, between Bond Street and Piccadilly, in the heart of London's most fashionable district, to differentiate it as much as possible from the working-class boxing gyms that already existed in the poorer suburbs of the capital. He marketed it to the upwardly mobile and very class-conscious skilled working and middle classes. Although no membership records survive from the Institute, Chapman believes that it was comparable to an American gymnasium of the same period for which we do have membership data: a quarter of the membership were blue-collar workers, including soldiers and policemen, a quarter were high-school and college students, and the remainder were white-collar workers and professional men.[27]

Sandow modelled the Institute's interior and facilities on the exclusive private gentlemen's clubs that are still a feature of London's St James's and Pall Mall. Chapman describes luxurious wood-panelled rooms, with suites for changing, bathing and relaxing after a workout. The gymnasium itself was a large, high-ceilinged room with a hardwood floor, with a Persian rug marking each exercise station. The exerciser would stand or lie on the carpet and be instructed by Sandow himself, or one of his trained instructors, in the use of the weights racked nearby. At the height of his success, Sandow had twenty institutes nationwide, catering to both men and women, and he had ambitious plans to open a chain of institutes in the U.S.

The Institute was only the first of Sandow's many business ventures. He published a series of training manuals, including Strength and How to Obtain It; he started the first health and fitness magazine in England, Physical Culture, in 1898, renamed Sandow's Magazine the following year; using the magazine as his platform, he sold a mail-order Half-crown Postal Course for those who could not afford to join his gymnasia; and he manufactured and sold his own branded home fitness equipment, including 'Sandow's Own Combined Developer' and the 'Spring-Grip Dumbbell'.[28] In 1901 he organized the first major bodybuilding competition open to all Sandow students in the UK. The event, for which he used all the showmanship at his disposal, was held in front of a sell-out crowd at London's Royal Albert Hall. The prizes for the winner and two runners-up were casts of Frederick Pomeroy's statue of the young Sandow holding a globe barbell, in gold plate, silver plate and bronze (1891).[29] In the decade before the outbreak of the First World War, Sandow knew his greatest worldwide fame. He toured the U.S. once more, meeting President Theodore Roosevelt, and travelled the length and breadth of the British Empire, spreading the Sandow message and training system wherever he went. But as early as 1907, Sandow's business empire was in trouble. He was forced to close many of his institutes, as well as Sandow's Magazine. By the end of the First World War, the fitness craze that he had single-handedly started in the UK and U.S. had waned. Although Sandow did not die penniless and disgraced like Triat, he was quickly forgotten. He died in comfortable but obscure suburban retirement at the comparatively young age of 58.

The Showman's Sport

The kind of showmanship that was such an important part of Triat's and Sandow's success has remained an important element in the world of strength and physique athletes. The feats of strength that Sandow and other Vaudeville strongmen performed on stage for fee-paying audiences became the basis for the sport of Olympic weightlifting, which was among the events of the first modern summer Olympics, held in Athens in 1896, and remains the only strength discipline on the programme of the summer Olympic Games. Compared to other forms of weight training, the sport requires very little equipment: an Olympic bar with rotating ends and collars, which has become the standard adjustable barbell in many gyms, and a stack of rubber-coated weights to practise the two Olympic lifts – the clean and jerk and the snatch, in which the bar is brought from floor to arm's length where it is held for three seconds.[30] Whereas bodybuilding employs exercises performed slowly, concentrating on one set of muscles and usually acting on one joint at a time, the Olympic lifts are compound exercises that are performed dynamically at speed, and which involve most of the body's musculature and joints.

I owe my introduction to the sport to 'Big' Nick, whose attitude to other forms of weight training, such as bodybuilding and power lifting, was that their practitioners were 'training lying down'. I had been introduced to conventional bodybuilding and learned the standard weight-training exercises before meeting Big Nick, but once I had seen him lift in excess of his own bodyweight in one explosive but incredibly smooth movement, and with little apparent effort, I was instantly converted to the sport. Compared to the slow-motion heaves of conventional weight training that pressed, pulled or curled a barbell or dumb-bell a few feet, the Olympic lifts looked fun, challenging and also quite dangerous. Weightlifting, I went on to discover, developed timing, coordination, posture, proprioception and balance – skills that bodybuilding barely addressed. Although technique has a lot to do with succeeding in the Olympic lifts, they are impossible to achieve with any significant weight without considerable strength and muscular endurance.

Big Nick had a perfectly proportioned physique without a spare ounce of fat, and as far as I knew, he had never trained with standard bodybuilding exercises. Fifteen years in the construction industry combined with weightlifting and underpinned by a genetic makeup that predisposed him to low body fat and pronounced muscular development had given him a physique that all the bodybuilders and power lifters in the gym envied. He had the size and definition sought by the former, and the brute strength that was the aim of the latter. In addition, he was extremely limber with lightning reflexes, and had a grip that could crack walnuts. Had he been born a century earlier, Big Nick might easily have found success on the stage as a strongman – displaying his outstanding physique and performing feats of strength for audiences whose own muscular development was stunted by poor diet, unsanitary living conditions, dull, repetitive work and long working hours that allowed them little time for any kind of sport or physical exercise.

The story of Big Nick, like that of the mythical Herakles who died after being tricked into putting on a shirt soaked in poison, does not have a happy ending. After I had returned from a stint working overseas, a mutual friend told me that Big Nick had died from a heart attack at the age of 55. As I was not living in London at the time, I never found out whether it was his smoking and drinking, combined with a diet that seemed to consist mostly of 'fry-ups' (the traditional English working man's breakfast, lunch and dinner, consisting of eggs, sausage and bacon, served with baked beans and, optionally, a large portion of chips), or a genetic predisposition to coronary heart disease that led to his premature death. I suspect it was the latter aggravated by the former, and paradoxically not helped by his extraordinary prowess in weightlifting, which would have put a considerable strain on his cardiovascular system.

A Question of Adjustment

The century that witnessed the invention of the commercial gymnasium also gave us the free and machine weight-training equipment that we now associate with the modern gym. The ancient Greeks used light metal or stone *halteres*, but principally as aids for the long jump and for warm-up exercises. Amoros and Jahn also used light handheld weights in their respective gymnastics, but they mainly used the exerciser's own bodyweight combined with different types of apparatus to develop strength and endurance. Anyone who has trained on the climbing rope, parallel bars, single bar or rings can testify that they require considerable strength, but as Sandow discovered when he was a turner, they did not develop the bulging muscles and brute strength that Vaudeville strongmen needed to impress their audiences.

Early modern strongmen understood the theory and practice of progressive weight training, even though the terms had not been thought of, and the medical opinion of the day decreed that this kind of exercise was not only counterproductive but also dangerous. Triat and Sandow's Renaissance forebears used improvised equipment, such as barrels that they could fill and empty, to train and perform their feats of strength. When Triat opened his gym in Paris in the mid-nineteenth century, fixed metal weights of different designs were commonplace. From his own muscular development, Triat understood progressive weight training, but for the *gymnastique de plancher* he limited his students to fixed *barres à spheres de 6 kilos* (6 kg/13.2 lb dumb-bells).[31] The problem with working with a fixed weight, as any personal trainer will tell you, is that once the exerciser succeeds in lifting the weight without effort, any subsequent repetition results not in major gains in muscle size or strength but only in muscular endurance. In order to stimulate constant muscle growth and make corresponding gains in strength, the exerciser must always increase his workload, keeping himself just on the right side of failure.

It is probably impossible to say who hit upon the idea of the adjustable dumb-bell, but it is a product that required not only a clever designer and willing consumer to purchase it, but also a certain level of technological sophistication to manufacture at an affordable price.

Early modern blacksmiths could have individually handcrafted sets of adjustable dumb-bells, but the cost would have been prohibitive. Hence, the casting and machining technology of the Second Industrial Revolution, combined with standardization and mass production, produced an affordable piece of weight-training equipment for use in the gymnasium and the home. In her essay outlining the development of the barbell and dumb-bell, Jan Todd rejects the claim that it was Sandow's mentor, Professor Attila, who devised the first adjustable dumb-bells, in the 1890s. She believes the honour should go to the early American bodybuilding pioneer George Barker Windship (1834–1876), who patented the plate-loading barbell in the u.s. in 1865.[32] Another type described by Todd was a hollow dumb-bell whose weight could be varied by adding or removing lead shot. However, this would have been much more complicated and time-consuming to adjust than a plate dumb-bell.[33]

The type of weight-training equipment that we associate with the modern health club (as opposed to the more traditional free-weights 'pumping iron' bodybuilding gym) is the adjustable machine-weight station. The most common arrangement of pulleys and weight stacks, which were once thought to date from the mid-twentieth century, are actually far older. Todd outlines the development of such machines from the simple harness and rope arrangements of the early modern period, through to more sophisticated machines of the late eighteenth century. Apart from its nineteenth-century design and wooden cabinet, James Chiosso's 'Gymnastic Polymachinon' of 1855 is not unlike the kind of multi-station weight-training machine that can be found in most gyms.[34] Handles and grips set at different heights and positions on the machine allow the exerciser to move the enclosed adjustable weight stack with cables and pulleys in order to perform a wide range of exercises. A foldaway seat allows the exerciser to perform seated chest and shoulder presses.[35]

A First Flowering

The simplest way to account for the appearance of commercial gymnasia in Europe in the mid-nineteenth century would be to say that there

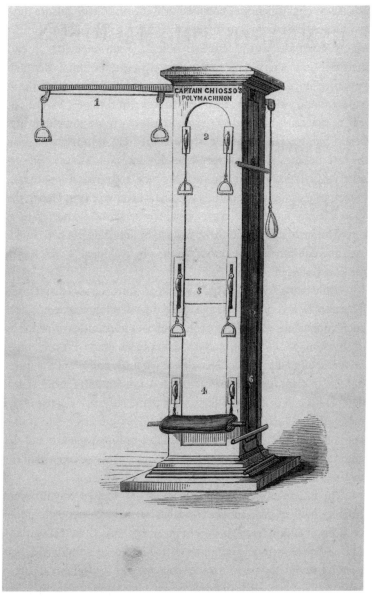

The multi-station weight-training machine is often thought of as a 20th-century invention, but Victorian ingenuity and mass-production methods, combined with a new interest in exercise, led to the invention of machines such as James Chiosso's (1789–1864) Polymachinon of 1855, for use at home and in the gymnasium.

was a new constituency of potential gym members with leisure time and disposable incomes to finance them, but that would not explain why, at this particular juncture, people suddenly decided to spend their free time, energy and money going to a gymnasium rather than pursuing more established athletic or leisure pastimes. Something had profoundly altered the social construction of the body, its relationship to the individual and its perceived role in private and public life. In stark contrast to the people who went to the state-run gymnasia in the early decades of the nineteenth century, individuals developed personal motivation to care for their health, fitness and physical appearance. In this, they found ready partners in a new breed of entrepreneur, the Vaudeville strongmen turned gymnasium owners, who did not just meet a need for instruction in aesthetic training by providing teachers, buildings and equipment, but embodied the physical ideal to which gym members aspired.

While many factors played a role in creating the social and intellectual space for commercial gymnasia, their development would have been impossible without the promotional opportunities provided by the medium of photography. Monarchs and generals were celebrated in heroic oil paintings and Neoclassical marble and bronze statues, but cheap photographic prints created a much more modest and democratic cult of celebrity. Sandow in particular made full use of the medium, and he owed much of his business success to the skilful management of his own image, which combined the fame of the entertainer with the prowess of the athlete and the sex appeal of the matinée idol.

The nineteenth-century gymnasium still looked very different from the modern gym, and most gymnasia remained essentially indoor versions of Jahn's Turnplatz. Although Triat's Paris Gymnase was furnished with barbells and dumb-bells, it more closely resembled a large exercise studio or a performance space where exercisers took part in synchronized gymnastic displays. Sandow's institutes, with their free weights and individual stations for exercisers, come closest to the modern health club, but again, much of the equipment that we take for granted on the main gym floor – adjustable benches, weight-training machines and cardio exercisers – was absent. Although

Triat's gymnases and Sandow's institutes helped to establish many aspects of modern physical culture, including progressive weight training, group exercise classes, health and fitness magazines, and bodybuilding and weightlifting competitions, they did not survive their founders. The nineteenth- and early twentieth-century commercial gymnasium remained a short-lived fad that was quickly superseded by other health and fitness pursuits, including cycling, outdoor sports, naturism and group callisthenics.

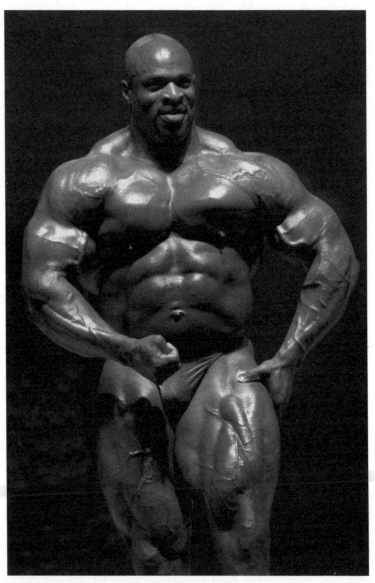

The differences between Sandow photographed in the 1900s (p. 108) and professional bodybuilder and serial Mr Olympia winner Ronnie Coleman (b. 1964) in the early 2000s demonstrate the extraordinary changes in muscularity made possible in the second half of the 20th century in part by changes in training practices and the professionalization of strength athletes, but mainly by the discovery and widespread use of performance- and muscle-enhancing substances. The appearance of the hyper-muscular 'supermale' had an impact on the training practices of amateur athletes in gyms worldwide.

5
PUMPING IRON

One of the first things you will experience when you start training is
the 'pump' – your muscles swell up well beyond their normal size, your
veins stand out, you feel huge, powerful and full of energy.

Arnold Schwarzenegger, *Encyclopedia of Modern Bodybuilding* (1995)

In the previous chapter I examined how the emergence of the Western
individual played a central role in the development of the nineteenth-
century gymnasium. Redefinitions of political citizenship led to the
appearance of state-sponsored gymnasia established for the functional training of schoolchildren and conscripts, but it was the
emergence of the fully fledged Western individual, whose civil rights
were guaranteed by a democratic state, that was a precondition for the
development of commercial gymnasia. The United States of America
was the first nation state to be founded on the principles of equality
and liberty, realized through elected representative assemblies, the
Houses of Congress and an elected head of state, the president. But it
took a century for the principles of equality and liberty to be extended
to African Americans, and a further century before women, minors
and all other ethnic and sexual minorities won the full protections and
rights afforded by the Constitution to adult heterosexual white men
during the nineteenth century.

As good followers of the Enlightenment, the Founding Fathers
cited classical models when they searched for political precedents to
underpin the organization of their new polity. If Jahn and the turners
had sought to resurrect the ancient gymnasium in an attempt to promote a more representative form of government in a unified Germany,

it was the existence of individual freedom guaranteed by democratic institutions that would ensure that it was in America that the gymnasium would have its greatest modern flowering. I commented above on the similarities between the political situation in early nineteenth-century Germany and the divisions that existed in the ancient Greek world, but in this chapter, the similarity to which I would like to draw the reader's attention is not between political and social systems but between individuals: ancient Athenians and twentieth-century Americans.

The freeborn Athenian citizen could freely pursue the realization of his physical, moral and social potential – his *arete* – as long as his actions did not incur the wrath of the gods or of his fellow citizens in the *Ekklesia*. When one looks at the modern American citizen, it is a well-worn cliché to say that the highest goal of American life is to achieve one's full potential – self-actualization through material success being the American version of ancient Greek *arete*. Just as physical beauty had moral implications about the individual in ancient Greece, the attainment of wealth and success is similarly invested by Americans with moral valediction. In both meritocratic Athens and America, in theory at least, inherited wealth, status and power were outweighed by intelligence, ambition, hard work and personal appearance. But the second ingredient central to both ancient Greek and twentieth-century American life was competition: freedom and equality, which reduced the advantages of birth, naturally led to a high degree of competitiveness between individuals. For heterosexual men in twentieth-century America, it was not appearance for its own sake that was the main motivation for going to the gym. What motivated them was the desire to excel and to be better than the other men there – which could have included looking better than them – but was really about being the dominant alpha male in the gym: the biggest, strongest and fittest.

Man and Superman

During the early twentieth century, the U.S. was not only the most politically advanced nation on earth in terms of individual rights, but was fast becoming the world leader commercially, technologically and industrially. Although the internal combustion engine and the automobile were invented in Europe, they were perfected in the United States, creating a new lifestyle based on greater individual mobility. It was an American, Henry Ford (1863–1947), who understood the enormous transformative power of the automobile when he set out to manufacture 'a car for the great multitude', the Model T Ford, first produced in 1908. In order to achieve his automotive revolution, Ford adapted and improved the assembly-line production methods first developed by Oldsmobile, reducing the production time of a Model T from 12.5 hours in 1908 to 93 minutes in 1914.[1] The assembly-line worker had a physically less demanding job than his predecessors, and he benefited from better conditions and a higher disposable income. He had the leisure time, the money and, more importantly, the energy to work on his body, and he also had the motivation to do so. According to Michael Budd in *The Sculpture Machine* (1997), the nineteenth century was the century of man versus the machine, of flesh versus metal.[2] By the early twentieth century, however, it was no longer a conflict between man and metal, but a fight for survival as humans were becoming integrated into industrial machinery itself – a subject highlighted cinematically in very different ways by Fritz Lang in *Metropolis* (1927) and by Charlie Chaplin in *Modern Times* (1936).

Although Budd's argument is political and external, concentrating on the use of the muscular Caucasian body to project European imperial, racial and colonial power, his argument can also be adapted to a more personal, internal dimension, where the individual is using the most fundamental aspect of his self – his flesh, sinews and muscles – to assert his independence of and power over the new world of machines that threatens to engulf him. Power, or *pouvoir*, which has the additional meaning in French of 'agency' and the verb 'to be able to do', is a major theme in recent sociology, and in particular in the works of social constructionists Michel Foucault and Jeffrey Weeks. Their notions of power do not repeat the classical theories of the use of brute force by the state or the individual, but involve attempts to redefine power and how it acts through social discourse throughout society, disciplining, constraining and regulating individual actions, and at the same time creating new forms of human agency through resistance to the established forms and structures of power.[3]

Bodybuilders are not usually noted for their philosophical or sociological insights, but I was particularly struck by something Arnold Schwarzenegger (b. 1947) said in the documentary film about competitive bodybuilding, *Pumping Iron* (1977), about what had drawn him to the sport: 'I was always dreaming about very powerful people – dictators and things like that. I used to always be impressed by people who could be remembered for hundreds of years, or even like Jesus, for like thousands of years.' Although Austrian by birth, Schwarzenegger embodies the competitive American alpha male who wants to be the best in whatever he does: lifting weights, competing in bodybuilding, starring in films or running the State of California.

In 1938 a new character appeared in the pages of America's comic books who embodied the U.S.'s masculine, heterosexual, cultural and military power against the forces ranged against 'truth, justice, and the American way'. This hero was literally an *Übermensch* – a superhuman: Superman, of course, who was represented as a hyper-muscular male. Although he is not depicted heroically nude like an ancient Greek athlete, warrior or demigod, his muscular physique is clearly displayed in a skin-tight suit, while his modesty is preserved by an external pair of underpants. Superman would be the first of many generations of similarly square-jawed, buff, male superheroes who fought America's enemies – real and imagined; human, alien and mechanical – and who would be as impossible to tell apart as Egyptian pharaohs, were it not for their trademark costumes, powers and accessories. Superman and other superheroes are updated versions of medieval knights in shining armour, defending truth and justice, except that in their case, the armour is no longer an external metal casing but an impressive layer of inbuilt muscles.

It is not a coincidence that Superman made his appearance just as the United States was preparing to go to war against the militaristic Axis powers, Nazi Germany, Fascist Italy and Imperial Japan. He was a projection of American power against the totalitarian war machines that were about to attack the U.S. and her liberal-democratic allies. Although Superman was naturally gifted by virtue of his birth on the planet Krypton, and did not need to go to the gym to develop his physique, those among his human fans who aspired to his hyper-muscularity needed to work out with weights. Comic-book heroes, later to be portrayed onscreen by real-life musclemen, would provide the first images of what Harrison Pope calls 'hyper-muscular supermales', and which would become the models for heterosexual men working out in the gym.[4]

In Sandow's Footsteps

When Sandow toured the U.S. in the closing decade of the nineteenth century, he made a considerable impact, sparking a craze for the muscular 'Grecian ideal' among American men who were relative latecomers to physical culture and aesthetic training with weights. On his second visit to the U.S., he published an American version of Sandow's Magazine and developed ambitious plans to open a chain of American institutes, but the U.S. market was not yet ready for his style of gym-based fitness. The magazine folded after four issues and the institutes never materialized.[5] Sandow was not alone in trying to exhort the American male to take up physical fitness. The YMCA had operated gymnasia and athletics facilities in the country's major cities since the 1860s, and the promoters of an American brand of 'Muscular Christianity' exhorted young men to develop true Christian manliness through regular exercise in the gym and on the basketball court. Sandow also had an American counterpart, the eccentric Bernarr Macfadden (1868–1955). Although Macfadden did not open a gymnasium, he published the U.S.'s first health and fitness magazine, Physical Development (1898), and organized America's first bodybuilding contest in 1903.[6]

It is to Macfadden that we owe the discovery of one of the early apostles of American muscular development, Charles Atlas (1892–1972), whom he dubbed 'The World's Most Perfectly Developed Man'. Born Angelo Siciliano in Calabria, southern Italy, Atlas emigrated to the United States as a child with his parents, settling in Brooklyn in 1905. Famously skinny as a teenager, Atlas overcame bullying by taking up weight training. He later developed his own training method, 'Dynamic Tension', which was marketed with comic-strip ads in which an underweight victim has sand kicked in his face by beach bullies, builds himself up with Atlas's training method and, once big and buff, gets his revenge on his tormentors. Although Atlas's method was sold as a correspondence course for home use, and the gymnasium that he opened was forced to close because of financial difficulties in 1928, Atlas played an important role in popularizing weight training in the U.S. and laid the groundwork for the postwar flowering of American gym culture.[7] He also provided a link between the last of the generation of Vaudeville strongmen – he worked as a performer at Coney Island – and the new breed of fitness entrepreneurs who followed a quite different career path on the other side of the country.

The Southern Californian Dream

It was in the United States that the commercial gymnasium was reinvented in the postwar period, and from where it would be exported to the rest of the world along with other aspects of American consumer culture. But it was not the America that Sandow had toured at the end of the nineteenth century – the industrial cities of the East Coast and Midwest – but Southern California, which at the time was an impoverished region of large cattle ranches, vineyards and vast agricultural estates. Formerly a backwater of the Spanish-American Empire, California came relatively late to U.S. statehood, in 1850. An area still famous for its vineyards and citrus orchards, Southern California's industrial economy took off at the beginning of the twentieth century after the discovery of a major oil field in Long Beach. The area's mild climate attracted another kind of turn-of-the-century entrepreneur, film-makers and producers, who settled in and around Hollywood. This inflow of wealth and people created a demand for new leisure facilities and resorts, which were established on the coast, giving birth to LA's beach cities: Long Beach, Santa Monica and Venice. The coastal fringe of any major city creates a very special kind of community: the seaside attractions and businesses need a steady supply of transient labour – young men and women who often have time off during the day to go to the beach – as well as wealthier visitors taking a break from the pressures of city life. The combination of warm weather and beach resorts created a laid-back but body-conscious lifestyle, in which spending your days between the gym and the beach replaced the relentless American drive for material success at whatever personal cost.

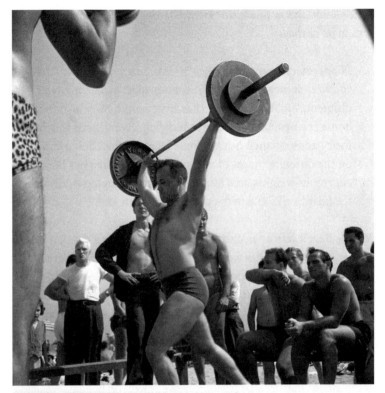

Established during the Great Depression as a new family-orientated amenity, Santa Monica's Muscle Beach became the birthplace of a new laid-back, hedonistic, body-conscious sub-culture, whose denizens divided their time between training in the city's new gyms and showing off their bodies and acrobatic skills on the beach. A weightlifter demonstrates his moves on Muscle Beach in its heyday during the 1950s.

In 1934, with the U.S. in the grip of the twentieth century's worst economic recession, the Great Depression (1929–41), the Works Project Administration funded a beachfront refurbishment project in the seaside town of Santa Monica to provide work for the local unemployed. Originally conceived as a multi-use public recreational facility and park by the city's Recreation & Parks Department, the area south of Santa Monica Pier quickly became known as 'Muscle Beach', attracting bodybuilders, acrobats, Hollywood actors and stuntmen, off-duty military personnel, and on busy holiday weekends up to 1,000 hangers-on and sightseers who came to gawp at the display of flesh on the beach, and marvel at the feats of strength and acrobatic stunts.[8] In his book

Muscle Beach (1980), Ed Murray gives a flavour of the atmosphere of the area in its heyday:

> When you came to Muscle Beach you knew straight away that you were somewhere special; the atmosphere was completely different. You'd see muscles that most people never imagined human beings could have, acrobats flying around, balancing on their hands, on their heads, alone, on each other, doing tricks on the different pieces of apparatus. There were guys lifting enormous weights, and Muscle Beachniks dancing wildly on the boardwalks and in the park. It was a circus.[9]

Muscle Beach was open to all, regardless of age and gender, free of charge, and divided into two sections: the weight-training area, with the equipment often provided by the exercisers themselves and stored in a makeshift hut; and the gymnastics equipment that the reader will be familiar with from Jahn's *Turnplatz* – the high bar, parallel bars, rings and so on. The Parks Department built platforms on the beach for weight trainers, weightlifters, gymnasts and acrobats, and these developed into stages for acrobatic displays and weightlifting and bodybuilding competitions that drew large, appreciative crowds on holiday weekends. The bodybuilder Steve Reeves (1926–2000), who would later become Hollywood's leading sword-and-sandal epic movie star, was typical of the young men drawn to Muscle Beach immediately after the war. In an interview given a year before his death, he described his early days in Santa Monica after having been discharged from the military. He lived on the '52/20' – that is, $20 a week paid to former servicemen for 52 weeks until they went to college or got a job.[10]

Reeves and fellow bodybuilder George Eiferman (1925–2002), who both went on to win major bodybuilding titles, shared a room in a muscle house, and spent their days between the gym and Muscle Beach, living comfortably on the small military stipend paid to them by the federal government. In a reversal of Triat's and Sandow's careers, which had begun on the stage, and which they had used as springboards to launch their fitness businesses, Reeves used his fame and success as a competitive bodybuilder to launch his Hollywood acting career. He was the most successful bodybuilder-turned-actor of the 1950s, but he was not unique. A flesh-and-blood version of the fictional Superman, Reeves embodied the projection of American power as the hyper-muscular heterosexual male. Reeves, Eiferman and other Muscle Beach regulars starred in Hollywood B-movies as Herakles and Samson, stripped to the waist with oiled muscles. This started a trend that continued into the next generation of bodybuilders, when Arnold Schwarzenegger played Conan the Barbarian and the Terminator and Lou Ferrigno (b. 1951) the Incredible Hulk.

Although Reeves and Eiferman were stalwarts of Muscle Beach during the year they spent in Santa Monica, Reeves explained that he and most of the serious bodybuilders trained at the gyms that had opened in the town to cater for the bodybuilders and muscle heads.[11] Murray describes one of the types of gym that operated in the area at the time, which was nicknamed 'the Dungeon':

> A descending staircase at the sidewalk entrance led to a huge, somewhat dirty, equipment-filled room. One small iron-grated window gave a tiny view of the sidewalk above. There were holes in the floor, of various sizes, because guys had dropped weights, and some of them would gather water when it rained, due to leakage in the walls and ceiling. Rats lived in the gym, and muscleniks, too, from time to time.[12]

This is perhaps the image that many readers will have of the early gym: a male-only environment, with only the most basic facilities, and low levels of cleanliness matched only by the poor standard of personal hygiene of the patrons. One of the first gyms I went to after college was a traditional muscle-head hangout, where every square inch of available floor space was occupied by racks of oversized dumb-bells, stacks of 45 and 55 lb (20/25 kg) black cast-iron weight plates, barbells, collars, benches, squat racks, power cages and ancient pulley machines with exposed weight stacks. Rather than the sleek, clean, hi-tech look that most twenty-first-century health clubs aspire to, this cavernous underground facility looked like a collision between a mechanic's workshop, a warehouse and an iron foundry, whose larger-than-life patrons put one in mind of words such as 'hewn', 'carved' and 'constructed'. My enduring memory of the place is its distinctive smell – a not entirely pleasant combination of rubber, rust, chalk dust, stale sweat and raw testosterone. Predictably, this gym did not have a women's locker room, or even a women's bathroom.

I had gone to the place with a friend who had a couple of years' head start in bodybuilding, and who himself worked out with a couple of training partners. It was not just that you needed partners to 'spot' you when you did heavy bench presses or squats, it was just how people trained in that kind of gym: as a group activity – with banter and a certain amount of horsing around, but mainly with an undercurrent of friendly rivalry about the amount of weight lifted and the number of reps achieved. It also helped to be in a group in order to lay claim to a corner of the gym and whatever equipment you needed for that day's workout. There were a few guys training on their own, and in their case the term 'muscle monsters' sprang to mind. Even the lifting gym novice that I was then instinctively knew that these were not men you disturbed or exchanged pleasantries with, let alone asked, however politely, for the loan of a weight plate or a piece of equipment.

I did not stay long at this particular gym, but it did teach me a couple of important lessons: first, it confirmed to me that progressive weight training worked, either on its own or, as was clearly the case with many of the gym's patrons, aided by legal and illegal supplementation; and second, that before joining a gym, you should look at the other members and staff, and ask yourself if you want to look like them. Whatever your original goals and intentions, if you go to a muscle-head gym for any length of time, you will sooner rather than later adopt the muscle head's ethos and training methods (and the illegal supplementation that is flavour of the month), and you will end up as a muscle head yourself – the peer pressure is just too great. In my subsequent fitness career, I have trained in many different types of gym: from the sanitized corporate health club, with chrome-plated free and machine weights, wood-panelled lockers and fluffy branded towels for use in the marbled wet area, to much more basic gyms with a strong muscle-head constituency and a single shower stall for the whole gym. Wherever I have worked out, however, I have always encountered a version of that heterosexual male rivalry-camaraderie that is not just a by-product of training with weights in a gym but is a vital part of what makes it work.

While Southern California had its dungeons, it was in Santa Monica that a new kind of gym opened that would transform weight training from a niche activity for competitive bodybuilders and muscle heads into an international business that would not be a short-lived craze dependent on the fame and success of a few celebrities but would become an integral part of the Western lifestyle. Even in California, however, there was considerable resistance to new notions of exercise, although when Santa Monica Muscle Beach was forced to close in 1959, it was more moral concerns that motivated the authorities. At a court hearing when the beach's supporters tried to stop the city from closing down Muscle Beach, the judge ruled in the city's favour, condemning it and the activities taking place there as 'freakish', 'homoerotic' and 'unbalanced'.[13]

Having won the legal challenge, the city sent in the bulldozers to demolish the gymnastics equipment, weights hut and competition platforms. But Muscle Beach had made a deep and indelible mark on the national psyche and had spawned an imitator a few miles away in Venice, where in 1951 the Los Angeles Recreation & Parks Department opened a similar outdoor weightlifting facility for the city, the Venice Beach Recreation Center.[14] For many tourists, it is Venice's Muscle Beach and its weight-training cage, which still hosts bodybuilding competitions on holiday weekends, that is the original Muscle Beach, despite the reopening of training facilities in Santa Monica, and the erection of a sign emblazoned with 'Muscle Beach' belatedly installed and paid for by the Santa Monica Recreation & Parks Department.

The Birth of the All-American Health Club

If the Dungeon described above was representative of the kind of gym where men trained in the early decades of the twentieth century, three fitness entrepreneurs, Vic Tanny (1912–1985), Jack LaLanne (1914–2011) and Bob Delmonteque (1926–2011), were determined to transform them from dark, dirty, smelly, dingy, all-male preserves populated by bodybuilders and muscle heads into comfortable recreational facilities that would attract the general exerciser. Although we are now used to the idea of men and women of all ages using weights for therapeutic and aesthetic training, in the 1930s it was a radical idea that many people found morally suspect, and that doctors warned could be dangerous. Coming from completely different backgrounds and parts of the country, Tanny and LaLanne faced resistance early on in their careers, until they made their way to the place that was fast becoming the Mecca for America's new health-and-fitness culture – Santa Monica, California.

Born Victor Iannidinardo in Rochester, New York, Vic Tanny opened his first gym in his home town in 1935 at the age of 23. He wanted to create a completely different training environment from the kind of gym that was the norm at the time by providing a clean, well-lit, comfortable workout space, with piped music, carpeted floors and mirrored walls, and equipped with rust-free chrome-plated free weights and weight-training machines that would facilitate and enhance the training experience, and make it accessible to the vast majority of the population that the professional bodybuilding gyms excluded. In a photograph illustrating a *Life* magazine feature of 1958 on the emerging American health-club industry, the besuited Tanny is shown standing proudly in one of his new health clubs. The three exercisers in shot are not hulking, sweating male bodybuilders but shapely young women in fashionable, figure-hugging 1950s workout wear, each training on a Smith Machine – a cage-like piece of apparatus halfway between a squat frame and a weight-training machine that enables exercisers to train alone without a spotter much more safely than when doing the equivalent exercises with a loaded barbell.[15]

Tanny's initial East Coast venture failed to attract sufficient members. In 1939 he sold up and with $700 in his pocket he moved west to Santa Monica, where he opened a gym to cater for the patrons of Muscle Beach. In the interview quoted earlier, Steve Reeves explained that he and 90 per cent of the other serious bodybuilders trained at Tanny's gym in Santa Monica.[16] Although probably not as luxurious and well-appointed as many of the 83 gyms that Tanny would open nationwide between 1950 and 1960, the Santa Monica gym was a significant improvement on the other training facilities available there in the 1930s and '40s. The Second World War had a serious impact on Tanny's first two health clubs, which were forced to close, but by 1947 he had opened several new gyms in the Los Angeles area.

In addition to a much more comfortable, attractive environment, Tanny offered a structured approach to aesthetic training that was aimed at members of the general public, and in particular was designed to appeal to women. In an early reference to America's ongoing struggle against obesity, the gym's motto was 'Take it off, build it up and make it firm.' Tanny's target market was not the muscle heads and competitive bodybuilders, though they played a role in his early success in Santa Monica, but men and women with work and family responsibilities who could not afford to spend their days on the beach and evenings in the gym, and who had much more limited fitness goals. New members were put on a three-day-a-week programme, with thirty-minute workouts consisting of 24 Tanny-approved weight-training exercises. In order to maintain the right atmosphere in his gyms, Tanny cautioned members not to over-train and asked them to refrain from grunting and groaning during workouts.[17]

Our second fitness entrepreneur, Jack LaLanne, was also a Muscle Beach habitué, who was often pictured with his second wife, Elaine (née Doyle), performing acrobatic feats of strength on the beach. LaLanne, like Tanny, wanted to transform the training experience and make it accessible to a much wider audience. A self-confessed sugar and junk-food addict as a teenager, LaLanne turned his life around at the age of fifteen after hearing a lecture by the nutritional pioneer Paul Bragg (1895–1976). He followed Bragg's advice to reform his diet and began exercising, dramatically improving his mental well-being and physical health. Fired by the zeal of the convert, LaLanne embarked on a major programme of self-improvement, working both on his body and his mind. He wrote:

I became a voracious reader and I absorbed everything that would help me to improve myself. *Gray's Anatomy* was my bible. During college, I studied pre-med to become a medical doctor and I also went to Chiropractic College and graduated; however, I was more interested in helping people by convincing them to take preventative measures, before they became ill.[18]

He opened his first health club on the upper floor of an old office building in his home town of Oakland, California, but, like Tanny in Rochester, he initially had trouble attracting enough members. He later wrote that the club was 40 years ahead of its time, and that the medical profession was against him, condemning him as a dangerous health nut and a charlatan, and claiming that working out with weights would give people heart attacks, cause sexual dysfunction in men, turn women into men and cause muscle binding in athletes.[19] A black-and-white photograph of LaLanne's Oakland health club available on jacklalanne.com shows a remarkably minimalist, modern interior, complete with potted plants spaced out around the walls. The large, spotlessly clean, open-plan training area has strip lighting for the evening and, unlike the dark subterranean gyms of the period, has large windows that would have flooded it with light during the day. A parquet floor surrounds a tiled central weight-training area where dumb-bells and barbells are neatly stored on racks by weight; a pulley-machine, one of the many weight-training machines designed by LaLanne, is visible on one wall.

With sports coaches forbidding their athletes to weight train, LaLanne had to give members sets of keys to the gym so they could train in secret at night. Like Tanny, LaLanne recognized that to be successful, gyms needed to appeal beyond the small bodybuilding fraternity to the wider community. His list of innovations included the first mixed-gender gym in the U.S.; the first to have women athletes, the physically challenged and the elderly working out with weights; and the first health club to provide health foods and nutritional advice. His equipment firsts included such gym standbys as leg extension machines, cable and pulley machines and Smith machines.[20] LaLanne would go on to establish a chain of over 200 health clubs nationwide, but his main claim to fame was The Jack LaLanne Show, a television health-and-fitness show that began as a fifteen-minute slot on a local TV station in San Francisco in 1951, was picked up by ABC in 1959 and ran for 34 years until 1985.[21] The first fitness entrepreneur to make full use of the medium of TV, LaLanne reached millions with his message of physical and mental well-being through regular exercise and a healthy diet. The Jack LaLanne Way to Vibrant Good Health, published in 1970, reads like a contemporary guide to healthy living, with warnings about processed 'foodless' foods that contain too much fat and sugar, recommendations about vitamin supplementation and exercise, and warnings against smoking, drinking and crash dieting.[22] Like his mixed-gender health clubs and his promotion of weight training for all, LaLanne's advice was decades ahead of its time and was considered faddish and even dangerous by doctors, but in the past few decades it has become health and fitness and medical orthodoxy.

Our third Southern California health-and-fitness and gym pioneer is the naturopath Dr Bob Delmonteque, who began his career training Hollywood stars, including John Wayne and Errol Flynn. In the 1950s, together with his business partner Ray Wilson, Delmonteque founded the American Health Studios, which were modelled on German postwar rehabilitation centres and European health spas. Initially equipped with weight-training facilities, the chain, which grew to around 300 clubs nationwide with a further 200 overseas, later featured wet areas with whirlpools, dry saunas and steam baths. The Health Studios were also the first gyms to offer therapeutic facilities to members. Like Tanny and LaLanne, Delmonteque and Wilson's vision was to repackage the training experience. They provided air-conditioned, carpeted gyms with full-length mirrors, and chrome-plated weights that, in Delmonteque's words, 'flavored exercise and made it taste good'.[23]

Ray Wilson has another important claim to fame in terms of the development of the modern gym. In about 1970, he and his business partner Augie Nieto acquired the rights to the first commercial stationary electronic cycle exerciser.[24] Although very different from today's multi-function electronic aerobic exercisers with their graphic-rich programmable functions, docking ports for smartphones, iPods and tablets, and screens for TV, games and Internet access, the Electronic Cycle Exerciser established Lifecycle Inc., today's Life Fitness, as one of the world leaders in the manufacture of cardio equipment for the home and professional markets.[25]

Although as businessmen the pioneers of the American health club industry sometimes left something to be desired, they established many of the elements of the modern gym that we now take for granted: clean, brightly lit and well-decorated spaces with music, featuring a range of equipment apart from free weights, such as machine weights and cardio equipment, and with good ancillary facilities, such as changing rooms, showers and wet areas, cafés offering healthy food options and nutritional advice, and therapy rooms. The muscle-head gym, however, was far from dead and gone, and in the 1970s and '80s it was to have a renaissance through the combination of competitive bodybuilding and Hollywood razzmatazz: the 'Age of Arnie' had arrived.

Mecca of Bodybuilding

The 25 years between 1950 and 1975 were a period of incredible contrasts in the United States. Triumphant in the Second World War, from 1947 the country was nevertheless plunged into the protracted Cold War against the Soviet Union and her ally, the People's Republic of China, against which the U.S. fought two proxy wars in Asia – the Korean War (1950–53) and the Vietnam War (1955–75) – the former a still unresolved stalemate, the latter a humiliating defeat. At the same time, the U.S. led the world economically, technologically and industrially, exporting its brand of consumerism worldwide along with its cars and domestic appliances, while it also led in youth culture and counterculture. For any trend, from the sexual revolution to civil rights reform, the world looked to the U.S. to see what was going to happen next.

What had started on a beach in Southern California had burgeoned into a nationwide phenomenon. And although Muscle Beach had been bulldozed in 1959, the coastal cities were still setting trends for the U.S.'s nascent health and fitness industry. In 1965 Joe Gold (1922–2004), who had trained on Muscle Beach and at Vic Tanny's gym in Santa Monica, opened the first branch of Gold's Gym in Venice, California, soon to become the self-styled 'Mecca of bodybuilding'. With its unrivalled location next to the new Muscle Beach and close to the heart of the film industry, Gold's Gym could not fail to attract both the musclemen and the movie stars, often one and the same. Just as Steve Reeves had launched his film career from the posing platforms of Muscle Beach, Arnold Schwarzenegger used his fame as a six-time winner of the Mr Olympia title to break into the movie business. He first made a name for himself with *Conan the Barbarian* (1982), but he established himself as a Hollywood superstar with *The Terminator* (1984).

Although the iconic Gold's Gym building in Venice was demolished in the summer of 2014, anyone wishing to see what it was like in its heyday need only watch *Pumping Iron* (1977), starring the leading body-builders of the day, including Arnold Schwarzenegger, Franco Columbu (b. 1941) and Lou Ferrigno.[26] The documentary follows their prepara-tions for Mr Olympia 1975, and features the contest held that year in Pretoria, South Africa, which was won for the sixth year in a row by Schwarzenegger. If Tanny and LaLanne wanted to attract general exer-cisers and make them feel comfortable with music and carpeting, Gold's was self-consciously aimed at competitive bodybuilders and their admirers and imitators. The hangar-like space had a concrete floor, with plenty of benches, and the occasional rubber mat for floor work and kneeling exercises; the walls were lined with racks of heavy-duty dumb-bells and barbells, while the centre of the room was occupied by pulley and cable machines, ab benches, weight stacks by the ton, power cages and squat racks. This was a functional no-frills workout space, whose only concession to health-club design were the mirrored walls – a necessary luxury for bodybuilders who are judged on the symmetry, proportion, size and definition of their muscles. In the 1970s Gold's Gym there was no motivational music, no personal trainers, no group exercise classes, no juice bar and very few women, though several occasionally stray into shot in *Pumping Iron*, caught admiring the testos-terone-fuelled display in the gym and, in one scene, featuring as makeshift weight-training props when two slender, blonde-haired Californian groupies sit on Arnie's back as he performs calf raises.

One of the striking aspects of the idealization of the male bodybuilder is how strongly differentiated the genders have become in the world of hyper-muscular strength athletes. In *Pumping Iron*, the only women present are Lou Ferrigno's mother and the Californian nymphets men-tioned above. According to the Harvard medical researcher Harrison Pope, this is not a coincidence. In *The Adonis Complex* (2000), he com-pares the milestones of feminism with those of the changing male body image and gym culture. He argues that as women won greater rights and therefore became a greater threat to male dominance, men responded by training at the gym to become physically stronger, bigger and more muscular.[27]

Pumping Iron inspired a generation of men and boys to start body-building and the dedicated few to compete. In terms of its ethos and image, Gold's Gym was something of a throwback to an earlier generation of gyms – an updated and sanitized version of the all-male 'Dungeon' – though bigger, better equipped, better lit and swept clean at the end of the day. When Gold's Gym became a chain, Gold quickly realized that he could not limit its membership to professional and amateur strength athletes, and that he would have to attract a much broader membership base, including general exercisers and women, to remain in business. Disillusioned with his lack of commercial success, Gold sold out in 1970, but he returned to the business in 1977 with a new brand, World Gym.[28] Both Gold's Gym and World Gym are still major players in the industry, and although they still capitalize on the all-male bodybuilding image in their promotional material and logos, they now offer the same facilities as all the other major corporate chain gyms in the U.S., including large cardio zones, personal trainers, piped music and group exercise classes.

If the all-male dungeon-gym has been superseded by a more comfortable, modern and inclusive training environment, something of its single-sex, testosterone-fuelled atmosphere persists in the free-weights area of many contemporary gyms – the friendly rivalry that heterosexual men use to motivate themselves as they train. Of course, the pressures of modern life being what they are, once through college, there is much less time to go to the gym with your friends who, like you, have to juggle work and conjugal commitments. Nevertheless, in all contemporary gyms you will see workout partners in twos and threes, motivating one another. Sometimes, friends will arrange to meet at the gym and train at the same time but not together, chatting during the breaks in their respective workouts. Thus for the heterosexual man the gym is not just a place to exercise but an extension of his social life, because it might be the only time that he can share with a particular male friend or colleague.

'Turn on Your Life'

The first nationwide chains were founded and fronted by health and fitness enthusiasts and celebrities who had gravitated to Southern California between the 1930s and '60s. Tanny, LaLanne, Delmonteque, Wilson and Gold established the look, facilities and ethos of the modern American health club, while also creating the market for facilities aimed at general male exercisers and women. But with the exception of Ray Wilson, who had a stellar career and established a number of successful gym chains, California's gym pioneers were not gifted businessmen. Despite Wilson's flair, his and Delmonteque's American Health Studios went out of business in 1959; Tanny overreached himself in the late 1950s and was forced to close many gyms and in 1962 to sell those that remained; LaLanne's TV career gave him little time to oversee his health clubs and he, too, sold his gyms in the early 1960s; and, as we saw above, Joe Gold sold his business, lock, stock and name in 1970.

Despite this litany of business failures, by the early 1960s there existed a sound business model for the health club industry, and the existence of hundreds of gyms nationwide confirmed that there was not only the demand but also a great deal of money to be made from selling fitness to increasingly health- and appearance-conscious American men and women. What was needed was the right product at the right price, tailored to the 1960s American consumer. In 1962, in a first move towards corporate consolidation, Health and Tennis Corporation of America bought out struggling gym chains, including Vic Tanny and Jack LaLanne's health clubs.[29] But the first major player in the business, and the ancestor of all today's corporate gyms, was Bally, now known as Bally Total Fitness.

Founded in 1931 in Chicago as Lion Manufacturing, but quickly renamed Bally Manufacturing, the company specialized in coin-operated arcade games. For the next half century, Bally continued to grow, manufacturing slots, pinball machines and arcade video games. As a natural progression, it entered the casino industry by purchasing several gaming hotels. In 1983, as part of a plan to diversify the company's portfolio and become a leader in the U.S. leisure industry, Bally purchased the

Health and Tennis Corporation of America, creating Bally Health and Tennis Corporation, a division of a new parent company, Bally Entertainment.

The company also bought Lifecycle (Life Fitness), renaming it Bally Fitness Products. By 1995, Bally had become the world's largest owner and operator of fitness centres, with 325 health clubs in the U.S. and Canada. That same year the company launched the Bally Total Fitness brand, renaming many of its clubs that had kept their original Tanny and LaLanne branding, in order to capitalize on the Bally image and name. The actor Teri Hatcher of *Lois and Clark* and later *Desperate Housewives* fame was hired to front Bally's 'turn on your life' promotional campaign. It is significant, in a business that had such a masculine self-image, that Bally chose a woman, though, of course, we should remember that Hatcher in her Lois Lane persona was Superman's girlfriend and faithful sidekick.

Although Bally experienced serious financial problems during the late 1990s, it remains one of the U.S.'s leading gym chains. The turn-around was achieved through a radical redesign of the clubs themselves: increasing the space allotted to the cardio and weights areas and cutting space for expensive and less-used swimming pools and basketball and racquetball courts. Another innovation was to introduce shops into the gyms to sell branded clothing, supplements and protein products to members.[30] Where Bally had trailblazed, many others followed – in the U.S., Europe, Australia and Japan, and now in the emerging economies of the former Soviet Bloc, Asia and South America.

The Evolution of the Muscleman

For many heterosexual men training between the 1970s and '90s, the bodybuilder physique was the ideal to be achieved: the broad shoulders and inflated chest forming a tapering triangle to the waist, with bulging arm and leg muscles. In one scene in *Pumping Iron*, at Gold's Gym Schwarzenegger tutors a younger man – who, while he clearly works out, is never likely to achieve anything like the master's size, symmetry and definition – in the finer points of posing best to display his burgeoning muscles. As with Sandow's books eight decades earlier, the message that the scene conveys is mixed: the top competitive bodybuilders are genetically superior supermen whose achievements and physiques mere mortals can never hope to equal, but at the same time, there is the slim hope that with enough hard work, they might be able to come close.

In the real world, the cult of the hyper-muscular supermale led to some rather odd results. When I began working out, I often came across men who suffered from what was dubbed 'chicken-leg syndrome': exercisers who had extremely well-developed arms, shoulders and chests, but whose bodies tapered to skinny, non-existent buttocks and legs, as they never worked out their muscles below the waist, hiding their undeveloped lower halves under layers of baggy workout gear. Another early gym denizen was the man who was only interested in developing strength in a limited number of lifts – often the bench press – with no regard for overall muscular development. Notionally identified as power lifters, these men developed very strange disproportionate physiques, often being as broad as they were tall, and nicknamed by some bodybuilders 'poison dwarves'.

Although many writers have remarked on the homoerotic aspects of the bodybuilding competition, as it gives men licence to admire other men wearing little more than minute briefs and posing pouches on stage, from its earliest days its ethos has always been and has remained self-consciously and aggressively heterosexual. As such, it has played a role in defining how heterosexual men see themselves, and what they aspire to in terms of their own physical development. But it is not just how the man in the street sees the strongman that has changed since Sandow's day; the past century has also seen an evolution in the ideal and reality of achievable muscular development. In order to appreciate the radical transformation of the bodybuilding ideal, readers need only compare the physique of Eugen Sandow, photographed at the turn of the century, with that of eight-time Mr Olympia winner Ronnie Coleman (b. 1964), photographed during a bodybuilding competition in the early 2000s (see pp. 108, 136). The reason for the marked difference between nineteenth- and twentieth-century competitive strength athletes is the use of anabolic steroids and other performance-enhancing drugs in the world of professional bodybuilding.[31]

The first anabolic steroid, the male hormone testosterone, was first identified in Germany in 1935. It had been synthesized by the late 1930s, and its role as an 'anabolic' compound that builds muscle was quickly realized in animal experiments, and confirmed when it was given to human patients to treat various diseases including cancer. Its 'androgenic' effects that impart masculine characteristics were also noted when testosterone was given to pre-pubescent children and women.[32] According to the expert Charles Yesalis, steroids could have been used to enhance the performance of German athletes as early as the Berlin summer Olympics of 1936, but their first securely attested use in international competitive sport was by Russian strength athletes who triumphed at the world weightlifting championships held in 1954 in Vienna. It is likely that by this time, West Coast bodybuilders, always at the cutting edge of weight-training developments, were also experimenting with synthetic anabolic steroids. Despite bans by the International Olympic Committee and most other sporting governing bodies, paralleled by moves by governments across the developed world to make their sale and purchase criminal offences, steroid use continued to increase through the 1960s, '70s and '80s.

Yesalis estimates that by the 1990s about one million people in the U.S. had used steroids to enhance sporting performance and physical appearance. Many users were adolescents, with 5 per cent of adolescent males and 2.5 per cent of adolescent females admitting to steroid use.[33] Pope cites two studies of twelfth-grade (aged 17–18) male students, the first from 1988, which showed that 6.6 per cent had used steroids, and one from 1995, which recorded an almost identical prevalence of 6.5 per cent. He used this figure to estimate that up to 1.5 million Americans had used steroids in the twelve years between 1988 and 2000.[34] From the late 1980s, a series of high-profile scandals across a number of sports revealed that steroids were only one class of banned substances used by athletes to enhance their performance; others were the blood-doping hormone EPO and synthetic human growth hormone (HGH).[35] Pope lists over 50 steroids and other compounds that are available to professional and amateur bodybuilders on the black market, which they take along with the legal supplements such as protein powder, amino acids, creatine and ephedrine to increase muscle mass and reduce body fat.[36]

Steroid use is more prevalent in gyms where competitive body-builders and muscle heads train. Bodybuilders use steroids and other illegal substances as part of their yearly training cycles, and they can be extremely effective when used in the right combinations (known as 'stacks' in the trade) and at the right time. However, taking steroids without a proper training regime and diet will achieve little or no gains in muscle mass. They are not magic bullets or miracle shortcuts to achieve a muscular, defined physique. The only way an aspiring body-builder is going to look like Arnold Schwarzenegger or Ronnie Coleman in their prime is if: a) he trains as hard as they did; b) he strictly controls his diet; c) he does not stay up late drinking and partying; and d) he makes use of steroids in a disciplined manner under medical super-vision. Over the years I have known strength athletes who have suffered from the adverse side effects of steroid use: early onset male pattern baldness, acute skin problems (whole-body acne), sexual dysfunction (impotence) and extreme mood disorders ('roid rage'), as well as more serious medical complications involving serious impairment of the liver, bladder, heart and kidneys from the high level of steroid toxicity, which unfortunately occasionally leads to fatalities.

It is obvious why competitive bodybuilders use anabolic steroids – because they know that their rivals are also using them. Quite apart from the ordinary level of competitiveness found in American life, which is carried into the gym, top bodybuilders can now make considerable sums in prize money when they win a major competition run by the IFBB (International Federation of Bodybuilding and Fitness), estab-lished in 1946 by Joe Weider, and the more fitness and modelling-orientated WBFF (World Beauty Fitness and Fashion Inc.). To give an example of prize-money inflation in the past four decades, when Arnold Schwarzenegger won the IFBB Mr Olympia title from 1970 to 1975, he scooped between $1,000 and $2,500; Ronnie Coleman, who won the title from 1998 to 2005, took home between $110,000 and $150,000; and Mr Olympia 2011, 2012 and 2013, Phil Heath (b. 1979), won $250,000 to $350,000. A title such as Mr America, Mr Universe or Mr Olympia also wins an athlete lucrative commercial sponsorship.

In addition to the major competitions, the sport is promoted by the muscle press (and now numerous spin-off websites). The grandfather of muscle publishing, Joe Weider (1919–2013), who established the Mr Olympia contest, founded a range of health and fitness and bodybuilding titles aimed at male bodybuilders and their fans. He launched his first muscle title, Your Physique, in 1936, and it became Muscle & Fitness in 1980. The Weider stable of publications features several of the leading muscle and fitness magazines, including Flex and Men's Fitness, and has now broadened out to include titles for the general exerciser and women.[37] With its own media, competitions, lucrative sponsorship deals and large amounts in prize money, the world of professional bodybuilding has become a big business with a global reach that has had a tremendous influence over the goals and training practices of heterosexual men.

Many bodybuilders and physique athletes cash in on their success in competition by promoting their own training systems. This is nothing new: Sandow published Strength and How to Obtain It, spicing up his training tips with anecdotes, real and imagined, from his colourful past. On the opening page of this chapter, I have used a quotation from Schwarzenegger's Encyclopedia of Modern Bodybuilding, one of many weight-training titles written by the great man. The latest breed of training advice, however, comes via the Internet, packaged in slick, high-end websites, with photographs and video clips of the promoter of a particular weight-training system, promising his potential disciples that if they follow his advice, they will look exactly as muscular and ripped as he does. There usually follow pages of complex workouts, nutritional advice and lifestyle tips, most of which are repackaged information about progressive weight training and healthy eating that has been available since Sandow's day. This kind of glossy programme, however, appeals to a certain type of aspiring male bodybuilder who, along with information about how to train, needs a role model to follow.

One such is Allan, a recent gym acquaintance who trains six or seven times a week with a grim, sweat-soaked determination that is quite impressive. With earphones permanently pumping motivational music into his ears, he is not someone you can casually engage in conversation between sets. After about six months of seeing him daily, I noticed that he was making real progress. But what alerted me to it was not just the change in his body shape but the way he came into the gym one day, when he not so much walked as strutted across the weights area, with the rolling gait affected by bodybuilders who swing their chest and shoulders as if they were too wide to fit through the available space. In other words, he marched in triumphantly as if he owned the place, which told me immediately that he had achieved a major personal goal, in terms either of his bodyweight or his body composition, or that he had succeeded in lifting a weight that he had once thought well beyond his reach.

Allan was not always so triumphant. On another morning a few weeks later I found him sipping his post-workout protein shake, disconsolately leafing through a sheaf of printed pages. I asked him what was wrong, and he admitted that he was exhausted from the new training programme that he was trying out. He handed me a printout that he had downloaded from the Internet. The programme title consisted of several initials. I had reviewed many of these programmes when I worked as a fitness journalist, and I knew that a combination of the initials H (hyper), M (massive), S (strength) and M (muscle) would feature in the title – which they did. The pages contained several weeks' worth of workouts and advice about diet and legal supplementation, recommending one of the author's product sponsors who manufactured protein powder and other supplements, and were peppered with encouraging interjections along the lines of 'You've done it!' and 'You're the best!' I turned to the front page, which showed a picture of the programme's creator: impossibly good-looking, hyper-muscular and 'shredded' (that is, with abnormally low body fat), he beamed confidently, assuring his readers that if they followed his programme they would achieve the same results. Although this was true to a degree, what was not made clear in the printout was that this would require an exerciser to train twice a day, seven days a week, leaving little time for a full-time job or family life; to follow the author's complex regime of legal and illegal supplementation for several years; and finally to pose for a photo shoot after several weeks of strict dieting and immediately before a contest, when he would have stripped off 20–30 lb (9–13.5 kg) of body fat and water.

It is an open industry secret that many of the physique and strength athletes who promote their own training programmes online and in the muscle press use illegal supplementation while at the same time claiming to be 'natural' or 'clean', that is, non-users of banned substances (understandably, as the use of steroids to improve performance and appearance is illegal), creating a gap between what is achievable without supplementation and the expectations of ordinary exercisers. This not only risks discouraging those exercisers who fail to achieve the promised results, turning them off the gym altogether, but may also encourage others to experiment with illegal supplementation. According to the findings of several researchers, unrealistic expectations about what is possible with unsupplemented gym-based exercise and growing pressure from the media and advertising for men to conform to certain ideal body types are the cause of a hidden epidemic of image-related disorders among heterosexual men.

The Trouble with Adonis

The story of the gym until the mid-twentieth century has been a largely positive one. The provision of facilities for different forms of exercise has been a social good, empowering individuals and improving their mental and physical well-being. But according to Dr Harrison Pope and his colleagues at Harvard Medical School, 50 or so years ago something changed in the relationship between heterosexual men and physical exercise; and the gym, rather than being a source of health and personal empowerment, became a place that was potentially dangerous to the average exerciser's psychological well-being. One of the unwanted side effects of the concentration on the hyper-muscular supermale image in competition and the muscle media has been the appearance of a psychological disorder known officially as 'muscle dysmorphia', and more colloquially as 'bigemia' or 'bigorexia', which Pope et al. have christened 'the Adonis Complex'.[38] In ancient Greek myth, Adonis was so good-looking that two goddesses fought over his affections, and he died at the hands of a third disgruntled female deity.

Bigorexia is a dangerous disconnection between what an exerciser sees in the mirror and his real size, muscularity and fitness. The condition can be seen as the mirror image of the eating disorder anorexia nervosa, in which sufferers feel that they are overweight, no matter how much weight they lose. Suffering from the opposite delusion, the bigorexic, who believes that he is underweight and out of shape, will continue to train even when it becomes dangerous or self-destructive, when he is injured or ill. He may also damage his health through ultra-low-fat diets to achieve unrealistic levels of body fat, and he is more likely to experiment with dangerous supplementation with illegal muscle-building and fat-reducing substances.[39]

According to Pope, bigorexia has reached epidemic proportions not just in the U.S. but in most of the developed world. In order to explore the phenomenon, he conducted studies in the U.S. and Europe, interviewing gym-goers and asking them to take part in psychometric tests about body image. He cites the case histories of men whom the majority of the population would describe as living 'Adonises', but who themselves feel physically inadequate and thus train obsessively. Overall, men's dissatisfaction with their bodies is increasing. A survey taken in 1972 revealed that 15 per cent of men were dissatisfied with their bodies; this had increased to 34 per cent in 1985; and a survey carried out by *Psychology Today* in the U.S. in 1997 recorded a dissatisfaction level of 43 per cent. There were even higher levels of dissatisfaction recorded for specific parts of the body, the highest, 63 per cent, being expressed by men about their chests.[40]

Body-image dissatisfaction leading to psychological disorders is more usually associated with women, who are bombarded with images of impossibly thin and perfect models in fashion magazines or of equally improbably curvaceous big-breasted 'glamazons' in the popular media. For Pope, the causes of male bigorexia are very similar to those of the image-related disorders that affect women: exposure to unrealistic images of hyper-muscular supermales since childhood, including comic-book superheroes, action figures such as GI Joe or Action Man, Hollywood action heroes, WWF stars and the plethora of muscular male bodies that have appeared in the muscle press and increasingly in the mainstream media and advertising since the 1980s.[41] The second cause that Pope identifies is the rising power of women since the emergence of second-wave feminism that has challenged male dominance at every level of society. Hence the subtext of the heterosexual man's desire to become bigger and more muscular is to reclaim his threatened masculinity and project male power against the steady rise of women.[42] An additional but related factor that Pope does not mention is the increased visibility of gay men since Gay Liberation in the 1970s. In an earlier era heterosexual men could write off gay men as effeminate sissies, but post-Gay Liberation, the guy who is training next to them at the gym and might be bigger and better defined might also be an out gay man.

There is one possible impact of the higher visibility and presence of gay men in the gym, and that is in the kind of workout clothes heterosexual men now seem to prefer. In the gym scenes in *Pumping Iron*, there is quite a lot of flesh on display: muscle vests slit all the way down the sides so that most of the torso is on view, and very tight short shorts emphasizing the crotch and backside – styles of dress that would now be thought of as gay because they allow for an explicit, erotic display of the body which, in an environment that was largely all male, meant the viewers were other men. In the 1980s and '90s, when gay men went to the gym in skin-tight Lycra shorts and vests that left very little to the imagination, heterosexual men began to cover up, wearing baggy T-shirts and sweatshirts, and long shorts, often worn over a pair of Lycra under-shorts. I have never heard a heterosexual man articulate the idea that he took up weight training because of the rising power of women or the increased visibility of gay men, who both present challenges to heterosexual male dominance, but it does give a plausible subconscious reason why some men might want to become more muscular and 'masculine'.

According to Pope, what men need to challenge the Adonis Complex is not men's liberation from the tyranny of women but a way to resist hegemonic images of hyper-muscular supermales. He believes heterosexual men have particular difficulty when trying to come to terms with image-related disorders. Whereas women have developed strategies to resist the damage caused by image disorders and, if they do succumb to them, are able to discuss them openly and seek treatment, heterosexual men are in the double bind of having no resistance strategies to fall back on and feeling inhibited about discussing any problems relating to self-image because 'real men' are not supposed to be concerned about their appearance.[43] Often, they do not realize that the bodybuilders they see in the muscle magazines and posters are at the peak of their competitive cycle, when they have maximum size and definition and minimum body fat, but they can maintain this level of shredded hyper-muscularity only for a matter of weeks or even days. Outside competition, bodybuilders are 20–40 lb (9–18 kg) heavier, and this extra weight is made up mostly of body fat and water that they shed through extreme dieting in the final weeks before a contest. And, of course, whatever the competitor himself may claim, at a certain level of competition it is taken for granted by anyone in the fitness business that they will be using steroids and other illegal substances to alter their appearance, weight and body composition. The image that heterosexual men aspire to, therefore, is never natural, because it is always achieved with illegal supplementation and extreme dieting.

From my own experience of gyms all over the world, I think Pope's dire warnings about a bigorexia epidemic are somewhat exaggerated. Dissatisfaction about oneself, after all, is part of the human condition, and it drives men and women to better themselves. Although in a minority of men it can trigger an image disorder that leads to dangerous training practices and illegal supplementation, in the majority it helps them combat a far more dangerous and immediate body-related epidemic: obesity caused by unhealthy, over-rich diets combined with sedentary lifestyles. Ultimately, with growing awareness and more discussion of bigorexia, heterosexual men will develop their own resistance strategies to the hyper-muscular supermale image, taking their cue from women who have been resisting hyper-feminine images for decades, and also from gay men, who have shown the greatest capacity in rejecting externally imposed stereotypes and reinventing themselves.

It's a Man's World

We often think of the u.s. as the original home of the body-beautiful gym culture, but it was a latecomer when compared to Germany, France, Scandinavia and England. The difference between Triat and Sandow's gymnasia and Tanny, Delmonteque, Wilson and LaLanne's health clubs is that the former did not survive their founders, while the latter established a business model that would thrive in the u.s. and later be exported to the rest of the world. The American health club that targeted amateur male exercisers and women first appeared in the mid-1930s, was well established by the 1950s and had gone corporate by the 1960s. However, such is the power of the media that the enduring image of the gyms of the 1960s and '70s is of Gold's Gym in Venice, with its pumping-iron hyper-muscular supermale bodybuilder patrons. The core activity of the mid-twentieth-century American health club was progressive weight training on free and machine weights, and though in the real world contemporary gym weights share the available space with other types of equipment and training facilities, in the media and popular imagination (of non-gym members), going to the gym still means pumping iron.

The second half of the twentieth century witnessed the creation of two parallel gyms in the u.s.: the first imaginary, populated by hyper-muscular supermales – 'Team Muscle America' – who reigned supreme in a competitive, all-male, heterosexual environment; and the second, real gym, which heterosexual men shared with women and gay men and where social interaction was considerably more problematic. In terms of the social meanings attached to the heterosexual male body and embodiment during the twentieth century, there was a continuation and development of the trends that began in the nineteenth century. On the individual level, the transformation of the body through exercise in the gym became a competitive arena where heterosexual men could pursue self-actualization and empowerment through physical means. At the same time, the hyper-muscular supermale body, as exemplified by fictional superheroes, was used to project the West's national, military, cultural and political power. The difference from the previous century was that the hyper-muscular body was increasingly achieved in real bodies in the gym through the use of anabolic steroids. For several researchers this represents a dangerous development that threatens the psychological health of heterosexual male gym-goers.

The hyper-muscular supermale body continues to have a significant impact on the design and layout of the contemporary gym by placing progressive weight training as the mainstream gym's core activity. Unlike the open courtyard of the ancient Greek *gymnasion* or the gymnastics equipment of the nineteenth-century Turnplatz, the contemporary gym is still defined by the presence of free and machine weights. This, in turn, has sustained a gendered division in the gym. Although a small but growing number of women are choosing to pursue hyper-muscularity, the majority of women train to attain a bodily ideal that remains within what is considered to be 'feminine' and 'natural' in terms of the ratio of muscle to body fat.

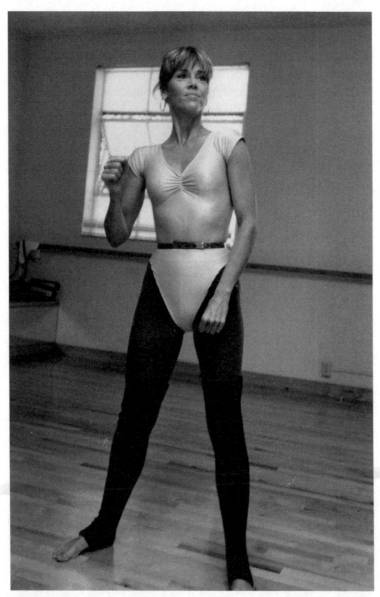

Political activist and actor Jane Fonda was the unusual poster child for the aerobics revolution that brought millions of women into the gym in the 1980s. Fonda's aerobic dance classes and videos combined scientific research into the best way to improve cardiovascular fitness and promote weight loss through exercise with the fun of disco dance performed to the latest club hits. Photographed at the opening of The Workout on 13 September 1979.

6
LET'S GET PHYSICAL

Refuse to be afraid that we will no longer be considered attractive and
acceptable when we are strong.

Jane Fonda, *Jane Fonda's Workout Book* (1981)

Women have been largely absent from the story of the gymnasium
as I have told it so far. Although I have not intentionally avoided
any mention of women, knowing that I was devoting one chapter to
them has allowed me to skip a detailed examination of the female contribution to and participation in the gymnasium from antiquity to the
early twentieth century. Women have always been present in health and
fitness and gymnasium culture, and not only as mothers, sisters and
helpers watering the wine, serving the beer or making the tea, but as
participants, even during periods when, for legal, cultural and religious
reasons, they were officially excluded from athletics and gymnasia.

It is a feminist historical cliché that the only roles open to adult
women until the modern era were 'wife, mother and whore'. Although
this makes for a good political sound bite, it is far from accurate, even
during periods when the freedom of women was most constrained.
During the Middle Ages, when women had lost the limited civil rights
they had enjoyed during the Roman period, they could still opt for
the monastic life instead of marriage, and work as wise women and
midwives, specializing in the care of women and infants. Widows, too,
because they had been married and could control the marital estate until
their sons were of age, could enjoy considerable power and independence. We should also remember that in the medieval and early modern
periods men's choices were also constrained by birth: Commoners

could be soldiers, artisans, clerks (priests and monks) or tenant farmers (if they were not already tied to the land as serfs – a form of indenture equivalent to slavery).

In terms of the levels of physical fitness expected of women, it is important to differentiate between periods and social classes. Evolutionary biologists like to explain the current physical differences between the genders by claiming that they evolved during the 240,000 or so years when *Homo sapiens* lived in small bands of nomadic hunter-gatherers – when man was the hunter, who put the meat in the cooking pot, and woman the gatherer, who collected the grubs, greens, nuts, fruits and roots, and brought up the children. However, looking at hunter-gatherer societies today, there is no marked physical difference between the genders. A weak prehistoric woman who fainted at the sight of a mammoth or sprained her ankle each time she ran away from a cave bear, and who could not forage or travel on foot for eight-hour stints while carrying an infant and a load, would not have survived very long. For most of human prehistory, there would have been little difference in the physical abilities of men and women, even if there was a division of labour made necessary by the fact that a woman of childbearing age would have been either pregnant or caring for an infant for most of her adult life.

Greater physical differentiation between the genders developed after humans became agriculturalists, but only among the wives and daughters of the elites, who had the luxury of not having to work in the fields. Hence, while a tiny minority of women had the luxury of becoming physically weak, the vast majority had to be as strong and active as their husbands in order to grow the crops they needed to survive. In addition, there are a few women in the historical record who challenged men's dominance directly, not by virtue of being socially superior, richer or more powerful, but physically, but these are extremely rare, and they usually came to unfortunate ends. One such was the fifteenth-century French military leader Joan of Arc, who could not have been a weakling because she went into battle wearing iron-plate armour and carrying equally heavy medieval weaponry. She was burned at the stake as a witch but, one suspects, just as much for challenging the dominant gender stereotypes of the period as for her claim of hearing angelic voices telling her to liberate France from the hated English.

The definition of the ideal female body as physically weak and slightly corpulent is a social construct of relatively recent historical vintage, and one that applies only to women of a certain social status. According to Germaine Greer and other second-wave feminists, its impact has continued to be felt in the present day in the often difficult relationship that women have with their bodies.[1] The second aspect of embodiment in the modern period raised by feminists is the commodification of the female body, which long predates the commodification of its male counterpart. Women's bodies have been used to sell and advertise a wide range of products and services, some aimed at women, such as fashion and makeup, and others that have no obvious link with the human body or female gender, such as the Pirelli calendar, which has used bare-breasted or naked female bodies in suggestive poses to sell car tyres since 1964.[2]

The dominant female body images used in the media and advertising can be divided into two archetypes: the very young, size-zero waifs of the fashion magazines, who are meant to represent the female ideal of women, and the more curvaceous, large-breasted and broad-hipped 'glamazons', who are supposed to represent the female ideal of heterosexual men. Unlike the male bodies used in advertising, neither of these is muscular or obviously gym-trained. Women, unlike heterosexual men, however, are much more likely to challenge and reject hegemonic images as artificial, unrealistic and oppressive, but even Jane Fonda (b. 1937), who represented the liberated, empowered, and physically active woman of the 1980s who was 'doing it for herself', still conformed to many of the traditional canons of feminine beauty.

Hidden Bodies

The central role of the gymnasium in the lives of boys, adolescents and adult men in classical Greece, and the prevalence of same-sex friendships and sexual relationships – between *erastes* and *eromenos* and adolescents and boys – would seem to exclude women and girls completely. Although this was certainly true of Athens at the height of the democracy, it was

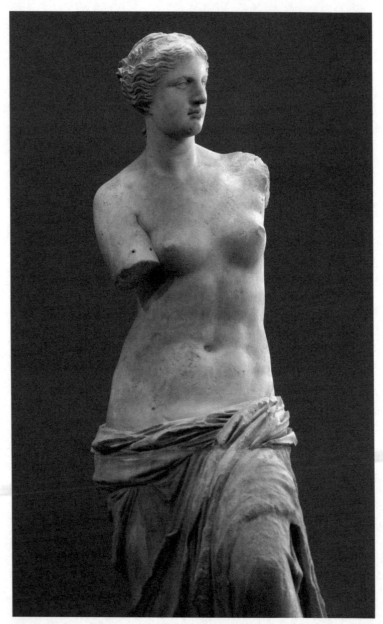

Voluptuous but verging on the corpulent, the world's most famous cult image of Aphrodite, the Venus de Milo, represents a feminine ideal that is neither muscular nor physically empowered; she remains the passive object of male desire caught in the act of undressing. Parian marble, c. 130–100 BCE, by Alexandros of Antioch.

not the case in all parts of classical Greece, or during the whole of antiquity, and there were changes in post-democratic Athens, especially during the period of Macedonian and Roman rule. Freeborn women in classical Athens had no civil rights, and they had no role in the government of the city alongside their fathers, husbands and sons. They had the status of family chattels that were passed between the male members of patriarchal clans. Although the wives of peasants and artisans worked in the fields and workshops and went to the market in the Agora to sell their produce, the womenfolk of well-to-do and aristocratic families were expected to stay cloistered in the harem-like *gynaikeion*, the women's quarters, which they left only for major family occasions and religious festivals. A freeborn Athenian boy left his mother's side at the age of seven to begin his education in the gymnasium or *palaestra*, but his sisters remained at home until they married, when they moved to their husband's home.[3]

The different conceptions of male and female embodiment were made plain in the artistic representations of women in archaic and classical Greece. Whereas the votive and funerary statues of young men known as *kouroi* are always nude, the female versions, *korai*, are dressed in floor-length gowns.[4] This extended into the later periods, in representations of goddesses who, with the exception of cult images of Aphrodite, the goddess of love and sex, were depicted fully clothed. The social conventions that expected or required nudity of freeborn men and boys during certain private and public occasions did not extend to freeborn women and girls. However, the reader should not be fooled into thinking that Athenian men had no sexual interest in women and wanted only to court adolescent boys.

Athens' great lawgiver Solon established state *porneia*, brothels, to meet the sexual needs of his fellow male citizens. High-class courtesans known as *hetairai*, the luxury call girls of the classical world, were much in demand at the symposia and in the beds of Athens' rich and powerful.[5] A quotation attributed to the Athenian philosopher Demosthenes explains the Greek male's attitude to the different sexual and social roles of women: 'We have courtesans for the sake of pleasure, but concubines for the sake of daily cohabitation, and wives for the purpose of having children legitimately, and of having a faithful guardian of all our household affairs.'[6] The tripartite division of women into sex workers, mistresses and wives may have continued into the modern period in the developed world, but many women, through good fortune or talent, succeeded in exercising considerable power and freedom of choice.

During classical antiquity the exception that broke the rule that the freeborn naked female body should be invisible in public was to be found in Athens' great political and military rival, the polis of Sparta. The leading city of the Dorian Greeks in the Peloponnese, Sparta was the antithesis of everything Athens stood for: oligarchic where Athens was democratic; frugal where Athens indulged in luxury; and militaristic where Athens, though also warlike, saw itself as the commercial and cultural capital of the Greek world. The ruins of Sparta are particularly unimpressive when compared to those of Athens, Corinth or Delphi. The city had no grand marble temples or civic buildings. Yet for centuries its warriors were the most feared in the eastern Mediterranean, and their legendary courage and self-sacrifice were recently celebrated in a fantastic re-telling of one of the ancient world's greatest victories, the Battle of Thermopylae (480 BCE), in which a small band of Spartans held off a much larger Persian force at a narrow defile of the Hot Gates, thus giving Athens and her allies enough time to organize resistance and save Greece from Persian domination.[7]

Classical Sparta was a city-sized armed camp where every able-bodied male citizen was expected to become a warrior. Like the Athenian boy, the Spartan youth began his education and military training at the age of seven or eight, though the Spartan system was far more brutal than the Athenian one. Instilling absolute obedience to one's superiors, devotion unto death and a courage that was proverbial, Spartan education was also unique in classical Greece in that it trained girls alongside boys. Although girls were not completely naked, period sources speak of them training, running, wrestling and throwing the discus javelin bare breasted, like the mythological Amazons. Although they trained with their brothers in the gymnasia of Sparta, girls were not expected to become warriors and fight for the city; their role was still to be the wives and mothers of warriors.[8]

The Games Women Played

Women were banned not only from competing in the Pan-Hellenic competitions at Olympia, Nemea, Delphi and Corinth, but from attending them as spectators. Only one woman escaped punishment when she was caught breaking this rule: Kallipateira of Rhodes, who was the wife, mother and aunt of famous Olympians. During one Olympiad after her husband's death, she entered the Olympic stadium in the guise of her son's trainer to watch him compete. She was unmasked when, after he won his event, she was so excited that she leapt over a barrier, catching her *himation*, which was pulled away, revealing her gender.[9] There was another way women could participate in the ancient Olympic Games: by entering horses and riders in the equestrian events. According to the ancient writer Pausanias, the Spartan Princess Kyniska (b. c. 440 BCE) not only entered teams of male riders and charioteers in the games, but also competed and won twice as a competitor, and dedicated a statue of herself in the temple of Olympian Zeus – a privilege normally reserved for male athletes.[10] She was followed by other royal equestrian competitors of the Macedonian Ptolemaic dynasty of Egypt, who took part in the Olympic chariot-racing events in the third century BCE both as patrons and as competitors.[11]

If women were all but invisible at the all-male athletics events, they had their own all-female contests at the four sites of the Pan-Hellenic games, and there is limited evidence from decorated ceramics that women and girls trained in gymnasia for these events.[12] The best known of the all-female games was the Heraia, held at Olympia in honour of the goddess Hera, wife of Zeus, which is thought to have begun between the sixth and fourth centuries BCE. According to Pausanias, the games were held every four years, and were organized by sixteen married women. As with the first ancient Olympiad, in 776 BCE, there was only one event: a foot race held in the Olympic stadium, in which only unmarried girls could take part. Unlike their male counterparts, female athletes did not run naked but in a short tunic that left one shoulder and breast exposed.[13]

During the Roman period women would have attended the public *thermae* that had been added to or replaced older men-only gymnasia in Greece's cities. Although exercise was still an option in these mixed establishments, their principal functions were as bathhouses and social centres rather than as places where the patrons went to exercise. Women did exercise, however, and a mosaic floor found in a Roman villa in Sicily shows women dressed in an ancient version of a bikini, exercising with light dumb-bells (*halteres*), though because of the lack of accompanying text, we do not know whether these represented the ladies of the house performing their daily exercise routine, or an erotic display by professional entertainers.[14]

In volume three of *The History of Sexuality*, Michel Foucault describes how female sexuality replaced same-sex relations between men and boys as the main locus of controversy during late antiquity and the Middle Ages. In the taboos and prohibitions of the Christian Church, Foucault identifies the origins of our modern conceptions of sexuality.[15] During the medieval period, the naked female body, like the naked male body, disappeared from artistic representation, only to make its reappearance during the Renaissance. Women do not feature in the works of Mercuriale and other Renaissance physicians who revived ancient theories of therapeutic training. The illustrations of *De Arte Gymnastica* do not feature any female athletes, and the text does not address any specifically female complaints, or make any mention of pregnancy and childbirth. The entire discipline of obstetrics and gynaecology appears to have been excised from the Western medical canon until the modern period.

The idealized classical female nudes that became the model for Renaissance art do not display the strength, confidence or muscularity of their male equivalents. The most sexualized ancient images of women are those of the goddess Aphrodite, who was often represented with her clothes slipping off, exposing her naked torso, as in the Venus de Milo, or as the *Venus pudica*, the modest Venus, whose hands are carefully placed to shield her breast and pudenda, as in the Medici Venus. The female equivalent of Michelangelo's *David* is Sandro Botticelli's *Venus pudica*, depicted in *The Birth of Venus* (1486). Like its ancient models, the female Renaissance Venus was neither athletic, muscular nor physically empowered; she remains an object of male desire and appears to be totally under male control – caught in the act of being discovered nude or protecting her modesty from the all-powerful male gaze.

Revolutions of the Waist

The Enlightenment educational reformers Locke, Rousseau and Pestalozzi recommended educating boys and girls together, while at the same time giving greater prominence to physical exercise. Rousseau, however, saw women's role as limited to being wives and mothers, and in *Emile* recommended a less athletic programme for girls than for boys. Nevertheless, with the fall of the old monarchical order in Europe, women experienced a brief moment of political emancipation. The French revolutionary activist Olympe de Gouges wrote the *Déclaration des droits de la femme et de la citoyenne* ('Declaration of the Rights of Woman and the Female Citizen') as a riposte and reproach to the Declaration of the Rights of Man (1789), which ignored women's rights, but she was guillotined during Maximilien de Robespierre's brief reign of revolutionary terror. In 1792 Mary Wollstonecraft published *A Vindication of the Rights of Woman: With Strictures on Political and Moral Subjects*, but with little active support from male politicians and no major feminist constituency among women, these early feminist stirrings were largely ignored and quickly forgotten.

If the late eighteenth-century political movement for women's rights was stillborn, there was a more practical sphere in which women could claim a measure of emancipation: fashion. Pre-revolutionary elite court dress with its corseted bodices constricted at the waist, over voluminous skirts made of heavy patterned fabrics, padded out with cumbersome underwear and panniers, and worn with absurdly large wigs, turned women into doll-like mannequins who were just able to walk, simper and sit.[16] Caught up with the rest of society in a fascination for all things ancient in the 1790s, women adopted what became known as the 'Empire line' in France and the 'Regency style' in England, which consisted of a fitted bodice gathered just below the bust, leaving the ribcage and waist free from constriction, and with the arms left bare, over a straight, fitted floor-length skirt made from a light, pale-coloured material.

Released from the tyranny of heavy, restrictive garments, elite women and girls achieved a physical freedom that they had not enjoyed since antiquity, which meant that they could take part in the new styles of gymnastics that were being developed for men. Jahn, Ling and Amoros, however, emphasized functional military training for men and boys, thus relegating women and girls to the status of spectators, as can be seen from period illustrations of early nineteenth-century *Turnplätze* and gymnasia. Women, however, were not completely ignored or excluded, but it was men who prescribed and regulated the physical exercise that women could perform. According to Jan Todd, the three figures most involved in women's physical culture in the early part of the century were Phokion Heinrich Clias, whom we first met in chapter Three when he came to England in the 1820s at the invitation of the British army, and, in particular, the Italian G. P. Voarino and the Frenchman J. A. Beaujeu (both n.d., but *fl.* 1820s –'30s), who devised exercise systems specifically aimed at women.[17]

Voarino's *A Treatise on Calisthenic Exercises, Arranged for the Private Tuition of Young Ladies* (1827) features 64 exercises performed without apparatus or with two simple pieces of apparatus: a bamboo cane and an indoor version of the 'Flying Course'.[18] The book's target readers were the female members of the sedentary elite classes, to whom it offered a combination of aesthetic and therapeutic training. Voarino claimed that his callisthenics would correct spinal deformities, instil grace and promote 'a regular and complete circulation of the blood'.[19] The illustrations in the book depict young women in Empire line dresses ending at the mid-calf, worn over a pair of pantaloons. Although Voarino's exercises were an advance on doing no exercise at all, they could be seen as the bare minimum of physical activity suitable for a genteel young lady.

A much more ambitious and strenuous exercise programme for women was put forward by Beaujeu in *A Treatise of Gymnastic Exercises for the Use of Young Ladies. Introduced at the Royal Hibernian Military School, also at the Seminary for the Education of Young Ladies under the Direction of Miss Hincks in 1824*, published in 1828. After preparatory exercises that feature shadow boxing, Beaujeu makes full use of Jahn's high bar and parallel bars for dips and chinning exercises, and includes other strenuous exercises for the flying course. When Beaujeu wrote *A Treatise of Gymnastic Exercises*, his wife managed a women's gym in Dublin, and she later moved to the U.S., opening a similar institution in Boston in 1840.[20] An illustration of a women's gymnasium from 1838 shows a similar arrangement to a Turnplatz, with ropes, trapezes, ladders, balance beams and other apparatus, on which women in dresses and pantaloons disport themselves, showing a level of strength and stamina not usually associated with the weaker sex.[21] Although it was not unique in terms of the level of fitness expected of women in the first quarter of the nineteenth century, Todd comments that Beaujeu's gymnastics was unusually strenuous, and challenged the established view of the types of exercise available to women at the time.

We cannot be sure how many European and American Amazons went to all-women gymnasia to climb ropes and ladders and perform dips and chin-ups, because they have left almost no trace in the historical record. We can be pretty certain, however, that they did not pass on their athletic skills and ambitions to their daughters and grand-daughters, because by the 1850s, the physical freedom of women was once again constrained by the dictates of fashion. Standard female attire in the mid-Victorian era was a dress with full-length sleeves and a tightly corseted bodice that constricted the ribcage and waist, over a hooped skirt that would expand into the absurdly large crinoline, which was not only cumbersome in crowded Victorian interiors, sweeping up small pieces of furniture and decorative items, but the cause of industrial accidents when the outsized skirt was caught in machinery, leading to serious injuries and fatalities among female workers.[22]

Les 'Reines' de la Force

Hippolyte Triat and Eugen Sandow used their fame as strongmen to launch their careers as gym entrepreneurs. A by-product of the strong-men's fame on the stage, and of their use of photography to promote themselves, was the creation of a new muscular ideal for men which could be attained by training in a gymnasium. Triat's Parisian Grand Gymnase offered classes to gentlemen, boys and small boys, as well as to ladies, girls and small girls. As Triat did not make a great play of any distinction between the genders, the exercises offered to women followed the same pattern as the men's classes, though they were taught not by Triat himself but by female trainers, several of whom had been stage strongwomen. Although there is no complete descrip-

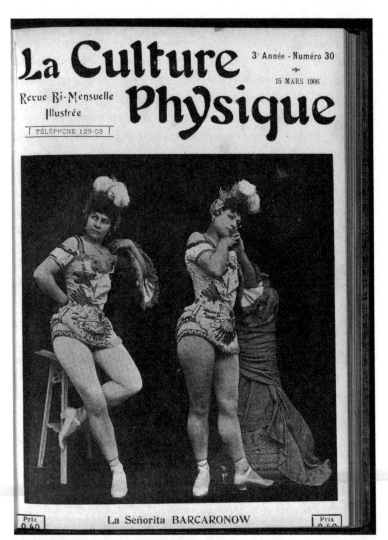

La **Culture** Physique

3ᵉ Année - Numéro 30

15 MARS 1906

Revue Bi-Mensuelle Illustrée

TÉLÉPHONE 128-09

La Señorita BARCARONOW

Prix 0.40

Prix 0.40

Although female strongwomen rivalled strongmen in popularity on the stage, none managed to capitalize on their fame to open gymnasia or start fitness-orientated businesses of their own. They, like the female bodybuilders of today, remained suspect as freakishly unfeminine 'man-eaters'. Cover of *La Culture Physique*, March 1906, showing a *reine de la force*, La Señorita Barcaronow.

tion of a women's class at the Gymnase to match that of the men's workout provided by Edmond Desbonnet in *Les rois de la force*, it is likely that it followed the same pattern, with free movements and exercises with dumb-bells and Indian clubs, followed by a cold bath and a vigorous rubdown by the female instructor.[23] Around the same time, in the U.S., the temperance campaigner, homeopath and advocate of physical culture for all Dio Lewis devised a system using lightweight dumb-bells, Indian clubs and weighted wands in *The New Gymnastics for Men, Women and Children* (1862), which he recommended for use by those not fit enough or too young to train on Jahn's gymnastic apparatus.[24]

Half a century later, Sandow actively canvassed women to become members of his twenty British institutes, in which he created separate women's gymnasia. Like Triat, he realized that for his business to thrive he could not afford to ignore the female half of the population. But in order to accommodate the sensibilities of Victorian Englishwomen who, unlike their French sisters at the Gymnase Triat, did not want to be observed while exercising, the stations in the women's sections were curtained off, allowing members to remove their corsets while working out, and also shielding them from the prying eyes of any friends or acquaintances who might be exercising in the adjoining cubicle.[25] As Sandow's training system was principally based on progressive weight training, we must assume that it was an adapted version of his programme for men that he prescribed for the female members of his institutes.

In the closing year of his life, Sandow became increasingly interested in the promotion of physical culture for women. He adapted his home fitness equipment for their use, and he designed and marketed a 'health corset', as he considered the compression of the ribcage and waist to be one of the greatest dangers to women's health. He also promoted the career of the Vaudeville strongwoman Katie Sandwina (b. Katharina Brumbach, 1884–1952), who, legend has it, defeated her mentor in a weightlifting contest in New York.[26] Sandwina was one of several strongwomen who won fame on the stage in the late nineteenth and early twentieth centuries. In *Les rois de la force*, Desbonnet included an account of the careers and feats of strength achieved by several *reines de la force*, female strength athletes, including the Belgian

'Miss Athléta' (married name: Mrs van Huffelen, b. 1868), who performed on stage with her three daughters, Anna, Brada and Louise, the English Kate Roberts (a.k.a. Miss Vulcana, b. 1885) and the Austrian Eugenie Werkme.[27]

Although Vaudeville strongwomen attracted a good deal of attention in the press, there was no female Triat or Sandow who was able to capitalize on her fame as an entertainer to open a gymnasium, or start a fitness-related business. Although strongwomen used the same promotional techniques as strongmen, being photographed in what were, for the period, extremely revealing outfits, they did not start exercise crazes among Western women or establish a more muscular, gym-trained ideal for them. In period cartoons, strongwomen such as Miss Athléta and Katie Sandwina are shown as giantesses carrying men at arm's length and tossing them around as though they were rag dolls. The subtext of these images is clear: strongwomen were freaks of nature, mannish despite their curves, and not physical models to be emulated by ladylike women and girls.

The 'Barbelle' of Santa Monica

As we have seen, the revolution that brought Americans to the gym in ever-growing numbers began in Southern California with the combination of the laid-back, body-conscious lifestyle of Santa Monica's Muscle Beach with a new type of clean, brightly lit and well-equipped health club designed to attract amateur exercisers. Pioneers such as Jack LaLanne, Bob Delmonteque, Ray Wilson and Vic Tanny realized that gyms had to come out of the dark, dingy basement dungeons and appeal to a much broader constituency than the professional bodybuilders and muscle heads. After difficult beginnings, the instincts of Tanny et al. proved to be correct, and they succeeded in creating the world's first national and international gym chains. Although these had all failed by the early 1960s, they had established a business model that was sound enough to attract the heavyweight American corporate dollar into the gym industry.

In addition to the appearance of the proto-corporate health club, a smaller-scale but no less far-reaching development was transforming the image of weight training and bodybuilding for women. If Vaudeville strongwomen were considered mannish and freakish, a new type of fit, muscular but feminine strength athlete appeared on the sun-kissed beaches of Southern California, whose exemplar and maven was Abbye 'Pudgy' Stockton (1917–2006). At 5 ft 2 in. (1.58 m) and weighing 115 lb (52 kg), the curvaceous, blonde Stockton was described as the 'barbelle' of Santa Monica.[28] Stockton began her working life as a telephone operator, but, worried that she was putting on weight from her sedentary job, she took up exercise on the advice of her boyfriend and future husband, Les Stockton (1916–2004). She began working out with light dumb-bells and practising acrobatic stunts on Muscle Beach with Les and another male friend, and together they performed on the beach's platform under the name of 'The Three Aces'. During the 1940s, Stockton appeared on the covers of health and fitness magazines and mainstream titles such as Life magazine. In 1948 she opened an all-female gym, the Salon of Figure Development, on Sunset Boulevard in Los Angeles, and she followed it with another women's gym in Beverly Hills with Les managing a men's gym next door.[29] Stockton sold her gyms in 1960 to concentrate on raising a family, but she returned to the industry in 1980. Assessing her legacy, her friend and biographer Jan Todd wrote:

> If Pudgy had power over men, she had equal, perhaps greater, influence on women. When she and Les Stockton began working out on Santa Monica's beaches in the late 1930s, she almost immediately attracted major media attention. And, as the photos and stories about Pudgy and Muscle Beach appeared in Pic and Laff and Life and Strength & Health, other women began to see that muscles could be feminine, strength an asset, and working out fun. This was her great and enduring gift to the game.[30]

Stockton was the progenitor of the female bodybuilders and physique athletes who compete in the IFBB and WBFF contests today. The women's competitions, like the men's, include different body types beyond the hyper-muscularity that was the hallmark of the original

Mr Olympia and Mr Universe titles. For example, to broaden the range of competitions and their fan bases, there is now also Mr Olympia 'Physique' alongside the Mr Olympia 'Professional' and '212', in which definition and symmetry are the main criteria, rather than size. Women can enter the IFBB 'Physique', 'Figure' and 'Bikini' competitions, which cater for different levels of size, muscularity and definition, and the WBFF features the 'Women's Figure', 'Diva Fitness Model' and 'Diva Bikini Model' categories, which, as the names imply, are more geared to fashion modelling than pure physique competitions.[31] The different names of the male and female categories imply that a double standard operates in the world of physique contests: while the men are judged on their bodies alone, the women appear to have extra criteria to meet in terms of their femininity and physical attractiveness. A recent gym acquaintance of mine, Pilates instructor Natalie, decided to enter a physique competition, but, despite her strenuous training regime, dieting and contest preparation, she was not placed in her category. After the contest the judges advised her that she had not made the final cut because she was too muscular for the bikini category and she should have entered the more muscular fitness competition.

Although I agree with Todd that women like Pudgy Stockton were extremely influential in encouraging women to follow men into the gym to weight train, it was not the image of the strong, muscular woman that would capture the imagination of millions of women and make them go to the gym in the 1980s. Although female strength and physique athletes, and muscular elite sportswomen such as the current generation of sprinters, swimmers and track-and-field athletes, are visible in the muscle and sports media, they are largely invisible in the mainstream media and advertising. Despite decades of feminism and the example of generations of gym-trained female athletes, the hegemonic image of women as the 'weaker sex', dependent on a larger, stronger and more muscular male partner and protector, seems remarkably difficult to overturn.

'Feel the Burn'

The gymnasium industry has always maintained close links with the world of show business: Vaudeville and nineteenth-century gymnasia, and Hollywood and the postwar gyms of Southern California. The next transformation of the gym business combined Hollywood movies with a new musical phenomenon that would take the world by storm – disco. In 1977, cinema audiences were enthralled as they watched John Travolta and Karen Lynn Gorney slip, slide, shimmy and shake their way across a flashing, multicoloured Brooklyn dance floor in *Saturday Night Fever*. The film's enormous box-office success created a new synergy between Hollywood, pop music, discotheques and exercise that would sweep across the world like an unstoppable mega-tsunami: the dance class. Before *Saturday Night Fever*, a dance class meant a classical ballet class, accompanied by a live pianist in a ballet school; a ballroom dancing lesson in a dance academy; or a tap class in a talent school. But what a growing number of young men and women wanted to do now was dance freestyle to loud, pulsating disco beats, which would make them feel, in the words of the anthemic title song from the hit film *Fame* (1980), that they were 'gonna live forever'.[32] Not only was disco dancing fun, but women quickly realized that it helped them stay to fit and shed surplus pounds. Soon women and the younger generation of recently emancipated gay men were donning Lycra leotards and leg-warmers and flocking to disco classes in dance studios to get fit and lose weight.

Disco dancing might have been fun and an effective method of weight control, but in order to enter the conservative gym mainstream, wedded to progressive weight training, it needed to obtain the seal of scientific respectability. The nineteenth-century pioneers of physical culture had concentrated on underweight, weak men who needed to increase their muscle mass by developing progressive weight training systems with free and machine weights. In the affluent 1960s and '70s, changes in lifestyle caused by a combination of increased car use, the availability of labour-saving appliances in the home, the multiplication of fast-food outlets and sedentary office work presented doctors, personal trainers and exercisers with the beginnings of what would become the developed world's obesity epidemic, bringing with it a Pandora's Box of degenerative diseases, including coronary heart disease, high blood pressure, type-2 diabetes, cancer and osteoarthritis, all of which could be alleviated or avoided altogether with a regime of regular therapeutic exercise.

Ever since classical antiquity, athletes had trained for both muscular strength and stamina by combining muscle-building exercises with running, swimming, wrestling and jumping. Triat's group workouts, which were designed to make his pupils break into a sweat and get them short of breath, achieved the same combination of muscular strength and endurance training with bodyweight drills and exercises with light dumb-bells. What was lacking was a scientific understanding of what was happening physiologically during different forms of exercise. During the 1960s, a U.S. Air Force colonel and physician, Dr Kenneth Cooper (b. 1931), conducted studies of the cardiovascular fitness of 5,000 military personnel by using a bicycle ergometer – a stationary bicycle – which he combined with equipment to measure the oxygen intake of the exerciser. He discovered that depending on the intensity and duration of exercise, the human body adjusted its energy metabolism by using different quantities of oxygen and of the two main types of fuel available to it: glycogen (glucose stored in the muscles) and body fat. During bursts of high-intensity exercise, such as sprinting and heavy weight training, the body used much less oxygen and little or no body fat and quickly depleted its stores of glycogen, but less intense forms of exercise such as jogging, cycling and swimming, which were strenuous enough to raise the heart rate and respiration, not only improved overall cardiovascular fitness but, if performed for long enough, 'burned' considerable amounts of stored body fat. Cooper christened this new understanding of traditional endurance training 'aerobics', to underline the role played by oxygen in the energy metabolism.[33]

Cooper popularized his findings in several books intended for the lay exerciser, including The New Aerobics (1970) and The Aerobics Way (1977), and continued to publish title after title throughout the 1980s, including those specially targeted at women readers, such as Aerobics for Women (1982) and New Aerobics for Women (1988). Cooper's starting point was therapeutic training. During his medical career, he witnessed the alarming increase in heart disease that was costing the U.S. tens of thousands of lives of middle-aged men and billions of dollars in annual healthcare costs. He had begun his research in order to answer the questions that were being increasingly asked by patients and physicians – how much and what kind of exercise would be the most beneficial to the health of the American public?[34] But Cooper also understood the social impact of exercise, especially on women. He contrasted former female archetypes of weak, sedentary women and of more curvaceous but corpulent matrons with what he saw as the ideal woman of the 1970s and '80s:

> The emancipation of women in the twentieth century has given rise to a new ideal of feminine beauty. Today we admire women whose appearance shows that they are competent and capable – women with lean but strong bodies moving with the natural grace of a healthy creature.[35]

Aerobics would enter the gym in two ways: through the aerobics dance class and through the first generation of aerobic exercisers – stationary cycles, treadmills and rowing machines – which began to appear on the gym floor, competing for space with free and machine weights. Jacki Sorensen (b. 1942) was among the first teachers to commercialize the link between Cooper's aerobics and dance in the 1970s, but the person responsible for starting the worldwide aerobics craze was the Hollywood actor and political activist Jane Fonda, whose 'No pain, no gain' and 'Feel the burn' mantras, popularized in best-selling books and videos, started a one-woman revolution in the fitness industry.[36]

In her autobiography, *My Life So Far*, Fonda explains that what initially attracted her to the fitness industry was not an interest in fitness or aerobics per se, but its potential as a means of funding her political activism. In 1978, recovering from an injury and needing to get in shape for her next film role, Fonda went to the Gilda Marx Studio in Century City, Los Angeles, where she attended Leni Cazden's dance class. The two women immediately established a strong rapport, giving Fonda the idea that women's fitness might offer the fundraising opportunities she had been seeking. Fonda remembers that Cazden's class was not aerobic but mainly a strengthening and toning class that incorporated many dance and ballet moves, all performed to the latest disco music. Fonda learned the class and began to teach it when she was on location, getting enormous personal satisfaction from teaching and from the enthusiastic responses from her female pupils, who felt empowered by the simple fact of taking control of their bodies through exercise.

Fonda and Cazden found premises on Robertson Boulevard, Beverly Hills, where they opened in 1979 as The Workout, a small fitness space, with three dance studios and changing facilities. The classes were immediately oversubscribed, and The Workout accommodated up to 2,000 clients a week. Its success led to the publication of *Jane Fonda's Workout Book* (1981), which immediately went to the top of the *New York Times* best-seller list. Hooked on this new style of exercise, Fonda studied physiology and fully absorbed Cooper's aerobics message, which had now penetrated the medical mainstream. In 1982 she was approached to make an exercise video for the home market. Although produced on a shoestring budget, unscripted and with Fonda 'winging it', *Jane Fonda's Workout* remains the biggest-selling exercise video of all time, with 17 million copies sold worldwide. The success of the book and video enabled Fonda to open two further studios, in Encino, California, and San Francisco. She went on to produce five further exercise books, twelve exercise audio tapes and 23 exercise videos, featuring different styles of exercise, including aerobics, step aerobics and yoga.[37]

But aerobics was not just about getting fit, burning calories and shedding pounds, it was about personal growth and empowerment. Although aerobics itself was the brainchild of a man, with aerobic dance it was for the first time women who were devising an exercise method specifically for other women. The image of the fit, self-confident woman was not being imposed on women from the outside, it was something they were choosing of their own free will, and in the process they were challenging a whole range of female stereotypes imposed on them by men. Fonda herself expresses this most clearly in the following passage:

> Working out can mean different things depending on where a
> person is at a given time in her life. Working out can be narrowly

about armoring ourselves in muscle or about striving for toxic, elusive perfection. But it can also, for a more conscious person, be about breathing energy and life into the core of the body, building chi, communicating on a deep level with your cells. For me it started off in the former categories and later developed into the latter as I began moving more frequently out of the gym and into nature, climbing mountains, biking, doing meditation and yoga. That's when I began adding working in to my working out.[38]

With the worldwide success of the aerobics dance class, there emerged two types of gym: BJFW and AJFW – before and after Jane Fonda's Workout. Around the time Fonda's books and workout tape came out in the UK, I was a member of the London Central YMCA, then a large new sports complex built on four underground levels, with a swimming pool, weights room and squash, badminton and basketball courts, and several rooms that were used for other activities, including rather static, staid group exercise classes such as yoga and ballroom dancing. What these rooms did not have were floors suitable for high-impact aerobics classes, which meant that many of the early aerobics practitioners – who trained in lightweight dance shoes or, like Fonda in her first workout video, in bare feet – suffered injuries to their ankles, knees and hips, and from the inflammation of the lower leg known as shin-splints, because their leg joints were not supported by athletics shoes or protected by the give of a sprung wooden floor. After Jane Fonda's Workout, newly built gyms had to include one or more studios with sprung floors, sound systems and mirrored walls, and many older gyms converted sports courts and unused rooms into similar facilities. The aerobics dance revolution not only brought millions of women into the gym, but transformed the appearance, layout and equipment requirements of the standard gym. Henceforth a health club would have to provide a range of cardio equipment, a dedicated warm-up and stretching area, and studios for group exercise classes, alongside the free and machine weights areas.

Although Fonda was extremely influential in teaching many women how to use exercise to take control of their bodies, liberating them from the image of the inactive and physically passive weaker sex, she was giving voice and shape to an idea that many women of her generation had already come to independently. Soon after joining the YMCA in 1979, two years before Fonda brought out her first book, I met Sue, who spent her time on the mats in the area at the gym set aside for members to stretch and warm up before they went on to other forms of training. She, however, had transformed this preparatory activity into a workout in its own right. In the same way as a bodybuilder would spend hours working on each major muscle group, she worked on stretching her joints with just as much concentration and dedication, training for several hours a day, as well as attending and later teaching group exercise classes with a strong stretching element. Instead of aiming to lift a 220-lb (100-kg) bench press or to get 24-in. (60-cm) biceps, she wanted to achieve the side and box splits, positions only achieved perfectly by gifted and dedicated dancers and gymnasts.

I never asked Sue why she had chosen this particular goal, and I am not sure she would have been able to give me an answer much beyond the mountaineer's 'because it's there'. It was a physical challenge that she had set herself, and one that was no less impressive than wanting to win a bodybuilding competition by developing huge muscle mass and extreme definition. I met Sue when she was in her late twenties, and well on her way to achieving her initial set of stretching goals. She had begun attending dance classes at a nearby dance studio, where she had got hooked on the stretching exercises at the start of the class, and decided that she had found what was going to transform both her body and her life. She quit her job and started assisting class teachers, and within a year was teaching her own class, concentrating on flexibility and muscle toning.

When Sue started training, a few women, mainly in the U.S., had begun bodybuilding, trying to compete directly with men with progressive weight training and the use of anabolic steroids. Although they, too, were achieving spectacular results, it was at the cost of what many saw as their femininity. Sue was not interested in challenging men in this way. Not wanting to follow the men into the weights room, and with experience of group exercise classes, she had defined her own fitness goals and then devised her own methods to achieve them. In doing so, she reinvented herself, and found a new career. Although Sue, like Fonda, was a true female fitness pioneer, she never codified her method, wrote a book or brought out a hit video. She was a one-woman revolution, but the only person she was interested in liberating through exercise was herself. Although what Sue practised and preached in her classes was just as radical as any second-wave feminist manifesto, in her case, the political remained fundamentally personal.

Seen and Heard

When discussing the visibility of women in gym culture, we have to distinguish between two related issues: the presence of women of any physical type and age in the gym, and the visibility of athletic, muscular women who challenge the dominant social constructs of the female body. Since classical antiquity, a few women have challenged prevalent female stereotypes: the Spartan princess who triumphed in the equestrian events of the all-male Olympics was no blushing *Venus pudica*; Vaudeville strongwomen were no fainting Victorian blooms; and Muscle Beach barbelles no simpering Barbie dolls. In the eyes of mainstream media, however, today's hyper-muscular female bodybuilders and female elite athletes remain problematic and suspect. Although they have many admirers among both men and women, there are also many who believe that their desire to acquire physical strength and muscularity beyond what is considered to be feminine automatically pushes them into freakish mannishness. Women have been able to challenge negative feminine archetypes, and have achieved a measure of empowerment through their participation in exercise in the gym, but they have not banished the size-zero waif and the busty glamazon. We have only to look at the criticism aimed at the entertainer Madonna, whose 'unfeminine' muscularity has been the subject of much media discussion and criticism.

If they were excluded from gyms for centuries, either by law or by custom, when women finally began to go to the gym, they initiated its complete transformation. At first, it was not at their own instigation, but through the active encouragement of male gym entrepreneurs and of a few female pioneers who realized that for their businesses to succeed, they would have to find a way of attracting the 50 per cent of the population that gyms had so far excluded or ignored. In the mid-twentieth century, the entry of women into the fitness market forced gyms to clean up their act. To appeal to women and to general male exercisers, gyms had to come out of dark, dingy basement dungeons and turn themselves into clean, brightly lit and welcoming health clubs. But the greatest transformative impact women made came during the 1980s in the wake of the aerobics revolution, when gyms had to make space for aerobic exercisers on the gym floor and to build group exercise studios for a wide range of classes that were initially aimed at women. Thus the greatest female contribution to the modern gym has been to bring diversity to the training on offer there, challenging the dominance of progressive weight training. In practical terms this meant that henceforth the floor space of a contemporary health club would be split three ways: weights area, cardio zone and exercise studios.

7
MACHO MAN

During prime gym time (4 to 8 pm) if you were to dim the lights, the scene would resemble a busy nightclub – minus the cocktails.

Erick Alvarez, *Muscle Boys* (2008)

According to the historians of sexuality Michel Foucault and Jeffrey Weeks, modern sexual identities were created in the late nineteenth century by the proliferation of sexological and psychological descriptions of sexual 'aberrations', 'paraphilias' and 'perversions' such as homosexuality, lesbianism, sadism and masochism. Contrary to the 'repressive hypothesis' that presupposes that Victorian sexuality was so regulated and constrained by taboos, customs and laws that it was stifled, they see the Victorian period as one of supreme invention and creativity in the sexual sphere.[1]

To cite one example, same-sex relations between men, long condemned by Church and State as a set number of wilful, sinful, sodomitic acts, were given a shape and voice with the invention of homosexuality in the 1860s, allowing, in Foucault's words, the homosexual man to appear as a 'separate species' of human for the first time. Although the distinction might be lost on the modern reader, there was a great advance for a man who had sex with other men in being recast from a sinner in the eyes of the Church and a criminal in the eyes of the State, into a person suffering from a biological or psychological illness, which by flicking some internal switch made him desire a man rather than a woman. But that was only the beginning of a century-long journey that would culminate in the birth of the Gay Liberation movement and the emergence of modern gay identities.[2]

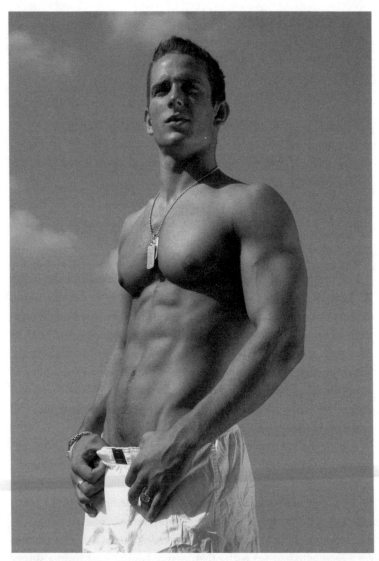

Both aspirational ideal and object of desire, the 'fitness body' is one of the dominant male archetypes of the 21st century that is used to sell a wide range of consumer products to both male and female consumers. Rather than signifying the triumph of the gay aesthetic as applied to the male body, it is the result of a long collaboration and cross-fertilization between gay and straight men that began in the gym during the late 19th century. The Czech model Jakub Stefano, 2005.

Gay men might have come out of the homosexual closet in the 1970s, but they were laden with a good deal of psychological baggage from a century of characterization as males whose sexuality was inverted – 'inversion' being the term Sigmund Freud preferred to 'homosexuality' – and who were seen as suffering from biological or psychological feminization. It is a testament to the power of this social construct of same-sex relations that many men who self-identified with the label homosexual accepted that they must also be, in some fundamental way, feminine, and behaved accordingly, adopting effeminate mannerisms and patterns of speech, and refusing to take part in 'manly' activities such as manual labour, sport and the gym. The sodomite might have made way for the homosexual, and now the gay man, but for many, being gay still meant being an effeminate sissy. That this was a nineteenth- and twentieth-century social construct is clear when one compares recent Western homosexuality with same-sex relations between men in classical Greece, when what defined a man's masculinity was not the gender of his partners but the sexual role he adopted with them. A freeborn adult Greek man could only ever be the active partner with a younger man, adolescent or a slave; to do otherwise would have been unthinkable and would have incurred the opprobrium of other men who were happy to engage in same-sex relationships themselves.

Even before Gay Liberation, there were men who had sex with men who did not identify with the homosexual label and its associated effeminacy. When the pioneer sex researcher Alfred Kinsey (1894–1956) published the first of his two ground-breaking studies of human sexuality, *Sexual Behavior in the Human Male* (1948), he dropped a bombshell on Western society when he revealed that over one-third of American men had had a sexual experience with another man leading to orgasm, and that about 10 per cent of the male population saw themselves as predominantly or exclusively homosexual. What has emerged in the intervening six decades is not one monolithic gay identity, but many gay subcultures and identities, one of which, gay gym culture and the gay muscle boy, played a central role in the development of the contemporary gym.

The Muscle Mary

Gay muscle boys, or 'Muscle Marys' as they were christened in the 1980s, did not appear fully formed – preened, plucked and pumped – like butterflies emerging from their chrysalises. They underwent a long period of gestation that began at around the same time as contemporary heterosexual gym culture, in the gymnasia of the nineteenth century, and using the same raw materials but for very different ends. In his biography of Eugen Sandow, David Chapman refers several times to possible same-sex liaisons between Sandow and several close male friends, in particular the Dutch pianist Martinus Sieveking, who accompanied the strongman on his first tour to the U.S.[3] However, as Chapman correctly points out, there was no such thing as a gay identity at the time, and close friendships between two men did not fall under the kind of suspicion that they would in a more liberated age.

The formative period of gym culture in Europe coincided with the development of photography, which produced images of muscular naked men, some taken for entirely non-sexual purposes, such as Eadweard Muybridge's (1830–1904) scientific studies of naked men walking, running and performing simple tasks, and others taken by homosexual men for their own sexual gratification. Sandow and other strongmen made use of photography to promote their stage acts and health and fitness businesses, and though these were intended for sale to women and heterosexual male fans, many would have been bought by homosexual and homophile men.[4] At the same time, homosexual artists such as Wilhelm von Gloeden (1856–1931) were using the medium of photography to celebrate their appreciation of the naked male form, creating a new photographic aesthetic based on same-sex desire. Although von Gloeden's artistic studies of naked Sicilian boys would not now be classed as pornographic, they are clearly ancestral to later, much more eroticized and sexually explicit depictions of men and boys.[5]

The nineteenth-century pioneers of gymnasia and physical culture, Bernarr Macfadden, Eugen Sandow and Edmond Desbonnet, published the world's first health and fitness magazines. They featured, alongside articles on weight training and nutrition, photographs of bodybuilders posing in the heroic attitudes of ancient statuary, with the obligatory fig leaf, as in Sandow's many self-promotional photosets, or flexing very self-consciously, as in the photographs of amateurs who sent their pictures for inclusion in the magazines. Again, it is likely that these magazines would have had significant homosexual readerships who were beginning to regard the muscular men portrayed in their pages as exemplars of masculinity and therefore as objects of desire.

I Wish They All Could Be California Boys

In the 1940s, large numbers of young men displaced by the Second World War gravitated to the West Coast of the u.s., with Hollywood acting as a magnet for the unemployed and the ambitious, where a new type of body-conscious and socially and sexually more liberated culture was emerging in Southern California. Two of the results were Santa Monica's Muscle Beach and the invention of the modern American health club; a third development that was synergistic with the heterosexual muscle and beach culture of Southern California was a new same-sex subculture emerging in Los Angeles. This subculture was different from the self-identified effeminate homosexual milieu created by the medicalization of same-sex relations in the nineteenth century, but it was not yet the open, 'out and proud' post-Gay Liberation gay scene; it existed on the cusp between repression and persecution and resistance and liberation, and its sexual ambiguity allowed considerable interaction between men who had sex with women and men who had sex with men. Muscle Beach drew homosexual men who were attracted by the bodybuilders and acro-bats who were happy to display their bodies, and among the Muscle Beach habitués there must have been a significant number of men who, if we accept Kinsey's findings, though they were not self-identified as homosexuals, had had sexual experiences with other men.

Out of this melting pot of beach-bronzed and gym-trained bodies emerged the 'Beefcake' magazines of the 1940s, which were aimed at the homophile market. In 1946 the homosexual photographer Bob Mizer (1922–1992) began to take physique photographs of young men in Southern California. His first published photograph depicts a young athletic marine leaping across a beach dressed in a minimal posing pouch. Mizer realized that there was no shortage of young, attractive men who would be happy to pose for him for a few dollars, and of customers who would be interested in purchasing photosets from news-stands in Hollywood, which was home to LA's growing homophile and homosexual community. He set up a modelling agency, the Amateur Models Guild, which specialized in producing photosets of athletic young men and muscle boys – the beefcake. Initially he ran the AMG from his mother's kitchen table, but as the business prospered, he moved into an office in West 11th Street, in central Los Angeles.

Mizer promoted his photosets by taking out adverts in mainstream and muscle magazines, but in 1948 he fell foul of the U.S. Postmaster General, who had decided to clean up the Post Office by banning any mail-order business that sold what was then defined as pornographic material, especially artfully posed and photographed pictures of naked or near-naked men. Mizer's response was to publish his own magazine, *Physique Pictorial*, which was modelled on the muscle magazines of the day.[6] According to F. Valentine Hooven III, *Physique Pictorial*, which began publication in 1950, was the first overtly gay magazine, in which the models were not shown with the metaphorical fig leaf as being exemplars of physical culture, or presented under the labels of art or scientific studies, but as explicit objects of same-sex desire.[7] *Physique Pictorial*'s early success spawned several rival homophile publications, including *Vim*, *Trim* and *Grecian Physique Pictorial*, which followed Mizer's example of photographing the musclemen who congregated in and around Muscle Beach and the young hopefuls who were working in LA waiting for their big break in the movies.[8] One of these men, who competed in bodybuilding and posed for Mizer, and who later followed Steve Reeves to become a sword-and-sandal epic movie star, was the ruggedly good-looking, all-American Ed Fury (b. 1928).[9]

There was a considerable crossover between the straight physique and beefcake magazines; hence, in looking for the genesis of the gay muscle-boy aesthetic of the 1980s, we should not think of a nascent gay press copying the straight muscle press, but of a collaboration between the two between the 1950s and '70s, with constant exchanges of models and photographers, each contributing to images of young men with smooth, tanned, gym-trained bodies, who exuded an easy but ambiguous allure that was appealing to both heterosexual and homosexual men. It would have been a short step for some young homosexual men from admiring pictures of muscle boys in magazines to going to the gym to train alongside them. Sadly, there are no first-hand testimonies that describe this golden age of ambiguous frater-nization, when Muscle Beach physique athletes such as Jack LaLanne and Bob Delmonteque could appear in the pages of *Physique Pictorial* and other homophile magazines, and when homosexual and heterosexual men shared the same gyms, beaches and bars.

Out of the Closet and into the Locker Room

The America of the 1960s experienced a series of seismic shocks with the campaign for African-American civil rights, second-wave feminism and the anti-Vietnam War and anti-draft movements all combining in a countercultural moment that opened up hitherto uncharted possi-bilities of social reform and individual self-actualization. Radicalism was also reaching into the recesses of the homosexual and homophile closets, but what lit the Gay Liberation fuse was not a repressive Supreme Court decision or act of Congress but a disturbance in New York's West Village, when the very diverse patrons of the Stonewall Bar, infu-riated by heavy-handed NYPD raids and petty persecution by the city authorities, finally decided that their Rosa Parks moment had arrived and began to fight back. What had begun as a minor neighbourhood disturbance at a gay bar on 28 June 1969 quickly turned into a national and then an international movement clamouring for recognition of what would become known as LGBT (lesbian, gay, bisexual and trans-gender) rights. But the immediate consequences of Gay Liberation were not quite what the political activists had imagined or hoped for. For every Harvey Milk (1930–1978) who wanted to make the world a better and more equal place for gay men and lesbians, there were nine young gay men who had moved to New York, LA and San Francisco and who just wanted to party and have fun. Post-Stonewall, the innocent co-habitation between heterosexual and homosexual men that existed on Southern California's beaches and in its gyms could no longer con-tinue. The beefcake magazines made way for overtly gay, sexually explicit pornographic magazines, in which straight muscle men and handsome

Hollywood hopefuls could not appear without risking their reputations and future careers. During the 1970s and '80s, gay men explored their own identities and reinvented the gay male image in exclusively gay, men-only spaces.

In *Muscle Boys* (2008), Erick Alvarez attempts to reconstruct the early phases of gay gym culture, but he acknowledges that very little has been preserved from this early period of LGBT history. Before Stonewall, homosexual men could only engage in clandestine, anonymous sex in public spaces, such as cottages (tearooms, public toilets) and parks, during which, because of the very limited and furtive character of the encounters, they had to keep most of their clothes on. All this changed after Gay Liberation in the gay bars, discos and saunas (bathhouses), where gay men could display their bodies freely for the first time. Suddenly the gay male body had become an instrument of pleasure that could be appreciated and enjoyed in its entirety. At the same time, a new archetype was emerging to replace the homosexual sissy: the self-consciously masculine, moustachioed 'clone', whose unstated *raison d'être* was to reclaim masculinity on behalf of all gay men.[10] In the 1970s, a gym-trained muscular physique was not a necessary attribute of the clone, who advertised his newly rediscovered masculinity through his choice of rugged outdoor clothing – jeans, a checked shirt and work boots – together with luxuriant growths of facial and chest hair, and a general male swagger that announced to the world that he was what the Village People celebrated in the disco anthem of the same name, a 'Macho Man': out, proud, gay, yet masculine. The 1980s gay muscle boy, therefore, was the product of a collision of two male archetypes – the 1950s Californian muscle boy and the 1970s clone. As Alvarez points out, they fused in the sexually charged environment of gay bath-houses, several of which also provided the gay scene's first gyms.

Despite the lack of documentary evidence, Alvarez succeeds in providing his readers with a reconstruction of the evolution of gay gyms in New York, San Francisco and Los Angeles.[11] The first exclusively gay gyms appeared in metropolitan areas with large gay populations in the 1960s and '70s. These were small, gay-owned and -operated spaces, such as the Sheridan Square Gym in New York's West Village, the Solarium and Apollo Gyms in San Francisco's first gay neighbourhood in and

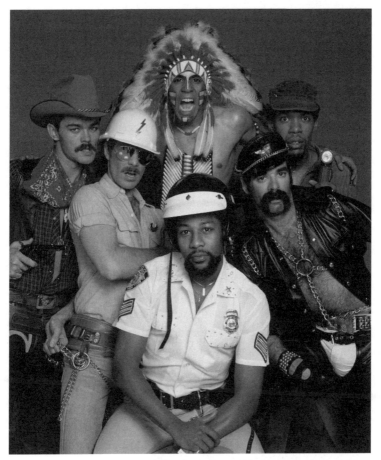

The Village People. Each member embodied a post-Gay Liberation masculine archetype. When gay men assumed the identities of the 'clone', the motorcycle cop and the leather-man, they were reclaiming a masculinity long denied them by their labelling as effeminate homosexuals.

around Polk Street, and Eastons on LA's Beverly Boulevard. Gay New Yorkers also went to the YMCA on East 48th Street, which inspired the Village People's song 'Y.M.C.A.' from their album *Cruisin'* (1978). In London, too, never far behind developments in the U.S., gay men were known to congregate at the London Central YMCA in Great Russell Street, which served as the community's first de facto gay gym.

With the growth of metropolitan gay communities, and the increasing self-confidence and visibility of gay men in the 1980s and '90s, gay gyms moved to larger premises, with equipment and facilities that rivalled the best straight gyms of the day. In Manhattan it was the Chelsea Gym that drew men to its upper-floor premises, and featured in a scene of the hit film *Jeffrey*, where the hero, Jeffrey, meets the hunky HIV-positive Steve while working out.[12] The gym in the movie is a traditional all-male bodybuilding gym, modelled on Gold's Gym in Venice, California, but with a completely different, sexually charged atmosphere. In San Francisco, with the move to the Castro, gay men trained at Muscle Systems, The Pump Room, City Gym and Market Street Gym, and in LA at Sports Connection on Santa Monica Boulevard, West Hollywood. In 1994 London's first American-style gay health club, Soho Gym, opened its doors in Macklin Street, Covent Garden.[13]

While one group of gay men were discovering weight training in exclusively male, gay gyms, another group who were not quite ready to pump iron were coming to the gym through a completely different route. When Jane Fonda released her workout video, there were many gay men whose sole contact with exercise was dancing in gay discos. They, too, were attracted by dance and aerobics classes, and began to frequent dance studios and to join gyms that offered dance and aerobics on their group exercise-class schedules. Once inside the gym, however, many would gravitate to the weights room where the muscle boys, both gay and straight, were working out.

At the height of the HIV-AIDS epidemic, which began in the U.S. in the late 1970s, many of the first- and second-generation gay gyms closed after their owners and many of their patrons died because there were no effective treatments for the disease. The epidemic, which reached crisis proportions in gay communities across the Western world during the 1980s and early '90s, made gay men much more health-conscious and more likely to go to the gym.[14] Hence the demand for places for gay men to exercise increased, and they joined gay and mixed gyms in growing numbers. One of the unexpected effects of the HIV-AIDS crisis and of the activism it triggered was to make the community much more visible to mainstream society. In a counter-intuitive way, the epidemic initiated a second 'coming out' of the gay community after Gay Liberation, and through the tragedy, it won a greater sense of acceptance.

The second unexpected result of the epidemic was the appearance of what Alvarez calls the 'poz jock' – the HIV-positive gay muscle boy. The first drug to have any effect on the disease, AZT, appeared in 1987, but it only slowed the condition marginally. Within seven years, however, new drugs had been developed that, given in combination, almost literally brought sufferers back from the dead. Men who had wasted away from 165–80 lb (75–82 kg) to 100–110 lb (45–50 kg), and were in the terminal stages of AIDS, recovered in a matter of weeks. To help them regain their lost bodyweight and wasted muscles, doctors prescribed the gym and courses of anabolic steroids. Within a few years, many of the buffest men in gay gyms were positive, transforming a group of unfortunates who had been outcasts and abandoned at death's door into the hottest and most desirable men on the gay scene.[15] For Alvarez, this represents an interesting paradox, in which men who had been seen as the least healthy and most dangerous by other gay men had become the most attractive and desirable men on the scene.

During the 1990s and 2000s, the corporate gym chains recognized the value of the pink dollar, pound and euro. Gay residents of Manhattan were spoilt for choice with several gay-friendly branches of David Barton gyms, the New York Sports Club and the Chelsea Pier Gym; in San Francisco gay men joined the World Gym in Potrero and Crunch in Van Ness; and in LA the main gay gyms were the West Hollywood branches of Gold's Gym and Crunch. In London, Soho Gym became plural when the franchise expanded with the opening of several new branches across the city. However, these had to compete with the major chains in Central London that were also actively canvassing gay members. Gay men had come full circle: in the 1950s and '60s they had started working out alongside heterosexual men in Southern California's health clubs; in the 1970s and '80s they developed their own exclusive exercise spaces where they were able to reinvent themselves; and by the 1990s they were coming back to mixed gyms, but completely transformed – no longer closeted and hiding, but out and proud, and often in better shape than the heterosexual men training alongside them.

Although many gay men prefer to go to mixed gyms, exclusively gay gyms continue to flourish. In *Muscle Boys* Alvarez describes the scene at a popular West Coast gay gym, enumerating the different types of muscle boy on the gay scene:

> During prime gym time (4 to 8 pm) if you were to dim the lights, the scene would resemble a busy nightclub – minus the cock- tails. This is one of the most popular, the largest, and most diverse gyms in San Francisco; it is home base to a mixture of muscle boys, circuit boys, muscle bears, athletes, poz jocks, and older males. The place draws the prettiest boys, the hottest men, and the buffest bears in the city.[16]

He explains that during the 1990s and 2000s, in cities with large gay communities, such as New York, San Francisco and London, for many men, gyms replaced the bars that had been the main social meeting places in the 1970s and '80s. This makes a predominantly or exclusively gay gym very different from a straight gym because of the sexualized nature of the interaction taking place there.

In their study of the Adonis complex, Harrison Pope et al. ask whether gay men are at greater risk from muscle dysmorphia than heterosexual men, and are therefore more likely to abuse steroids.[17] In this case, however, we have to differentiate between HIV-positive men who have been prescribed steroid therapies for muscle wastage, for which there are no reliable figures but which could be as low as 5 per cent or as high as 60 per cent of HIV-positive men, and the percentage of gay men who use steroids without prescription purely for aesthetic purposes, which could be as high as 28 per cent.[18] My own view is that, although gay men are bombarded with and influenced by the same hegemonic hyper-muscular supermale images in the media as heterosexual men, like women they have evolved resistance strategies to these images, and they are also more able to discuss image disorders than are heterosexual men. In the past century, gay men have successfully challenged the social construct of homosexuality as effeminate, and so they have access to resources and ways of resisting that are not available to heterosexual men. As the Alvarez quotation above makes clear, even within the gay muscle community there are a number of different archetypes: the standard-issue Muscle

Mary; the circuit boy who lives for a series of mega-party weekends across the U.S. and now the world; the muscle bear who, as the name implies, is much hairier and cuddlier; the poz jock; and the older man – each fit and gym-trained, but each with its own distinctive embodiment.

A Suitable Boy

Most readers, male or female, gay or straight, will probably agree that the Czech model Jakub Stefano (p. 194; b. 1985) embodies one of the dominant male archetypes in the media and on the Internet, which I have christened the 'fitness body'. Stefano is muscular and well proportioned, while at the same time his low body fat gives him excellent muscular definition. He has a symmetrical, boyish yet masculine face, with short hair; most of his body hair is shaved or trimmed, with the exception of a 'treasure trail' leading suggestively to the waistband of his shorts. In the 1950s this image could have been considered pornographic, and a beefcake magazine displaying it on its cover might have found itself in trouble with the U.S. Postmaster General. Today, such images are so commonplace in the media and on advertising hoardings that they barely attract comment.

We can be pretty sure that Stefano goes to the gym, where he performs aesthetic training with free and machine weights, as he could not have developed this level of muscularity from a sport or day-to-day physical activities. For a man only in his early twenties, he has an extremely well-developed physique, and partly because of his age and genetic makeup, combined with an intensive weight-training regime and a good diet, he also has enviably low body fat. Although not out of reach of any 20- or 30-something-year-old male, the fitness body requires a great deal of work and upkeep – probably as many hours of dedicated training as those performed by an elite athlete – but the event in which Stefano and other fitness models excel is not an athletic discipline or sport but consists of posing for the camera or walking down a catwalk displaying their finely honed physiques.

My aim is not to question or criticize the fitness body's undeniable charms, but to ask why it now represents the acme of masculine beauty in Western culture. What is it about the fitness body that makes it so marketable as a commodity? As with what makes a certain type of female body desirable, evolutionary biology might seek the answer in human prehistory in the evolutionary advantages of different physical characteristics. A biologist would point out that Stefano's youth, good health, physical strength and virility combine to make him an ideal mate for any human female seeking a male protector, provider and father for her offspring.

Even if we were to accept the evolutionary argument, I can immediately see several flaws. For example, if the desirable qualifications for a mate are masculinity and virility, would not a hairier male be even more attractive? And although youth is an attractive quality in a mate, might not experience, which implies a proven ability to survive, be an even more desirable trait? Thus would not the ideal prehistoric male be a few years older and considerably more masculine? In terms of Stefano's build, I can see several factors that would probably turn off a potential Neolithic female. Ancient hunter-gatherers lived on a knife edge between survival and starvation, and in terms of living through the lean times, the fitness body's total lack of subcutaneous fat would mean that he would have no reserves to fall back on. Nor does its well-developed musculature have any significant evolutionary advantage. The ability to bench press or squat 220 lb (100 kg) is not particularly useful in the wild, where cardiovascular fitness, essential for running away from something dangerous or for running down prey, is much more useful than brute strength.

The fitness body is a highly desirable but entirely manufactured artefact that could not exist in a prehistoric state of nature; it is clearly a product of aesthetic training in the gym, which itself is a product of civilization. Although the fitness body is very easy on the eye, functionally it probably leaves something to be desired. Without carrying out a series of physical tests, we cannot be sure of its cardiovascular fitness, flexibility, hand–eye coordination or proprioception, which are the qualities it would really need to survive in a prehistoric environment. When compared to the bodies of male models and Hollywood actors of a generation ago, the fitness body is already more muscular and defined, and if one goes back a couple of generations to action stars such as John Wayne and Errol Flynn, the fitness body is completely different in terms of body fat and composition. We should also compare the fitness body with other bodies considered to be ideal in Western and non-Western cultures. We have to go back only a century and a half in the U.S. to a time when underweight male exquisites and overweight men were considered to be masculine ideals. And in the present day, in parts of the world where food scarcity remains an issue, corpulent or even obese male bodies are still seen as attractive and desirable.

Therefore, to understand why the fitness body is considered ideal by many Western viewers, we must abandon any notions of evolutionary advantage and universal ideas of attractiveness based on the Vitruvian Golden Mean. It is a social construct that belongs very much to its time and place. First, we need to place the fitness body in its early twenty-first-century context, when the developed world is obsessed with three things: sex, age and fat. In rapidly ageing societies, where close to two-thirds of the population are either overweight or obese, Stefano's youth and leanness are particularly attractive by sheer contrast. His virility makes him desirable as a sexual partner to both heterosexual women and to gay men, and so he is a role model for both gay and heterosexual men. Finally, just as physical beauty had a moral dimension in ancient Greece, as expressed in the phrase *kalos kagathos* ('beautiful and good'), physical attractiveness carries moral connotations in the modern period. An overweight man is stigmatized as being lazy and unable to control his base appetites; conversely, an underweight man is seen as morally weak and lacking in masculinity – an echo of Charles Atlas's 97-lb (45-kg) weakling who gets sand kicked in his face. Thus their antithesis, the perfectly honed fitness body, can be seen as not only physically but morally superior to other body types: a contemporary expression of ancient Greek *sophrosyne* and *arete*.

Queer Eye for the Straight Guy

Now that we know a little more about why the fitness body might represent the dominant male ideal, we must ask what or who created it. Alvarez sees it largely as a product of media, fashion and advertising – Calvin Klein underwear and the Abercrombie & Fitch fashion label –

which are heavily weighted towards the youth and gay market and whose advertising, PR and marketing are produced by gay or gay-friendly photographers, PR and advertising executives, and art directors.[19] He goes so far to claim that, 'In terms of media and male image, the ideal image of modern heterosexual man is by and large built on the fantasies of gay men, not those of women.'[20] I agree with him that the sexual fantasies of women have very little to do with current male archetypes, but I would disagree that they are entirely the product of gay men's fantasies. What I have tried to explore and describe here and in chapter Five is the collaboration, synergy and cross-fertilization that have taken place between the fantasies that heterosexual men have developed about becoming hyper-muscular supermales and those that gay men have developed about their own bodies and the bodies they desire, which have been evolving in the gym since the late nineteenth century.

It would be impossible to ignore or deny the influence that straight men had on the formative period of gay male images, especially during the 1950s and '60s, and also the influence that gay men had on the heterosexual male image during the 1990s and 2000s. Although there are significant differences between the hyper-muscular body and the fitness body, they are both the product of aesthetic training in the gym, and there are also strong similarities between them, the most obvious being that they are both shaved smooth to show off the musculature and definition. The influence of ideal gay male body images is probably strongest on heterosexual men in their twenties and thirties, who do not necessarily aspire to the exaggerated size and extreme definition of the hyper-muscular competitive bodybuilder, which can be achieved only with illegal supplementation and can be maintained only for short periods. Their model is the more natural fitness body, which is a much more attainable physique that can be maintained all year round. The generation of younger heterosexual metropolitan men, often called 'metrosexuals', are also less concerned with the questions of sexual identity that troubled their fathers and grandfathers, and do not have to assert their heterosexuality by aggressive displays of masculinity or homophobia.

An important factor that has contributed to this change in attitudes is the commodification of the male fitness body, which is now used to sell an increasing range of products. Gym-trained bodies were first used to market underwear and male fragrances and grooming products, often specifically targeted at the gay market. However, like female bodies, their marketability is broadening to include products aimed at the general consumer, regardless of age, gender or level of fitness, such as a recent ad that features a young male gardener tricked into taking off his T-shirt after he sprays himself with a canned drink given to him by a group of female admirers. While the youthful model in the ad is not a hyper-muscular supermale, he has a lean, gym-trained fitness body. Even the Pirelli calendar, for decades a bastion of the sexual exploitation of the female form to sell car tyres, now features a more balanced male–female offering of naked flesh.

Style and Substance

The journey that gay men have undertaken over the past 150 years has been a complex one, with many redefinitions and reinventions, often in the face of the most violent prejudice, intolerance and repression. As is often the case, oppression triggers resistance, which ultimately leads to liberation. In the latter stages of the journey, from the 1950s onwards, the gym played an important role in shaping gay cultures and identities, helping men to leave behind the label of homosexual sissy and seek new ways of expressing and embodying what it is to be a man who desires and loves other men. The process has not always been easy or without cost. The burden of centuries of homophobia combined with a sudden moment of liberation resulted in a culture of sexual hedonism and excess, which had tragic consequences when many gay men succumbed to HIV-AIDS. However, gay men today are part of a vibrant community composed of many subcultures, which has gained acceptance and won its full civil rights, at least in most of the developed world.

If homosexuals in the late nineteenth and early twentieth centuries had looked longingly at strongmen like Eugen Sandow, by the mid-twentieth century they were training alongside their idols, equalling their physical achievements and helping to shape the masculine ideal. With Gay Liberation came a moment of separation, as heterosexual and homosexual men became divided by the need to define separate gay and straight identities. In both cases, they continued to do so in the gym. While heterosexual men modelled themselves on the hyper-muscular supermale, gay men explored a number of different physical images. Those who were not ready to pump iron in the gym started out in the much less daunting environments of the dance studio and aerobics class. Another group preferred to train in exclusively gay gyms, which became extensions of the gay scene, where men socialized and met potential partners.

Post-HIV-AIDS, with greater tolerance and integration into mainstream society, many gay men chose to return to mixed gyms, where they interacted once more with heterosexual men. Some gay men chose to pursue the same hyper-muscular supermale ideal, but it was only one of the gay muscle-boy archetypes available to them. Since the 1990s, the media, advertising and the Internet have combined to produce a hegemonic male image that I have called the fitness body, but rather than see this as having been imposed by gay men on heterosexual men, or vice versa, I would argue that it is the culmination of an evolving collaboration between the two that began in the late nineteenth century. In terms of impact on the gay community, it is clear that these images are capable of triggering image-related psychological disorders, but because of their past experiences, gay men are much better equipped than heterosexual men to develop resistance strategies that can protect them from harm.

The contribution that gay men have made to the contemporary gym is more subtle than that brought about by women but no less transformative. In the final chapter, I shall discuss the concept of 'extertainment' – the combination of exercise and entertainment that is an important feature of the contemporary gym. In the 1980s gay gyms became extensions of the bar and club scene where gay men met and socialized. In the 1990s gay men brought this sense of the gym as a social community and a place to have fun (in the broadest sense of the term) to mixed gyms. They encouraged diversification in the types of training on offer, as they were not completely wedded to the hyper-muscular supermale image, and they provided a bridge between the majority-female group exercise studio and the majority-male weights room, encouraging both men and women to emerge from their gendered

exercise ghettos. Although the gay contribution might appear to be more about style than substance, we should remember that the ways an activity is performed can often transform how it is experienced, and that if the gym has become less aggressive, exclusive and competitive, and more socially inclusive, welcoming and diverse, it will be able to attract and retain more members, and encourage existing gym converts to experiment with different forms of exercise.

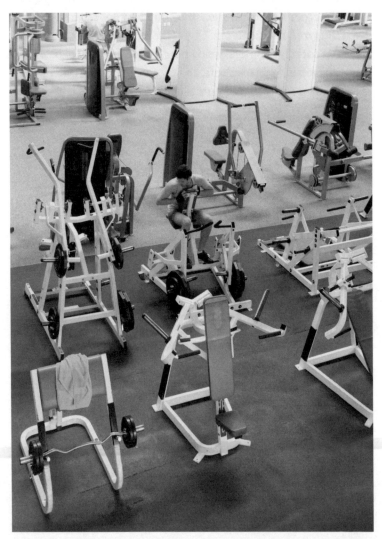

One of the defining characteristics of the contemporary gym industry is its global reach and standardization. The sports hall of Gold's Gym in Moscow, opened in 1996, is indistinguishable from those of other major chain gyms all over the world, featuring the same type of free and machine weights and cardiovascular equipment.

8
CONSUMING FITNESS

Exercise and rest are the cornerstones of improving your quality of life. It's not always easy but it's always worth it. When you find a fitness routine you enjoy, you'll feel better, look better and be happier in your own skin.

Fitness First, 'Regular Exercise – Looking After Number One'

While I was writing this book, I made a point of keeping track of the gender, age, weight, body composition and level of fitness of people I saw in the gyms where I trained. It was not intended to be an exact statistical exercise, more of a rough head count to confirm what I already knew. In terms of male–female balance, there is not a single gym I have visited where there is not a degree of gender segregation between different activities: the free-weights tends to be majority male and the group exercise classes tend to be majority female, while the machine-weights and cardio areas, spinning and circuit classes are fairly evenly split fifty-fifty. In terms of age profile, the majority were adults from their twenties to fifties, with a few outliers at either end of the age range – unless the gym was running an introductory course for teens or a group exercise class for seniors. When estimating the average weight and body composition[1] of exercisers, we have to remember that between 50 and 60 per cent of the population of the developed world have issues with their weight, ranging from being overweight to obese. In a twelve-month period, however, I saw only a handful of people who would fit the description 'obese', while the majority were within what is currently considered the normal range for bodyweight and composition, with a sizeable group being slightly to moderately overweight and a much smaller group being slightly to moderately underweight.

Perhaps most striking of all, however, was the level of fitness of gym-goers. As could be expected from a group of regular exercisers, they were fitter than people of the same age and weight in terms of basic criteria such as strength, flexibility and cardiovascular (cv) fitness. However, there was a significant number of gym members who excelled in one or more areas of fitness, and who could be classed alongside elite athletes as being super-fit. The one major problem this rough-and-ready reckoning reveals, and the one thing the fitness industry must tackle in order to continue recruiting and retaining new members at the current rate, is how to make itself relevant to the unfit and increasingly overweight majority that has never been to a gym. At present the industry is catering to the converted – men and women who acquired the exercise habit when they were children or teenagers, long before they joined a commercial gym as adults.

The Reflexive Exerciser

In 1992 the American academic Francis Fukuyama published *The End of History and the Last Man*, in which he argues that humanity reached the final phase of its economic, social and political development with the triumph of free-market capitalism and liberal-democracy over Soviet-style communism after the collapse of the USSR in 1991. Within a decade, however, the democratic West, which had been celebrating the end of 40 years of the Cold War, had declared the 'War on Terror' on militant Jihadist Islam after the Al-Qaeda attacks of 11 September 2001. A second but no less significant challenge to Fukuyama's theory is the runaway success of the People's Republic of China, which has defied all established socio-economic and political models by becoming the world's second largest economy, and the world's banker, while remaining firmly under the control of an anti-democratic, anti-liberal communist one-party state.

The West has been battered not only ideologically and militarily by these developments but economically, as it is only just beginning to emerge from the economic downturn caused by the financial crisis of 2007–8, which many economists characterize as having been even more damaging than the Great Depression (1929–41). Although these events have sapped the confidence and global political reach of the u.s. and other Western powers, in cultural terms the West's influence continues to grow, which could provide an explanation for the incidence of religious and cultural fundamentalism that has emerged in the Near East and other parts of the world during the past two decades. Non-Western cultures exposed to Western lifestyles and values through the global media and Internet feel under threat as never before, and their response has been to go on the offensive – even though it is with weapons developed for them by the hated, corrupt West: the Internet, the mobile phone and the IED. To give examples of this creeping process of globalization and Westernization, during trips to the Near East and China I visited gyms that were indistinguishable from those of the u.s. and Europe, with the same layout, equipment and group exercise-class schedules. The only major difference was the language of the staff and members, and sometimes their style of dress: for example, women in Muslim-majority countries exercise in what is considered to be 'modest' Islamic workout gear, with the hijab covering the hair and a tracksuit covering the arms and legs, worn with a short skirt around the midriff.

The Western gym is part of a cultural fifth column, along with pop music, fashion and fast food, which is transforming lifestyles in societies as diverse as India, China and the Islamic Near East. The gym re-emerged in the West at a time of intense political and social ferment during the nineteenth-century Age of Revolutions. It was not itself a cause of any major social dislocation but was a consequence of changing conceptions of the individual and his rights and duties within society. As individual rights came to the fore, every aspect of personal identity became more important, including embodiment. A similar process is now taking place in societies that once stressed communal values over individual freedom of choice. At the same time, immigrant and minority communities in the developed world are picking up the gym habit. In an interesting juxtaposition that I recently witnessed in a European gym, an older Jewish man who, while not ultra-orthodox, was readily identifiable by his kippah, was exercising on a cross-trainer next to a young woman in Islamic workout gear running on a treadmill.

Like Jahn's *Turnplatz*, the modern gym is a great social and cultural leveller that can bring together people of different faiths, nationalities and socio-economic groups. In the West, embodiment has become one of the key aspects of self-actualization, which is a modern version of the ancient Greek concept of *arete* – the realization of an individual's full potential in all areas of life. Beginning with the body as the visible expression of the empowerment of heterosexual men, the gym-trained body has also played a role in the emancipation of women and gay men. But going to the gym is not the only way humans can transform their appearance. Makeup has always played an important role in the presentation of women, and now increasingly of men, who are spending record amounts on grooming and beauty products. Anyone watching reality TV could not fail to appreciate the growing popularity of cosmetic surgery as a quick fix to a range of aesthetic concerns from an unsightly physical feature to unwanted midriff flab.[2]

The most powerful medium for disseminating discourses of physical attractiveness and fitness is now the World Wide Web. The significant difference between the Web and previous disseminators of idealized body images, such as the Hollywood movies of the 1940s and '50s and the television shows of the 1970s and '80s, is that it is what the British sociologist Anthony Giddens calls a 'reflexive' medium. The viewer of a film or television show is a passive spectator, but the Web enables a two-way flow of information between the creators and consumers of content.[3] The media, governments and multinational corporations disseminate their messages through the media and the Internet, but the individuals viewing them can undermine and resist them through their participation in social media and by creating their own Internet content. This unparalleled reflexivity has led humans into uncharted territory: with enough money they can, through cosmetic procedures, makeup, illegal supplementation and exercise, turn themselves into simulacra of Pamela Anderson or Jakub Stefano, no matter what physical characteristics they were born with. One need only watch the hit U.S. TV franchise *Real Housewives of . . .* to realize that many affluent citizens of the developed world have bought into these images of ersatz perfection.

For those who live in this brave new secular world of affluence, leisure and longer lifespans, embodiment has become the main marker of personal identity, replacing religious, cultural and political affiliation. But the other side of the reflexive coin is that humans have become empowered as never before to resist, transform and reject externally imposed images. The Internet has become a battlefield of conflicting constructs of beauty, fitness, desire and embodiment, each sustained by their own *pouvoir–savoir* nexus, meaning that it is still impossible for us to tell exactly which constructs will emerge as dominant and where they will lead humanity in its relentless pursuit of perfection. At present, it is encouraging a growing number of consumers to join the gym to engage in aesthetic and therapeutic training.

The Obesity Epidemic

Despite our culture's obsession with physical appearance (or maybe, in part, because of it), the major health problem affecting the population of the developed world, and increasingly that of the wealthier sections of emerging economies, is obesity. According to the U.S. Surgeon General, 61 per cent of the adult American population is overweight or obese, with a BMI greater than 25, and obesity among America's children and teens has nearly tripled in the past twenty years.[4] Although weight problems can affect people of all ages, racial and ethnic groups, and both genders, certain groups in the U.S. are more prone to the condition, in particular Hispanic and African Americans. Obesity-related diseases, including coronary heart disease, high blood pressure, stroke, endometrial, breast and colon cancers, type-2 diabetes, osteoarthritis and gall-bladder disease, contribute to the premature deaths of 300,000 Americans every year, at an estimated cost to the U.S. in the year 2000 of $117 billion, rising to $190 billion in 2012.[5]

Where America leads, it seems, the rest of the world appears doomed to follow. According to the World Health Organization (WHO), obesity has doubled worldwide since 1980, with 1.4 billion adults overweight in 2008, of which 200 million men and 300 million women were obese. In a reversal of trends going back millennia, 65 per cent of the world population now lives in countries where eating too much food kills more people than not eating enough. Most disturbing of all, more than 40 million children under the age of five were overweight in 2011.[6] Both the u.s. Surgeon General and the WHO agree that overweight and obesity 'result from an imbalance involving excessive calorie consumption and/or inadequate physical activity'. Along with dietary changes, they recommend a minimum daily exercise regime of 60 minutes for children and 30 minutes for adults. At present, less than one-third of American adults engage in the recommended amount of daily physical activity, and 40 per cent do not participate in leisure-time physical activity of any kind. Until the end of the First World War, governments in the Western world were principally concerned about the poor physical condition of new recruits, who were short and underweight. From the mid-twentieth century onwards, however, governments have had to come to terms with the opposite problem: a sudden increase in the diseases of affluence, as Western diets became increasingly calorific and Western lifestyles increasingly sedentary. Dr Kenneth Cooper's main motivation for devising aerobics was to tackle the epidemic of coronary heart disease that began to afflict the u.s. in the 1960s.

The nation state continues to have an interest in the fitness for purpose of its citizens, but now with a completely different emphasis. With President Barack Obama's Patient Protection and Affordable Care Act of 2010, better known as 'Obamacare', the u.s. is gradually adopting Europe's social care model, meaning that the state will increasingly have to find the resources to pay for the health crisis caused by the obesity epidemic. In order to combat obesity, governments across the developed world are openly or tacitly encouraging people to join publicly funded and commercial gymnasia. The percentage of the population with a gym membership has steadily increased, with the u.s. leading the countries of the developed world with 16 per cent, and the UK in the top ten with almost 12 per cent. Despite the increase, this leaves the vast majority of the population either completely inactive or insufficiently active, and this despite what a recent International Health, Racquet and Sportsclub Association (IHRSA) report on the fitness industry describes as hundreds of thousands of pages of free promotion in the mainstream media, and high-profile celebrity endorsements.[7]

In the BBC documentary series *The Men Who Made Us Thin* (2013), the British investigative journalist Jacques Peretti examines the causes of the ongoing obesity epidemic and tries to explain why the well-meaning and relatively simple messages about overweight and obesity issued by the WHO and Western governments have so far failed to have any impact on rising obesity rates.[8] According to Peretti, one of the main reasons is because positive messages are drowned out by the multi-billion-dollar advertising and marketing campaigns of the food, beverage and fast-food industries, which continue to deluge the world population with unhealthy, calorie-rich options at rock-bottom prices, making the ready-to-eat hamburger or fried chicken portions, with extra-large fries and extra-large soda or milkshake, followed by a deep-fried apple pie or ice-cream sundae, cheaper and more convenient than the healthier alternatives.

Peretti's findings correlate with data from the U.S. Surgeon General and European Commission that it is the lowest socio-economic groups in the developed world who suffer from the highest levels of overweight and obesity, creating an obese underclass condemned to consume the unhealthiest foods and with the least disposable income to invest in healthy dietary options, active leisure activities and gym memberships. He goes on to explore the claims made by the larger chain gyms that promote exercise as a way of losing weight. Although increasing physical exercise plays a part in controlling bodyweight and body composition, exercise alone will not reduce or even maintain normal bodyweight without an adjustment of daily calorie intake. However, Peretti argues that the marketing and advertising campaigns of many gyms imply that working out alone is sufficient, setting unrealistic goals and expectations that in the long run will prove to be counterproductive for both prospective gym members and the fitness industry.[9] The industry itself realizes that an over-reliance on therapeutic and aesthetic training for weight control is a dangerous course to pursue. In *The Future of Fitness* (2010), Suzie Dale and her colleagues present a scenario in which the pharmaceutical industry develops medication that successfully tackles obesity and the degenerative conditions associated with it. In their summing up, Dale et al. ask the question that must be troubling every gym manager and owner: 'Where will the fitness-as-hard-work ethic be if a pill is invented that creates muscle mass and definition with little or no exercise?'[10]

'Obesogenic' vs 'Exercisogenic'

Who are the current generation of gym converts? And how have they managed to escape the obesity epidemic that is fast overtaking the rest of the population? With a few exceptions, gym members are not members of a genetically gifted race of supermen and -women who train for elite sports; they are average individuals whose motivation for training is to attain or maintain a desired body shape or to improve an aspect of their health and fitness – that is, for aesthetic or therapeutic reasons. Another sizeable group of gym converts is accounted for by the growing number of health-and-fitness professionals – gym staff, personal trainers, group exercise-class teachers, nutritionists and complementary therapists – for whom the gym is their place of work. Although it is not a rule that fitness-industry employees should be physically fit, it is usually the case that they, too, train regularly, because they have free or discounted access to the facilities and the time to make use of them, and because they can use their physical fitness to market their services. Hence they exercise for a mix of work-related functional, aesthetic and therapeutic reasons.

As has been the case throughout the history of the gym, however, there are gym-goers who are physically and genetically gifted – the Milos, Triats, Sandows, Stocktons, Schwarzeneggers and Fondas – but they represent a tiny minority of gym members. There is a clear trend, however, promoted by some doctors and pressure groups, to medicalize obesity, redefining it as a disease or genetic predisposition and thereby absolving of all responsibility those who are unfit and overweight because of the poor lifestyle choices they have made. If we begin to accept that so many of our fellow citizens are overweight or obese primarily because of genetic factors, we will write off two-thirds of the population as somehow constitutionally unfit, creating a new kind of racism that would be just as insidious, objectionable and damaging as the nineteenth-century contention that all non-whites were inferior by virtue of their darker skin, and that the socially disadvantaged were poor because they were less intelligent, less able and less hard-working than the rich.

My own view of the causes of the current obesity epidemic is that environmental factors are much more significant than genetic ones. We have only to go back 60 years to reach a period when obesity was practically unknown, and the main problem facing the world was not obesity but malnutrition. I know of no theory of genetic adaptation that would account for the evolution of *Homo sapiens* from a majority slim-to-underweight group of populations to a majority overweight-to-obese group of populations in the space of three generations. The explanation of why so many of us are fat must be found in changes in society and behaviour, and in particular in the creation of an 'obesogenic' environment, which according to the u.s. Centers for Disease Control and Prevention 'offers ready access to high-calorie foods but limits opportunities for physical activity'.[11] For regular gym-goers, therefore, the gym is a response to the obesogenic environment, which they have successfully replaced with an 'exercisogenic' environment, where they often have access to healthier, more nutritious and less calorific foods than are generally available from family and fast-food restaurants. For many gym converts, therefore, going to the gym is not just about exercising for a few hours a week; it is part of a much broader set of lifestyle choices that also includes diet, smoking and drug-taking (including nicotine and alcohol).

There are several factors that set gym members apart from the non-exercising majority, but none of them are physical or genetic. The first is opportunity: in order to go to a gym, there needs to be one within easy reach of your workplace or home. If you live in the centre of a city, or in a well-to-do suburb, you are probably much better served in terms of gyms than someone living in a rural area or in a poorer urban neighbourhood; second, you need a certain disposable income and available leisure time to be able to pay for a gym membership and make full use of it. But perhaps most important of all is a pre-existing experience of and interest in physical activity and sport in childhood and adolescence that make it much more likely that you will continue to exercise throughout the remainder of your adult life. Many of the gym members and staff whom I interviewed when researching this book had been keen (though not necessarily gifted) sportsmen at school or college. Although most no longer took part in organized sport because of work or family commitments, their early participation had given them the 'exercise habit', which had made them much more likely to join a gym to keep up their fitness.

One final advantage that gym converts have over non-exercisers is the level of knowledge about exercise that they can obtain from the gym or a personal trainer, or that is readily available to them through printed media, exercise DVDs and the Internet. In the past two or three decades, there have been significant improvements in our understanding of how different forms of training and sport affect the human body. As a result, compared to the gym-goers of the 1970s and '80s, contemporary exercisers are far better informed, which means that their training is more effective in attaining their goals and maintaining any gains, and they are less likely to suffer from injuries that will interrupt their training. The gap between gym converts and the unfit majority can be seen primarily as socio-economic, but it is compounded by differences in life experience and knowledge.

A Visit to the 'Fit for Purpose' Gym

There is no standard contemporary gym, so the one that I am inviting my readers to visit is a generic twenty-first-century facility, with elements assembled from several gyms in which I have trained over the past decade. The 'Fit for Purpose' (FFP) gym is a medium-sized chain gym located in the centre of a major city in the developed world, and has a diverse membership, reflecting the population of the area. One of the most striking aspects of contemporary gym culture is how standardized it has become all over the world. You could step into a gym on any continent and find the same layout, equipment, facilities and schedules of group exercise classes, and increasingly the same multinational chains, and the only clue you would have to your location would be the language spoken by the staff and members. Hence the FFP gym could be in London, New York, Dubai, Shanghai, Rio or Sydney.

In terms of gym locations, in addition to large public or private purpose-built sports facilities, gyms can be found throughout the urban environment in a wide variety of building types. In the U.S. and many other countries, gyms are often found in malls, which are easy to access by car and provide ample parking. A mall I recently visited in the Near East accommodates two gyms. The first, part of a multinational chain, occupies a large basement retail unit, which was designed as a large open-plan space to house a clothing store or supermarket. The architect has outfitted it with a reception area and back office, changing rooms and two exercise studios, leaving the remainder for the main gym floor; the second, an independent gym built on the mall's upper floor, with a sundeck and an open-air pool on the roof, occupies a space that was designed to be a health club when the building was first planned and outfitted.

Whereas gyms in North American cities are often housed in purpose-designed premises, in the more crowded settings of older European city centres, where there is little free space and planning regulations make it difficult to demolish existing structures, gyms have taken over buildings whose original functions are no longer needed, such as old cinemas, deconsecrated places of worship, public swimming pools, covered markets and commercial and light industrial premises. The most common format in many countries, however, remains the basement gym, which occupies what would otherwise be dead space in an office, retail or residential building. According to the IHRSA, from the prospective member's point of view, the most important factors that influence gym choice are not price or facilities but convenience and accessibility. It is a much-quoted industry truism that 'closer is always better', and that the gym you choose should be ten minutes from your home or preferably your place of work, otherwise you will not use it. Another key aspect is that is has to be accessible at all times, so factors such as the availability of public transport links, parking and safety and security issues are also crucial in informing consumer choice.

The FFP gym occupies the basement of a mixed-use building with retail units at street level and office space on the upper floors in a busy part of town, close to a metro station, which complies with the IHRSA's convenience and accessibility criteria. Like many gyms today, it is part of an international franchise, with branches in Europe, Asia, Australia and North America. The point of access to the gym is the brightly lit and inviting street-level reception, which also features a small retail area, selling the chain's branded workout gear, accessories, protein bars and sports supplements. Behind the desk sit the first gym staff that members and prospective members will encounter, the gatekeepers of this modern shrine dedicated to the perfectibility of the human body.

To one side of reception, behind a glass partition, is a back-office area with several desks with their obligatory computers and phones for the staff in charge of the club's administration. In addition to the day-to-day running of the gym, the main business of the back office is to recruit new members and ensure the retention of existing members. Retention is one of the industry's major problems. In the U.S. almost a quarter of members leave their clubs within the first year of joining.[12] In order to attract new members, gyms offer attractive joining packages, while at the same time trying to lock in members for a twelve-month contract with a joining fee. Even with the high turnover of members, when compared to all other retail businesses that begin each month with a trading balance of zero, health clubs are in a unique position because they benefit from what the IHRSA describes as 'annuity-like' features. On the first day of every month, a gym will get an electronic transfer of funds amounting to anywhere from $40,000 (£25,000) to $400,000 (£250,000). And unlike restaurants and shops that have constant outgoings to replace stock, the gym has fixed upfront costs for fitting out the club and purchasing equipment, and much lower outlays for maintenance thereafter. In terms of the ratio of staff to customers, gyms are also in a much better position than other service-orientated businesses.

Once through the turnstiles, we descend to the mezzanine level that accommodates the locker rooms. In the past few years I have visited two gyms with mixed-gender changing rooms, kitted out with large individual cabins with showers, and with another separate area for lockers. This arrangement saves on space and the costly duplication of plumbing installations, but may not be socially acceptable in many cultures. The FFP gym has the standard set-up of separate male and female changing rooms. Although many premium gyms have luxurious spa and wet areas, with hot tubs, sauna, steam and pools, because of space constraints, FFP has only a small sauna cabin in each changing room. Sharing the mezzanine level with the changing facilities are several rooms that the gym sublets to other businesses. In any building that was not purpose-designed to be a health club, there will be dead spaces to fill, which a gym can use to generate additional income streams. At FFP, the tenants are divided into two types: four independent businesses that have their own products, branding, management, marketing and advertising – a tanning room, a cosmetologist, a self-contained Pilates studio and a hairdresser – and four therapy rooms furnished and equipped by the gym and rented out to freelance complementary therapists.

A typical example of this kind of synergy between the gym and free-lance therapist is the gym's longest-standing tenant, Dave, a martial arts teacher and specialist in Traditional Chinese Medicine (TCM), who offers a mix of traditional Chinese and Western therapies. This kind of arrangement is beneficial to both the gym and the freelance therapist: it helps the former diversify what it offers to members and attract non-members to the premises, while differentiating itself from its competitors; and the freelance tenant-therapists have access to a ready-made pool of potential clients for their services and on-site facilities such as changing rooms and showers, all at a much cheaper cost than if they had to furnish and equip their own treatment rooms. My choice of Dave to represent the current generation of gym-based therapists is not accidental, as the gym is particularly fertile ground for alternative exercise methods and therapies. Gym members are naturally health conscious – therapeutic training is an important motivation for joining a gym – but they are not necessarily well served by conventional medicine when it comes to sports injuries and the stress-related problems that many of us suffer from, which Western doctors treat with drugs and surgical interventions, both of which can be extremely debilitating. TCM and other alternative therapeutic systems, such as Indian *Ayurveda*, different forms of massage, osteopathy and chiropratic, offer non-invasive, holistic approaches to treating minor injuries and ailments and stress-related problems, without side effects, and often using exercise as a major component of the treatment. In the twenty-first century, many contemporary gym converts, like their ancient Greek forebears, are more likely to go to the gym for medical treatment than to a doctor's office or clinic.

The Main Gym Floor

Once changed into appropriate workout gear, we are ready to proceed into the gym proper. After the rather crowded arrangement of staircases and rooms on the mezzanine, the open-plan gym floor feels relatively uncluttered and spacious. Although we are in a basement, the combination of bright colours and a clever lighting scheme means that it does not feel like a dark, dingy, dirty subterranean space. The equipment is not brand new but it is spotlessly clean and well maintained. The upbeat music pumped into the room is at just the right volume and, combined with the video screens showing various TV entertainment, sport and music channels, creates an atmosphere of purposeful, fun activity known as 'extertainment' – a combination of exercise and entertainment.[13] Some gyms have taken this one step further, with theatre-sized screens in dedicated CV training areas where members can clock up the miles and burn up the calories while catching up with the latest movie releases.

At the bottom of the staircase is a health bar serving protein shakes, drinks and light meals, with a couple of tables next to a chill-out area with sofas and low tables. The main gym floor is divided into five areas: warm-up, core, stretching and functional training; CV; machine weights; free weights; and a weightlifting platform. As it is a quiet time of day, there are only about a dozen people working out, several on their own and others with their personal trainers. FFP employs its own in-house personal trainers (PTs), in branded uniforms, who double up as gym supervisors, as well as freelance PTs, who pay a monthly fee for the use of the facilities. The PT is a popular option for novice exercisers but it is not a cheap one. A freelance trainer charges an average of $100+ (£60+) per hour, so the option is really open only to the affluent or to those who enjoy a subsidized gym package from their employer or HMO (health management organization). According to the IHRSA around 31 per cent of the employees of large U.S. corporations now receive subsidized gym memberships, and many U.S. HMOs encourage their clients to train by giving them reward points each time they visit the gym.

In the developed world's service-orientated economies, personal training has become a popular career choice for young men and women with proven athletic abilities, and with the steady increase in the percentage of the unfit and overweight in the general population, there is an ever-expanding client pool for their services. The job, however, has its disadvantages. Clients want to train before and after work or at lunchtime, which means a long working day with dead periods mid-morning and mid-afternoon. Anyone frequenting FFP during off-peak hours will see trainers in between clients either working out themselves or sitting in the café and chill-out area. One of the gym's stalwart PTs, Julien, gets in to train his first clients as the gym opens at 6 a.m., and often leaves when the gym closes at 10 p.m. Like many other gym professionals, he has a background in sport – as an aspiring rugby player in his native France – but when professional sport did not work out for him he re-trained as a personal trainer.

We are visiting the FFP gym during an off-peak period that is quiet for most city-centre gyms, the majority of whose members come in the evening after work. This presents logistical difficulties for most gyms, as their facilities are heavily oversubscribed at peak times. There is also the issue of employing staff who have little to do for parts of the day, and although the setting up costs of a gym are fixed, there are expenses for heating, lighting and maintenance, which have to be paid whether the gym is empty or crowded. One of the challenges for gyms is to find ways of making sure that the facilities are used as much as possible during opening hours. FFP organizes subsidized classes for seniors from the local community several times a week. It also rents out studio space to special-interest groups, such as school glee clubs, actors and dancers rehearsing for performances, and organizations running courses to train the next generation of group exercise teachers and PTs.

About one-third of the FFP main gym floor is given over to the CV area, with ranks of treadmills, stationary bikes, elliptical trainers and climbers facing a wall of flat-screen TVs whose audio can be accessed by flicking through an earphone jack on the control panel. The latest generation of CV machines have their own built-in personalized screens for TV, radio, games and Internet access, as well as docking ports for every conceivable electronic device. For the social-media generation, wi-fi and Internet access is an essential part of the extertainment package. Three or four people are pounding away on various CV exercisers, listening to music on headphones, watching a favourite TV show, or catching up on their email or Facebook newsfeed.

On the far side of the cardio area is open space set aside for warming up, stretching, core and ab work and functional training. It is equipped with a range of portable and fixed equipment including a freestanding metal frame with ladders and chinning bars, abs exercisers (ab-rollers and ab-wheels), variable height steps, medicine balls, fitness balls (Swiss balls), BOSU (half a fitness ball on a plastic base used for balance training), TRX (a modern take on gymnastics rings with adjustable straps used for bodyweight and suspension exercises) and foam rollers (used for stretching and self-massage). A new hi-tech addition is a Powerplate – a vibrating device on which you stand, lie or sit to perform stretching and core exercises. Building on the media

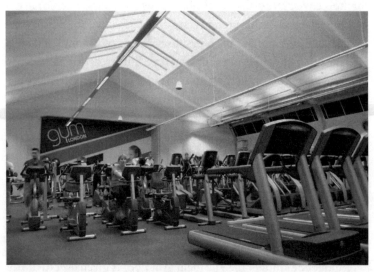

In the contemporary gym, ranks of treadmills, stationary bikes, climbers and elliptical trainers, each with their individual screens with TV, radio and Internet access, share the gym floor with weight-training equipment.

profile of athletic pastimes such as parkour (free running) and extreme sports, functional training is an increasingly popular option both in the gym, and in purpose-built cross-fit studios, as well as outdoors in parks and in the built environment, where exercisers can make use of whatever is on offer: stairs, low walls and outdoor gymnastics and fitness equipment.

Unlike conventional gym-based activities that concentrate on one aspect of fitness – for example, weight training builds muscular strength and size and CV machines and group exercise classes develop cardiovascular fitness – functional training aims to bring gains in strength and CV fitness and also to develop other aspects of fitness, including power, speed, balance, hand-eye coordination and flexibility. As such, it is particularly well suited to athletes and sportsmen, who are increasingly coming into the gym to perform complementary training to improve their performance and general fitness. Although they are relatively few in number, they are highly motivated, and during the off-season they will train five or six times a week, sometimes twice a day, and therefore are a highly visible presence in the gym. While they may use the same equipment and facilities as members training

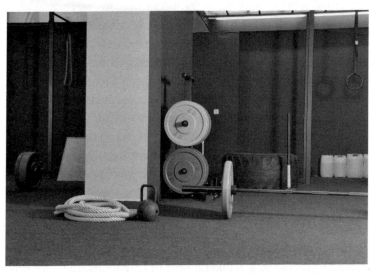

A recent addition to the gym floor is the functional training area where participants combine conventional strength-training exercises with weights and other types of equipment with bodyweight exercises borrowed from gymnastics and callisthenics.

for aesthetic and therapeutic reasons, they often use them in very different ways.

There is no typical user of this part of the gym but a regular in FFP's functional training area is Teemu, a Finnish pro triathlete who competes in Ironman races all over the world. As an extreme endurance athlete who puts his body through a 2.4-mile (3.86-km) swim and a 112-mile (180.25-km) bike race finished off with a 26.2-mile (42.2-km) marathon three to four times during the season (plus several shorter races), and who has a gruelling training schedule of daily runs, bike rides and swims, he does not have much time or need to spend in the gym working out on weights. Most of his training is functional for his events, but he usually does one hour-long session a week in the gym with light weights and, in bad weather, he will use the gym's treadmills and stationary cycles for interval training. Like all endurance athletes, he takes his body to the extreme in both training and racing, making him particularly prone to musculoskeletal injuries. In order to reduce the chance of injury and speed up recovery from minor stresses and strains, he does flexibility training five days a week in the gym's functional training area.

Crossing to the other side of the basement space, we come to what many people still consider to be the core of any gym: the free- and machine-weights areas, which at FFP are separate but contiguous. While there is a noticeable gender distinction between the two areas, there is also a certain amount of fraternization. Free weights include the full range of fixed and adjustable barbells and dumb-bells, Olympic weights and bars, and kettlebells.[14] These are used alone or in combination with different types of bench, squat racks, Smith machines, power racks and cages, as well as fixed-path free-weight machines.

Machine weights that started as simple pulley-and-weight-stack arrangements like the Polymachinon in the nineteenth century have evolved into superbly engineered pieces of equipment that control the exerciser's body position and guide him through the correct performance of the exercise. The most advanced electronic key-operated machines set the weight and number of repetitions (reps) for each exercise, and monitor the exerciser's speed and range of motion (ROM), correcting them if they train too fast or do not reach full ROM.

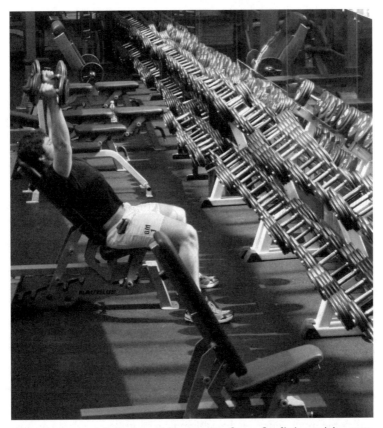

Although most gyms divide the available space into four or five distinct training areas, for many non-participants, the dominant image of the contemporary Western-style gym remains a place where predominantly male exercisers train with free weight to build bigger muscles.

Machines provide a safe and effective way to train, and they can be adjusted quickly and easily, making them ideal for the novice or the exerciser with limited time. Exercisers aiming for major increases in size and strength use free weights, and while there is an advantage in terms of the engagement of the core and other muscles when using barbells and dumb-bells, there is also a greater risk of injury, as well as an increased likelihood that the exerciser will cheat – that is, use his bodyweight or other muscles to lift a heavier weight in a particular exercise, or not complete the exercise within the full ROM. FFP has a standard set of machines that cover the whole body, with their weights encased in branded plastic cases, featuring adjustable seat heights and depths and a simple control to set the desired resistance.

There are several people working out in the weights area, either alone or with a trainer. As it is mid-morning, they are among the fortunate minority of gym members who can train outside peak times. Jack is a professional entertainer and photographic model who needs to maintain his physical fitness and a certain body shape for work, and as an out gay man, having a good physique is also a major social asset. An elite national squad gymnast until he was 21, he falls into that category of early gym converts who started regular gym training when at school. He follows a conventional programme of progressive weight training using free weights, doing one major body part per day. Nancy, who runs a retail business in the area, also uses what would be considered a conventional mix of resistance training using weight-training machines and light dumb-bells and endurance training on a cv machine under the supervision of her personal trainer. Together, Jack and Nancy represent what used to be the mainstream male and female gym exercisers from the 1950s to the early 2000s, each concentrating on weight training, but with a different emphasis: the men going for muscle size and strength, the women for muscular tone and endurance.

In the past decade, however, progressive weight training has been challenged by other activities, some new, such as functional training, and some much older, such as Olympic weightlifting, whose origins can be traced back to the stage shows of strongmen like Triat and Sandow. In response to renewed interest in weightlifting for general training, FFP has installed a weightlifting platform at one end of the free-weights area. It is an area about 8 ft (0.7 m) square whose floor has been reinforced and given extra protection with thick rubber mats. Using the lifting platform, as he does three times a week, is physiotherapy student Adam, whose session will include lifting in excess of his bodyweight in the two Olympic lifts, the clean and jerk and the snatch. Like many of the gym converts I interviewed while researching this book, his first experience of the gym was prompted by his participation in college sports, when his coaches told him he had to bulk up. He switched from progressive weight training to weightlifting precisely because its technical difficulty presents a much greater challenge than other forms of resistance training. Adam exemplifies the kind of gym member who is constantly pushing himself to his limits to excel in his chosen discipline, competing against himself as much as with other exercisers.

The Group Exercise Class Studios

The group exercise class is among the oldest forms of gym-based exercise: the ancient Greeks performed dances and group exercises to the sound of the flute; in the nineteenth century, Pehr Henrik Ling developed synchronized callisthenic routines (but without music, which he thought would be too distracting); and in his Paris gymnasium, Triat taught group classes that were very similar to modern circuit classes, performed to the beat of a drum. Unless they are extremely small or specialized, all gyms now make provision for group exercise classes, and many have purpose-built studios with sprung wooden floors, mirrored walls, bespoke sound systems and lighting rigs that rival those of the best dance clubs. It was the invention of aerobics by Dr Kenneth Cooper, and its later transformation into a new type of

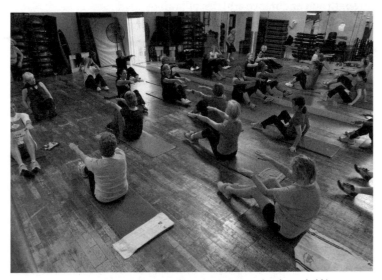

Originally devised to attract women into the gym, group exercise classes held in purpose-built studios now attract many more male participants. However, even today, different areas of the gym retain noticeable gender differences, with more men in the weights area and more women in group classes.

group exercise class by dance teachers, including Jacki Sorensen and Leni Cazden, and by actor Jane Fonda, that brought women into the gym in large numbers in the 1980s. The success of aerobics dance classes led to the development of new types of aerobics exercise class, such as step aerobics, devised by Gin Miller (b. 1960) in 1989.[15]

With the growing popularity of the group exercise format, gym members can choose classes based on a wide variety of physical disciplines, including yoga, boxing, Pilates, martial arts and dance. Yoga was the first alternative exercise system to reach a wide audience in the West after its introduction to the U.S. as a spiritual discipline at the end of the nineteenth century. Richard Hittleman (1927–1991) popularized it as a form of therapeutic exercise through his TV show *Yoga for Health*, which first aired in 1961.[16] With celebrity endorsements from actors and entertainers including Jane Fonda and Madonna, yoga remains a mainstay of the group exercise-class schedule. Once the preserve of older women who wanted to exercise but did not want to weight train or join more strenuous aerobics classes, yoga has broadened its appeal as a form of complementary flexibility training for strength and endurance athletes of both genders.

In addition to exercise classes, gyms increasingly offer other activities in their studios, such as classical ballet, traditional Western and non-Western dance styles, including line and folk dancing, ballroom, salsa, flamenco, classical Indian dance and burlesque. Equipment manufacturers have also entered the group exercise market, and many gyms now have dedicated spinning studios with bespoke spinning bikes, boxercise studios equipped with punchbags, and circuit-training studios with a range of different equipment and apparatus. An hour-long circuit class is probably one of the most exhausting things you can do (or watch) at FFP. The exercises are set up in a roughly circular course, and participants take turns at each station for a set period – usually a minute – with the teacher blowing a whistle when it's time to move on to the next station. A typical circuit class consists of free movements, such as push-ups, core exercises, burpees and sprints, combined with exercises that make use of different types of equipment: light barbells, kettlebells, steps, jumping blocks, mats, skipping ropes, medicine balls, fitness balls and so on, all performed to loud, heart-thumping music that is calibrated to the desired heart rate for each section of the class.

Circuit classes are not segregated by gender, and the ones at FFP have the same number of male and female participants. The atmosphere, however, is quite different from that of an aerobics or dance class, where the emphasis is on having fun as a group. If a dance class is like going to a party or a dance club with your friends, a circuit class is more akin to a race or athletics contest. Just as heterosexual men use competition and rivalry to motivate themselves when weight training, circuit-class participants not only push themselves to their own physical limits, but try to be the best in the class. A good teacher, like Chrissie, who has been teaching circuit classes at FFP for two decades, knows how to make her participants work harder by combining encouragement and fostering competition in equal measure. Looking at the participants as they leave Chrissie's daily lunchtime class, exhausted, soaked in sweat, but energized and high on their own achievements and endorphins, you can appreciate what Suzie Dale means by the 'fitness-as-hard-work ethic' that motivates many in the contemporary gym.

Our last stop in the FFP gym is also the latest addition to its facilities, a purpose-built spinning studio with state-of-the-art sound and lighting systems. Spinning, or indoor cycling, has existed as long as the bicycle itself, but it emerged as a popular exercise format in gyms in the past three decades. Participants use a specially designed, fully adjustable stationary cycle on which the resistance can be changed to simulate different riding conditions. The instructor leads the class through the workout, varying the resistance and cycling positions (sitting, standing, climbing, and so on), using music to keep his or her pupils motivated and to help them raise and lower their heart rates during different segments of the class. The brainchild of FFP group operations director John and FFP manager Oliver, the spinning studio is the gym's answer to established and new competitors in the area. With 46 health clubs within a mile radius, FFP's main problem is retaining and attracting members in a market that has become increasingly crowded and diverse, with the appearance of no-frills budget gyms, functional training, military training, boot camps, CrossFit and, a new entry into the market, the spinning-based Psycle studios.[17]

The Bespoke Gym

In my description of the FFP gym, I've gone for a fairly standard chain gym that could be found anywhere in the developed world in the first decade of the twenty-first century. In the century's second decade, which has been economically much more difficult than the first, particularly in the U.S. and Europe, the gym industry has bucked all economic trends and continued to grow. According to the Fitness Industry Association's 'State of the UK Fitness Industry Report' for 2011, between 2008 and 2010 the UK fitness industry grew its total market value by 4 per cent, increased its member base by 2 per cent to 7.3 million (11.9 per cent of the UK population) and increased its facilities by 1.7 per cent. The industry has proved itself recession-proof, sustaining growth during the worst economic downturn since the Great Depression, but as Dale et al. recognize in their report on the future of fitness, the greatest challenges to the industry are how to stay relevant to existing participants in a fast-changing exercise environment and how to reach out to the majority of the population that is not taking part in any form of recreational physical activity. The Dale report focuses on the emergence of two main trends – exergaming and extertainment – and also cites greater diversification and personalization of gyms to address the individual needs of members.[18]

Diversity has always been a feature of the industry. The development of the modern health club in the mid-twentieth century was quickly followed by the emergence of speciality gyms, such as all-women's gyms and gay gyms across the developed world. As we saw in chapter Seven, gay gyms had their heyday in the 1980s and '90s when, for a number of reasons, the gay exercise community was segregated from the heterosexual one. With the growing acceptance of LGBT lifestyles in the past two decades, however, many gay men have opted for mixed rather than gay gyms. We can contrast the experience of two gay men, one of whom, Jack, we met above training in the mixed FFP gym, and the other, Stefan, who prefers to train at an exclusively gay gym.

In understanding why the two men have made different choices, we have to take into account their ages: Jack is in his early thirties, while Stefan is in his late forties. Stefan came out as a gay man when homophobia was a much more serious problem than it is today, even in the major cities of North America and Europe. A secondary consideration for Stefan is his HIV status. He has been HIV positive for more than a decade, and though this would not be an issue in any gym, it is one of the reasons he gives for feeling more at ease in a gay environment. There continue to be exclusively gay gyms, especially in areas with very high gay populations, such as London's West End, LA's West Hollywood, Paris' Marais and New York's Chelsea and West Village. But in other areas, formerly exclusively or predominantly gay gyms have had to become more inclusive. For example, London's Soho Gyms, which began as exclusively gay with branches in Covent Garden and Earl's Court, has now opened in another four locations in the capital, marketing itself like any other mainstream chain gym.[19]

The contemporary gym can no longer be a one-size-fits-all product any more than a car, a pair of athletic shoes or a dishwasher can. Joining a gym has been transformed from a necessary chore, a hobby or a leisure activity into a branded lifestyle choice. The type of gym you go to says just as much about you as the car you drive or the fashion label you wear. The diversification of the fitness industry is already well under way in the developed world. In addition to the mainstream chains, new types of gym are opening with different price points and USPs. At one end of the scale is the no-frills budget gym, such as Blink Fitness in the U.S., with a monthly membership of $20, and Easygym in the UK, priced at £19.99 per month.[20] I asked a friend who had recently joined a budget gym what were its main attractions: value for money – when he was a member of a more expensive gym and he did not use it, he felt he was not getting his money's worth; convenience – the gym is close to his home; availability of equipment – the gym is no frills but much larger than most gyms, so he does not have to wait for equipment even at peak times; and, finally, bucking the trend for sociability, anonymity – he can go in and out without having to spend time socializing.

At the premium end of the scale are luxury gyms such as Equinox and celebrity gyms such as Madonna's Hard Candy Fitness.[21] Finally, for those, like the retiring Victorian ladies who trained behind curtains at Sandow's institutes, who do not want to be observed with their metaphorical corsets off, another increasingly popular option is the personal training studio – a private gym with PT that can be rented by the hour. The most recent trend is for the specialist exercise studio that offers drop-in classes in single activities such as Pilates or spinning without the need for membership. So far, because the overall percentage of gym members is still increasing, the chain gyms are not losing members, but in a fast-changing industry, they can no longer afford to take its members and their regular monthly income streams for granted, especially with the appearance of budget gyms that do not ask for a fixed-term contract or joining fee.

Working Gear

Throughout the book, I have described the typical workout wear of different periods, beginning with the ancient Greeks, who wore oil, dust and a 'dog leash'. During the eighteenth and nineteenth centuries, exercisers wore their everyday clothes and footwear to train. In the twentieth, with the emergence of Muscle Beach, it seemed that we were returning to a much more liberated era, with men in swimming trunks and women in bikinis parading their bodies unashamedly in public. Although gyms in gay bathhouses can be clothing optional, in most other exercise settings exercisers are expected to cover up, though how much has varied over time, with, for heterosexual men at least, a growing modesty in the past few decades. This might be a response to the greater visibility of out gay men, and a need for heterosexual men to differentiate themselves by their style of dress, but the trend for wearing baggier T-shirts and Lycra shorts under gym shorts is also visible among gay men. Hence, while gay men will often wear clothing that accentuates their best physical features, they, too, have followed heterosexual men in being much more modest than their gay and straight forebears in the 1970s and '80s.

A similar phenomenon can be observed in certain physique competitions. Although the bigger professional bodybuilders still pose in the smallest of briefs and posing pouches, made to look even smaller by their bulging musculature, some of the other physique categories now specify that men appear on stage in long shorts. Considering the importance given in our culture to the size of male genitalia, this seems to be a counter-intuitive development. In past centuries, men wore clothes that emphasized their virility, such as the Elizabethan codpiece and the tight breeches of the Regency buck – even Superman wears his underpants on the outside – but many heterosexual and gay men today, maybe worried that they will fail to match up to the hyper-masculine stallions that they see on Internet porn sites, or that they will appear to be too sexually predatory, go to great lengths to shield and disguise that part of their anatomy.

Women's gym wear, in contrast, has changed very little since the 1980s. Remove Jane Fonda's legwarmers and put her in the latest pair of Nike or Reebok shoes and she would not look out of place in a contemporary gym. Women's workout gear has remained figure-hugging and much more revealing of physical features, emphasizing the bust, waist and hips. The most significant change in workout gear for both men and women, however, is not in clothing but in footwear and accessories. I can still remember in the dark ages of fitness when many gyms allowed male exercisers to wear heavy-duty work boots to train. Since the 1980s, the introduction of treadmills and high-impact aerobics classes has made it necessary for exercisers to protect their joints with cushioned running and cross-training athletics shoes. In terms of gym accessories, the must-have item used to be the personal MP3 player or iPod, but it is now the smartphone with a built-in music and video player.

Taking the Gym Out of the Gym

A workout space outside the gym is something that we increasingly take for granted and now expect in a wide variety of settings. For example, on my way to an appointment, I cycled along a city-centre cycle lane flanked on one side by mid-sized office blocks and on the other by an urban waterway. As there was no automobile and little pedestrian traffic, the office windows did not have blinds or shutters, and I could look inside and observe the employees at work or in meetings. One set of ground-floor windows opened onto a small office gym. It was nothing fancy: a large carpeted room with three CV machines set in front of one window, a multi-use pulley machine against the back wall, one bench with a small selection of light dumb-bells, a couple of floor mats and several fitness balls. A solitary exerciser was clocking up the miles on the treadmill, listening to music on her smartphone. Many mid-sized or large companies in the developed world have gyms on their premises on the sound commercial grounds that providing exercise and stress relief for their employees will improve their health and concentration and prolong their working lives. New-build residential developments also usually include health-and-fitness facilities, operated by the building itself or by a franchise. Gyms are standard in hotels, at resorts and spas, and on cruise ships, and the latest travel option will soon include the 'gym in the sky', slated for the largest super-jumbos.

The home gym dates back to the nineteenth century, when fitness entrepreneurs including Eugen Sandow realized that though many people could never afford to join a gym, they could invest in home gym equipment, ranging from a set of adjustable dumb-bells and barbells to elastic-band devices designed to fit on doors. The home gym business is now a multibillion-dollar industry, with home versions of all the equipment you can find in a professional gym, as well as small single items for which infomercials make very big (and often quite misleading) claims. The home gym can consist of a corner of a room with a couple of pieces of equipment, like the weight-bench-and-dumb-bell combination found in many a teenage boy's bedroom, to full-sized professional set-ups built in the basements of luxury townhouses and apartments. A much more affordable home-gym option is the home workout DVD, popularized in the early 1980s by *Jane Fonda's Workout* video, which has spawned a huge number of celebrity imitators teaching every conceivable style of exercise, with recent market leaders including 'Zumba', a mix of Latin-American dance moves and callisthenics devised by Alberto Perez (b. 1970), and Tony Horton's (b. 1958) 'Insanity' cross-training workout programme.[22] The combination of TV screen and games platform and controller are the electronic exercise options offered by major games-industry players, PlayStation, Wii and Xbox, which industry analysts Dale et al. see as playing an increasing role in the future of the fitness industry by combining gaming, entertainment and exercise into exergaming and extertainment.

The increasing portability of the wi-fi Internet connection, through the smartphone or the smartphone-watch combination, means that

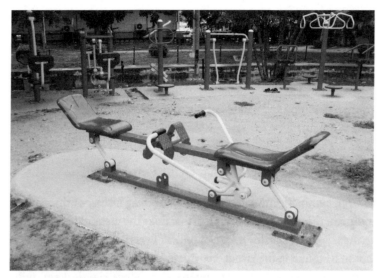

In part as a response to the growing popularity of the gym, and also in an attempt to combat the worsening obesity epidemic, municipal authorities worldwide have installed outdoor gym equipment, based on weight-training machines but that use the exerciser's own bodyweight in public parks, and on beaches.

you can carry the gym and a personal trainer with you wherever you go through a growing number of gym-related apps for use at home, in the park or in the gym. With the fast pace of development of the electronics and the apps sectors, it is difficult to gauge the impact these will have on the physical gym. In their present form, apps are just adjuncts to training that can be used to record and monitor progress and set programmes and goals. But in the future, they might have far greater capabilities, electronically docking with weights and cardio equipment in the gym, and providing constant feedback about the state of the body and its energy consumption.

At the low-tech end of the scale, there has been a trend in the past decade to install exercise equipment modelled on gym weight-training machines and cardio exercisers but which uses the exerciser's bodyweight rather than weight stacks in parks for public use – part of the 'green' or 'eco-gym' movement, which also sees personal trainers making use of the built environment and public parks to train their clients, singly or in groups. On a recent trip to Tel Aviv, Israel, I made use of the city's outdoor gyms set up in the city's parks and beaches, which because of the city's warm, dry climate are a popular and well-used amenity at most times of day by both genders, both children and adults. The growing interest in new forms of functional training has led to the appearance of mini Turnplätze in parks and on beaches all over the world, and because of the low-tech nature of their equipment – metal climbing frames, chinning and parallel bars – they are extremely cheap to install and maintain.

Gyms Past, Gyms Future

Having completed my survey of the 2,800-year history of the gymnasium, there is one very obvious fact that links the institutions known as gymnasia that I became aware of only as I was writing this book. It is not to be found in the layout, activities, equipment or social functions of the gymnasium, but in its membership. Since classical antiquity, going to the gym has been a minority and, often, an elite activity. In ancient Greece, approximately 20 per cent of the population had the right to use publicly funded gymnasia. In the nineteenth century, when the gymnasium reappeared in Europe, and during the twentieth century, when it took its contemporary form in the U.S., the percentage of the population using commercial gymnasia would have been much lower. It was only in the closing decades of the twentieth century that the proportion of the adult population of the developed world with gym memberships exceeded 10 per cent. Even today, in the U.S., which has the most private health clubs, gym members account for only 16 per cent of the population – for the most part its most affluent, best educated and most health-conscious citizens. While in previous centuries the poorer segments of the population would have been underweight and suffering from diseases associated with malnutrition and unsanitary living conditions, in the twenty-first century we have witnessed the emergence of an obese, unfit socio-economic underclass. Worse still, compared to health-aware gym converts, non-exercisers are more likely to smoke, drink and eat unhealthily, adding yet more risk factors that compromise their health and well-being.

Despite its elitist, minority status, the gym punches far above its weight in the collective Western consciousness with constant media coverage and celebrity endorsements. In addition to the advertising and marketing paid for by the gym industry itself, and the gym's high visibility in our urban environments, the institution also benefits from the support of the medical profession, government healthcare agencies and private HMOs. Despite this vast array of support and free promotion, gym converts do not yet make up one-fifth of the population, while the obesity epidemic affects around two-thirds of the population. The remaining 20–25 per cent, who are within what is considered to be the normal range for bodyweight and composition, could go either way, but the odds seem to indicate that a significant proportion will join the overweight majority, unless the pharmaceutical industry discovers a magic bullet that tackles obesity cheaply and safely.

Fit for What and Whose Purpose?

For the four ages of the gymnasium – exemplified by the ancient Athenian *gymnasion*, the early eighteenth-century Prussian Turnplatz, the mid-nineteenth-century commercial Parisian *gymnase* and the twentieth-century American health club – I have described how evolving notions of fitness for purpose have shaped and transformed the gym and the activities performed there. During each stage, the dominant gym ethos emerged from the interaction of four players: the individual, the state, the gymnasium and the media. Classical antiquity was the period when the aims of all four were most closely aligned. In democratic Athens, the individual citizen was the state, and the gymnasium was a state institution established to train the city's soldiers and future citizen rulers. The only discordant notes were voiced by dramatists and philosophers, but often these related to the institution once it had begun its long decline after the fall of the democracy.

When the gymnasium reappeared in the early nineteenth century it was part of a movement to empower the individual citizen, underpinned by ideas that had begun to emerge during the Renaissance and Protestant Reformation and developed fully during the Enlightenment. In the fractured world of European politics during the Revolutionary and Napoleonic wars, there was no coherent state response to the reappearance of the gymnasium. In some countries it was encouraged as beneficial, in others repressed as politically suspect. In most of Europe it took the best part of a century for the various states to realize the value of physical education, leading to the establishment of an infrastructure of school, college and military gymnasia. But these imposed a one-size-fits-all, state-sponsored version of physical fitness that ignored the aims and motivation of the individual exerciser. With the commercial gymnasium of the mid-nineteenth century, the balance of power between the state and the individual was reversed – in some cases fatally for the gymnasium, which was once again seen as the potential breeding ground for dangerous democratic radicalism.

As the century progressed, and the Western powers asserted their industrial, commercial, political and cultural might over the rest of the world, the gym-trained male Caucasian body was co-opted to project national, racial, military and cultural superiority. In a parallel movement, individuals went to the gymnasium to empower themselves against the brave new mechanized world created by the First and Second Industrial Revolutions, which was both a source of social and economic emancipation and a cause of greater personal alienation. The numbers of gymnasia and of people going to them remained so small, however, that if they had any impact at all, it was because of a temporary celebrity-driven craze that subsided as quickly as it had appeared. The twentieth-century American health club established a solid business model for the fitness industry that has been exported worldwide. Although gym membership continues to increase in the developed world, and is increasingly popular among the wealthier citizens of the emerging economies, the gym's survival is not assured if it does not keep pace with technological developments and if it fails to meet the needs and expectations of its current members.

A New Religion?

The gym industry has succeeded in attracting and retaining exercise converts, but it has so far failed to reach the inactive, overweight, unfit majority. In order to bring them into the gym, the industry must capitalize on the personal motivation of existing gym members. To explain what these might be will also answer the question that I asked in the

Introduction: do gyms now fulfil the individual and social functions that communal places of worship once did? From my own fitness career, as well as from my interaction with a large number of gym members over several decades, I would say that for its converts, training in a gym is one of the most important aspects of their individual identities. On the physical level, it provides very tangible benefits, in terms of appearance, health and general well-being, and we should not underestimate or ignore the sheer physical pleasure that exercisers get from moving and activating the body, recognized by the philosopher Jeremy Bentham as 'the pleasure of health, or, the internal pleasurable feeling or flow of spirits which accompanies a state of full health and vigour'. The gym also gives its members a sense of personal empowerment and agency that might not be available to them in other areas of their lives, as well as a sense of achievement when they accomplish the physical challenges they have set themselves. On the social level it gives them access to a ready-made community of like-minded people who are potential friends and partners. My conclusion, therefore, is that for the convert minority, the gym has once again become a quasi-religious space – a temple dedicated to personal identity and the perfectibility of the body, where members pursue and achieve their individual *arete*.

Only Connect

In the past three millennia the gymnasium has undergone several major transformations, but its greatest change is probably only just beginning, as we enter the brave new world of hi-tech consumer electronics and wi-fi connectivity. In the short term, the gym is already undergoing a degree of diversification as new book-online-and-walk-in specialized training formats seduce members away from one-size-fits-all health clubs. In response, chain gyms have started to diversify and personalize the types of training they offer, moving away from the standard cardio-weights-classes formula to more innovative cross-training and class options. Given sufficient space, they provide a wide range of services to members, including cosmetic treatments, nutritional advice and complementary therapies, and capitalize on the social aspects of the gym with better facilities for members, such as chill-out zones, restaurants and cafés, and social programmes that reach out to local communities.

In the medium term, the industry could go one of two ways. Many mid-sized gyms might close, squeezed out by new, smaller, specialized training formats and super-sized budget gyms. Alternatively, they might thrive by providing a combination of fitness, social and healthcare functions to their neighbourhoods. The long-term prospects for the industry, however, are potentially the most exciting. The gym is already one of the most connected retail environments in terms of the electronic and Internet services it offers as standard to its users. But in a century's time, a historian of the gym might invite his viewers to visit a virtual 3-D, holographic gym that will combine features from big-screen entertainment and gaming with physical input and feedback devices that allow an exerciser to go full circle and train in the ancient Athenian Akademia alongside his favourite *eromenos*, perform on the gymnastics apparatus of the Hasenheide *Turnplatz* with fellow turners, or be coached by Arnold Schwarzenegger in Gold's Gym in 1975.

REFERENCES

INTRODUCTION

1 See www.fitness.gov and www.acefitness.org.

1 THE PURSUIT OF *ARETE*

1 The Greek kingdoms of Central Asia and northern India endured until the first century CE.
2 See 'Homer, *Iliad*, Book XXIII', www.classics.mit.edu, accessed 10 December 2012.
3 Vitruvius, *On Architecture*, trans. R. Tavernor and R. Schofield (London, 2009), pp. 157–9.
4 Mark Golden, *Sport and Society in Ancient Greece* (Cambridge, 1998), pp. 30–32.
5 Ibid., p. 176.
6 Eric Chaline, *Traveller's Guide to the Ancient World: Greece in the Year 415* BCE (London, 2008), pp. 62–9.
7 Stephen Miller, *Arete: Greek Sports from Ancient Sources* (Berkeley, CA, 2004), p. 17.
8 See 'Pliny, XV', www.penelope.uchicago.edu, accessed 10 April 2012.
9 Miller, *Arete*, p. 18.
10 The adjective 'phlegmatic' is a survival of a Graeco-Roman humorism.
11 For example, the sculptural scheme of the temple of Athena-Nike on the Acropolis in Athens.
12 The definition of a metic, and the rights they enjoyed, varied from *polis* to *polis*. In Classical Athens a citizen was supposed to have an Athenian mother and father, but in practice the regulations were not always adhered to, and could be waived by a vote of the Assembly. A citizen could also be stripped of his citizenship.

13 Chaline, *Traveller's Guide*, pp. 22–3.

14 John Camp and Elisabeth Fisher, *Exploring the World of the Ancient Greeks* (London, 2002), pp. 154–5.

15 Golden, *Sport and Society in Ancient Greece*, p. 176.

16 The Theban poet Pindar (c. 522–443 BCE) celebrated the winning athletes competing in the Pan-Hellenic games with victory odes.

17 Golden, *Sport and Society in Ancient Greece*, p. 177.

18 Quoted in Girolamo Mercuriale, *De Arte Gymnastica*, trans. V. Nutton (Florence, 2008), p. 183.

19 Robert Flacelière, *Daily Life in Ancient Greece at the Time of Pericles*, trans. P. Green (London, 1965), pp. 91–4.

20 Chaline, *Traveller's Guide*, p. 104–5.

21 The use of the word 'school' does not imply the existence of permanent, dedicated buildings, as would be the case with later educational institutions. During the classical period these were informal gatherings of teachers and students who met at gymnasia, in public spaces in the city and private houses.

22 Robin Osborne, *The History Written on the Classical Greek Body* (Cambridge, 2011), pp. 52–3.

23 Jenifer Neils, 'The Panathenaia and Kleisthenic Ideology', in *The Archeology of Athens Under the Democracy*, ed. W. Coulson (Oxford, 1994), pp. 151–60.

24 Flacelière, *Daily Life in Ancient Greece*, p. 111.

25 S. L. Glass, 'The Greek Gymnasium', in *The Archeology of the Olympics*, ed. W. J. Raschke (Madison, WI, 1988), p. 158.

26 For a full discussion of this topic, see Michel Foucault, *History of Sexuality*, vol. I: *The Will to Knowledge*, trans. R. Hurley (London, 1998).

27 Michel Foucault, *History of Sexuality*, vol. II: *The Use of Pleasure*, trans. R. Hurley (London, 1992), p. 38.

28 Quoted in Thomas K. Hubbard, *Homosexuality in Greece and Rome: A Sourcebook of Basic Documents* (Berkeley, CA, 2003), pp. 95–6.

29 Flacelière, *Daily Life in Ancient Greece*, pp. 109–12.

30 Quoted in Foucault, *The Use of Pleasure*, p. 199.

31 For a full discussion of this topic, see ibid., pp. 204ff.

32 Quoted in ibid., p. 72.

33 Hubbard, *Homosexuality in Greece and Rome*, p. 85.

34 The aristocratic *erastes–eromenos* pairing of Harmodios and Aristogeiton assassinated the ruling tyrant's younger brother, Hipparchus, in 514 BCE), striking a blow that would lead to the establishment of democracy in

Athens, but for very personal motives: because Hipparchus had slighted Harmodios' sister and made sexual advances to Harmodios himself.

35 Thomas K. Hubbard, ed., *Greek Love Reconsidered* (New York, 2000), pp. 7–8.

36 Quoted in Hubbard, *Homosexuality in Greece and Rome*, p. 99.

37 Miller, *Arete*, p. ix.

38 Christopher Hallett, *The Roman Nude: Heroic Portrait Statuary 200 BC–300 AD* (Oxford, 2005), p. 17.

39 Glass, 'The Greek Gymnasium', pp. 162–5.

40 Chaline, *Traveller's Guide*, pp. 75–7.

41 After his conquest of the Persian Empire, Alexander the Great continued eastwards across Central Asia to the borders of modern-day Pakistan, founding several cities that bore his name, where he settled his veterans, intermarrying them with the local population.

42 Miller, *Arete*, pp. 126–9.

43 Waldo Sweet, *Sport and Recreation in Ancient Greece* (Oxford, 1987), p. 104.

2 THE REBIRTH OF VITRUVIAN MAN

1 Britannia (England and Wales), Gaul (France), Iberia (Spain and Portugal), Italy and Illyricum (Albania, Croatia, Montenegro, Bosnia-Herzegovina and Slovenia).

2 See 'Plutarch, *Moralia, Roman Questions*', www.penelope.uchicago.edu, accessed 1 December 2013.

3 Christopher Hallett, *The Roman Nude: Heroic Portrait Statuary 200 BC–300 AD* (Oxford, 2005), pp. 61–4.

4 Ibid., p. 82.

5 Ibid., p. 75.

6 Ibid., p. 218.

7 Ibid., p. 264.

8 Ibid., p. 74.

9 Michel Foucault, *The History of Sexuality*, vol. III: *The Care of the Self*, trans. R. Hurley (London, 1990), 'Boys', pp. 187–228.

10 Jeffrey Weeks, *Sexuality and Its Discontents: Meanings, Myths and Modern Sexualities* (London, 1985), pp. 89–90.

11 'Thou shalt not make unto thee any graven image, or any likeness of any thing that is in heaven above, or that is in the earth beneath, or that is in the water under the earth' (Exodus 20:4; King James Version).

12 'Demes' comes from *demos*, the citizens of Athens, or the people; originally there were four factions, the Blues, Greens, Reds and Whites,

which were later reduced to two.

13 John Julius Norwich, *Byzantium: The Early Centuries* (London, 1990), p. 185.

14 For a detailed account of this period, see John Julius Norwich, *Byzantium: The Decline and Fall* (London, 1996).

15 Norwich, *The Early Centuries*, pp. 392–3.

16 Eleanor English, 'Sport, the Blessed Medicine of the Renaissance', www.library.la84.org, accessed 8 August 2011.

17 Johannes Gutenberg's (*c.* 1395–1468) invention of moveable type is usually dated to about 1439, some 30 years before the publication of Mercuriale's text.

18 Girolamo Mercuriale, *De Arte Gymnastica*, trans. V. Nutton (Florence, 2008), p. 5.

19 Ibid., p. 23.

20 Jan Todd, 'The History of Cardinal Farnese's "Weary Hercules"', *Iron Game History*, IX/I (2005), pp. 29–30.

21 Quoted in John Adamson, *A Short History of Education* (Cambridge, 1930), p. 156.

22 Lewis W. Spitz, *Johann Strum on Education: The Reformation and Humanist Learning* (St Louis, MO, 1995), p. 62.

23 Quoted ibid., p. 248.

24 Eric Chaline, *Simple Path to Yoga* (London, 2001), pp. 46–50.

25 Eric Chaline, *The Book of Zen* (Gloucester, MA, 2003), pp. 12–15.

26 Ibid., pp. 26–7.

27 Peter Lewis, *The Martial Arts: Origins, Philosophy, Practice* (London, 2001), pp. 39–74.

28 Eric Chaline, *Tai Chi for Body, Mind & Spirit* (New York, 1998), pp. 6–11.

29 Chaline, *Simple Path to Yoga*, pp. 170–88; Ted Kaptchuk, *Chinese Medicine: The Web That Has No Weaver* (Victoria, NSW, 1983), pp. 35–40.

30 Gilbert Andrieu, *La gymnastique au XIXe siècle* (Paris, 1999) deals with the period 1789–1914, but he makes several references to the physical culture of the Ancien Régime throughout the text. See pp. 14–22.

31 Ibid., p. 18.

32 Kasia Boddy, *Boxing: A Cultural History* (London, 2008), pp. 26–54.

3 THE HEALTH OF NATIONS

1 Voltaire, *Essai sur l'histoire générale et sur les mœurs et l'esprit des nations*, chapter 70: 'Ce corps qui s'appelait et qui s'appelle encore le saint empire romain n'était en aucune manière ni saint, ni romain, ni empire.'

2 James Bryce, *The Holy Roman Empire* (London, 1871), p. 302.

3 Peter Gay, *The Enlightenment: The Rise of Modern Paganism* (New York, 1995), p. 3.

4 Quoted ibid., p. 20.

5 John Locke, *Some Thoughts Concerning Education* (Oxford, 1989), pp. 252–4.

6 Robert Quick, *Essays on Educational Reformers* (New York, 1896), p. 227.

7 Jurgen Glessing and Jan Todd, 'The Origin of German Bodybuilding', *Iron Game History*, IX/2 (2005), pp. 8–9.

8 Christian Salzmann and Johann Guts Muths, *Gymnastics for Youth, Or, A Practical Guide to Healthful and Amusing Exercises for the Use of Schools: An Essay Toward the Necessary Improvement of Education, Chiefly as it Relates to the Body* (London, 1800), pp. 168–9.

9 Ibid., p. 189.

10 Saket Tiwari, Chhote Rathor and Yogesh Singh, *History of Physical Education* (New Delhi, 2003), p. 144; V. K. Rao, *Teaching of Physical Education* (New Delhi, 2008), p. 2.

11 Friedrich Jahn, *Die Deutsche Turnkunst* (Berlin, 1816), p. 25.

12 Friedrich Jahn, *A Treatise on Gymnasticks*, trans. Charles Beck (Northampton, MA, 1828), pp. 156–70.

13 Ibid., p. 156.

14 Beck uses 'gymnick' in his translation, where I have preferred 'turner'. Ibid., p. 158.

15 Ibid., p. 157.

16 Glessing and Todd, 'The Origin of German Bodybuilding', p. 10.

17 Rao, *Teaching of Physical Education*, pp. 11–12.

18 The Sacramento Turnverein website, www.sacramentoturnverein.com, gives a fascinating insight into the history and continuing role of the turners in the United States.

19 Richard Mandell, *The Nazi Olympics* (Urbana, IL, 1971), p. 154.

20 Britain did not have the draft (conscription) until the First World War, but relied on a small professional standing army and volunteers in times of national emergency.

21 David Chapman, *Sandow the Magnificient: Eugen Sandow and the Beginnings of Bodybuilding* (Urbana, IL, 2006), pp. 44–5.

22 Rao, *Teaching of Physical Education*, p. 2.

23 Marc Le Coeur, 'Couvert, découvert, redécouvert . . . L'invention du gymnase scolaire en France (1818–1872)', *Histoire de l'education*, 102 (2004), p. 4, published online on 27 May 2009.

24 Hugo Rothstein and Pehr Ling, *The Gymnastic Exercises of P. H. Ling*, trans. M. Roth (London, 1853), p. 122.

25 Rao, *Teaching of Physical Education*, p. 6.

26 George Mélio, *Manual of Swedish Drill* (London, 1889), p. 18.

27 Ibid., pp. 24 and 30.

28 Ibid., p. 7.

29 Ken Worpole, *Here Comes the Sun: Architecture and Public Space in Twentieth-century European Culture* (London, 2000), pp. 43–8.

30 Gilbert Andrieu, *La gymnastique au xixe siècle* (Paris, 1999), pp. 14–22.

31 Johann H. Pestalozzi, *How Gertrude Teaches Her Children*, trans. Lucy Holland and Francis Taylor (London, 1938), p. 177.

32 Andrieu, *La gymnastique au xixe siècle*, p. 29.

33 Francisco Amoros, *Manuel de l'éducation physique, gymnastique et morale* (Paris, 1830), pp. 57–61.

34 Quoted in Andrieu, *La gymnastique au xixe siècle*, p. 30.

35 Ibid., p. 32.

36 Le Coeur, 'Couvert, découvert, redécouvert', p. 13.

37 Ibid., p. 19.

38 Georges Hébert, *La Culture Virile et les Devoirs Physiques de l'Officier Combattant* (Paris, 1913), pp. 11–12.

39 Kasia Boddy, *Boxing: A Cultural History* (London, 2008), chapter 4, pp. 76–109.

40 Rao, *Teaching of Physical Education*, p. 8.

41 Archibald MacLaren, *A System of Physical Education Theoretical and Practical* (Oxford, 1869), p. 505.

42 For illustration and the accompanying article, see 'Gymnasium', www. oxfordhistory.org.uk, accessed 6 September 2013.

43 Michael Budd, *The Sculpture Machine: Physical Culture and Body Politics in the Age of Empire* (Basingstoke, Hampshire, 1997), p. 20.

4 THE WORLD'S STRONGEST MAN

1 The Congress of Vienna was interrupted by Napoleon's 'Hundred Days' (20 March–8 July 1815), when he escaped from the island of Elba and tried to regain his throne.

2 Louis was the younger brother of the guillotined Louis xvi, and the uncle of the *dauphin*, posthumously known as Louis xvii by French royalists, although he was never crowned. France's flirtation with constitutional monarchy lasted until 1848, when it made way for the

short-lived Second Republic (1848–52). The republic was overthrown by the Second French Empire, which lasted until the establishment of the Third Republic in 1870.

3 Eric Chaline, *Fifty Machines that Changed the Course of History* (Buffalo, NY, 2012), pp. 84–110, covers the main inventions that defined the Second Industrial Revolution.

4 Ibid., pp. 90–93.

5 Gilbert Andrieu, *La gymnastique au XIXe siècle* (Paris, 1999), pp. 14–22.

6 Ibid., pp. 56–9.

7 In many countries, one could add white and members of the national or majority church.

8 Jeremy Bentham, *Selected Writings on Utilitarianism* (Ware, MA, 2001), pp. 87–8.

9 Ibid., p. 120.

10 John Stuart Mill, *On Liberty*, ed. Edward Alexander (Peterborough, ON, 1999), pp. 55 and 101.

11 Michel Foucault, *History of Sexuality*, vol. 1: *The Will to Knowledge*, trans. R. Hurley (London, 1998); Jeffrey Weeks, *Sex, Politics and Society: The Regulation of Sexuality since 1800* (Harlow, 2012).

12 Eric Chaline, *History's Worst Disasters* (New York, 2013), pp. 109–14. On the first day of the Battle of the Somme, the criminally incompetent British commander Field Marshal Haig sacrificed 57,470 British and imperial troops, considering the loss not 'severe'.

13 Andrieu, *La gymnastique au XIXe siècle*, pp. 14–16.

14 The term 'homosexual' came into use in the 1860s, and therefore is no longer anachronistic. At the time it defined a psychopathology also referred to as 'inversion', and not the lifestyle choice it would become in the twentieth century.

15 David Chapman, *Sandow the Magnificent: Eugen Sandow and the Beginnings of Bodybuilding* (Urbana, IL, 2006), p. 4.

16 Gilbert Andrieu, *Force et beauté* (Bordeaux, 1992), p. 64. The society's prospectus of 1847 was grandly titled *Société milonienne pour l'exploitation de la gymnastique appliquée à la réhabilitation physique de l'homme, d'après la méthode de M. Triat.*

17 Andrieu, *La gymnastique au XIXe siècle*, p. 65.

18 Chapman, *Sandow the Magnificent*, p. 127.

19 David Chapman, 'Hippolyte Triat. From: Edmond Desbonnet's *Les rois de la force*', *Iron Game History*, IV/1 (1995), p. 6.

20 Edmond Desbonnet, *Les rois de la force* (Paris, 1911), pp. 58–78.

21 Andrieu, La gymnastique au XIXe siècle, p. 35. Aerobic conditioning of the cardiovascular system would be understood only in the twentieth century, but Triat's gymnastique would certainly have developed heart–lung fitness and promoted fat burning, rather than building muscle mass. In this, Triat probably understood his market perfectly, as they were very likely more concerned with losing weight than with developing a hyper-muscular physique.

22 Ibid., p, 44.

23 Chapman, Sandow the Magnificent, pp. 8–10.

24 Ibid., pp. 18–19. Sandow had close male relationships during his youth, some of which, Chapman believes, might have gone beyond mere friendship. However, such was Sandow's and his partners' discretion that the stories were never confirmed. He later married, and fathered two daughters.

25 £500 would be worth an estimated $20,000/£12,000 today.

26 Chapman, Sandow the Magnificent, p. 77. The short film is available on youtube.com and wikipedia.com.

27 Ibid., pp. 101–2.

28 Ibid., pp. 114–16. The Combined Developer combined a chest expander, rubber bands and dumb-bells in one piece of multi-purpose equipment that could be fitted to a door. Similar home gym equipment continues to be sold today, but after a couple of uses usually ends up forgotten in the bottom of a cupboard, in the attic or under the bed.

29 Ibid., pp. 129–31. The statues were gold and silver plate, and not solid as advertised. A copy of the statue is still used as the prize for the Mr Olympia bodybuilding contest.

30 See www.olympic.org, 'Weightlifting Equipment and History', accessed 18 December 2013.

31 Jan Todd, 'From Milo to Milo: A History of Barbells, Dumbbells, and Indian Clubs', Iron Game History, III/6 (1995), p. 10.

32 Jan Todd, '"Strength is Health": George Barker Windship and the First American', Iron Game History, III/1 (1993), pp. 3–14. Windship started a one-man fad for bodybuilding in the U.S. in the mid-nineteenth century. However, his early death of a stroke at the age of 42, which was blamed on weight training, led many to abandon the sport for other health-related pursuits.

33 Todd, 'From Milo to Milo', p. 12.

34 Todd, 'Strength is Health', p. 5.

35 For a fully illustrated account of the Polymachinon and its use, see James Chiosso, The Gymnastic Polymachinon: Instructions for Performing

a *Systematic Series of Exercises on the Gymnastic & Calisthenic Polymachinon* (New York, 1855).

5 PUMPING IRON

1 Eric Chaline, *Fifty Machines that Changed the Course of History* (Buffalo, NY, 2012), pp. 104–9.

2 Michael Budd, *The Sculpture Machine: Physical Culture and Body Politics in the Age of Empire* (Basingstoke, Hampshire, 1997), p. 13.

3 Jeffrey Weeks, *Making Sexual History* (Malden, MA, 2000), p. 37.

4 Harrison Pope, Katherine Philips and Roberto Olivardia, *The Adonis Complex: The Secret Crisis of Male Body Obsession* (New York, 2000), pp. 12–13.

5 David Chapman, *Sandow the Magnificent: Eugen Sandow and the Beginnings of Bodybuilding* (Urbana, IL, 2006), pp. 148–9.

6 Ibid., pp. 109 and 135.

7 Sam Dana, 'The 97-Pound Weakling Who Became "The World's Most Perfectly Developed Man"', *Iron Game History*, IV/4 (1996), pp. 3–4.

8 See www.musclebeach.net, 'Santa Monica', accessed 30 September 2013.

9 Ed Murray, *Muscle Beach* (London, 1980), p. 9.

10 Jan Todd and Terry Todd, 'Steve Reeves: The Last Interview', *Iron Game History*, VI/4 (2000), p. 3.

11 Ibid., p. 6.

12 Murray, *Muscle Beach*, p. 47.

13 Ibid., pp. 13–14.

14 See www.musclebeach.net, 'Santa Monica'.

15 See www.iron-age-classic-bodybuilding.com, 'Vic Tanny', accessed 3 October 2013.

16 Todd and Todd, 'Steve Reeves: The Last Interview', p. 5.

17 See www.iron-age-classic-bodybuilding.com, 'Vic Tanny'.

18 See www.jacklalanne.com, 'Jack's Adventures – King of Fitness', accessed 3 October 2013.

19 See ibid.

20 See www.jacklalanne.com, 'Jack's Adventures – Firsts', accessed 4 October 2013.

21 See www.jacklalanne.com, 'Jack's Adventures', accessed 3 October 2013.

22 Jack LaLanne, *The Jack LaLanne Way to Vibrant Good Health* (New York, 1970), pp. 83 and 54.

23 See www.clubindustry.com, 'Fitness – Evolution of Health Clubs' and www.nationalfitnesshalloffame.com, 'Bob Delmonteque', accessed 7 October 2013.

24 A picture of the original cycle is available on www.lifefitness.com.

25 See www.lifefitness.com, 'Life Fitness Legends: Ray Wilson', accessed 7 October 2013.

26 *Pumping Iron* (1977), directed by George Butler and Robert Fiore.

27 Pope et al., *The Adonis Complex*, p. 52.

28 See www.bodybuilding.com, 'Golden Age Legends, Part 1: Golden Age Greats', accessed 6 October 2013.

29 See www.clubindustry.com, 'Fitness – Evolution of Health Clubs'.

30 See www.fundinguniverse.com, 'Company Histories: Bally Total Fitness', accessed 7 October 2013.

31 Although many top competitive bodybuilders, including Arnold Schwarzenegger, have admitted to using steroids and other forms of illegal supplementation, Ronnie Coleman has always denied using them. An Internet search on 'Ronnie Coleman and steroids', however, reveals that the topic is still the subject of a lively debate in the body-building community several years after Coleman's retirement from competition. In a short YouTube clip, Arnold Schwarzenegger discusses his steroid use in about 1977. Owing to the temporary nature of YouTube, this may no longer exist at the time of publication; however, a search for 'Arnold Schwarzenegger and steroids' will no doubt find the same interview.

32 Charles Yesalis, ed., *Anabolic Steroids in Sport and Exercise*, 2nd edn (Champaign, IL, 2000), pp. 21–38.

33 Ibid., pp. 118–19.

34 Pope et al., *The Adonis Complex*, pp. 103–4.

35 Yesalis, *Anabolic Steroids in Sport and Exercise*, p. 365.

36 Pope et al., *The Adonis Complex*, pp. 120–21.

37 See www.homegymsonline.info, 'Joe Weider: His Fitness Legacy', accessed 10 October 2013.

38 Pope et al., *The Adonis Complex*, p. 87. Muscle dysmorphia was recognized as a psychiatric disorder as defined in the American Psychiatric Association's *Diagnostics and Statistical Manual of Mental Disorders* IV (Arlington, VA, 1994).

39 Ibid., pp. 10–11.

40 Pope et al., *The Adonis Complex*, p. 97.

41 Ibid., pp. 40–44.

42 Ibid., p. 51.

43 Ibid., p. 5.

6 LET'S GET PHYSICAL

1 Germaine Greer, *The Female Eunuch* (London, 1971), 'Curves', pp. 33–5.

2 For a selection of calendars, see www.pirellical.com.

3 Eric Chaline, *Traveller's Guide to the Ancient World: Greece in the Year 415 BCE* (London, 2008), pp. 28–9.

4 Ibid., p 51. The most famous *korai* are the caryatids that support the porch of the Erechtheion in Athens.

5 Ibid., pp. 116–17.

6 See www.attalus.org, 'Athenaeus, 13b', accessed 16 October 2013.

7 For a fantastic modern re-telling of the story, see *300* (2007), directed by Zack Snyder and starring Gerard Butler as King Leonidas of Sparta.

8 Robert Flacelière, *Daily Life in Ancient Greece at the Time of Pericles*, trans. P. Green (London, 1965), p. 84.

9 Stephen Miller, *Arete: Greek Sports from Ancient Sources* (Berkeley, CA, 2004), p. 105.

10 Ibid., p. 106.

11 See www.ancientolympics.arts.kuleuven.be, 'Female Olympic Victors in the Horse Races', accessed 16 October 2013.

12 Waldo Sweet, *Sport and Recreation in Ancient Greece* (Oxford, 1987), pp. 134–8.

13 See www.ancientolympics.arts.kuleuven.be, 'The Heraia', accessed 16 October 2013.

14 Jan Todd, 'From Milo to Milo: A History of Barbells, Dumbbells, and Indian Clubs', *Iron Game History*, III/6 (1995), pp. 4–5.

15 Michel Foucault, *The History of Sexuality*, vol. III: *The Care of the Self*, trans. R. Hurley (London, 1990). See 'The Wife', pp. 145–86.

16 Panniers were wickerwork basket armatures that extended the skirt to the sides.

17 Jan Todd, 'The Classical Ideal and its Impact on the Search for Suitable Exercise: 1774–1830', *Iron Game History*, II/4 (1992), pp. 6–16.

18 A flying course was a pole with ropes attached at the top that allowed gymnasts to run and leap in a circular course, while supporting their full bodyweight with their arms.

19 Todd, 'The Classical Ideal', p. 10.

20 Ibid., pp. 11–12.

21 Reproduced on p. 101 of Jan Todd's *Physical Culture and the Body Beautiful: Purposive Exercise in the Lives of American Women, 1800–1870* (Macon, GA, 1989).

22 For a romanticized Hollywood version of the crinoline, which is nevertheless accurate in terms of its size and physical limitations on the women who wore it, see *The King and I* (1956) directed by Walter Lang and starring Yul Brynner and Deborah Kerr.

23 Edmond Desbonnet, 'Le gymnase Triat', in *Les rois de la force* (Paris, 1911), pp. 60–78.

24 Jan Todd, 'The Origins of Weight Training for Female Athletes in North America', *Iron Game History*, 11/2 (1992), p. 4.

25 David Chapman, *Sandow the Magnificent: Eugen Sandow and the Beginnings of Bodybuilding* (Urbana, IL, 2006), p. 103.

26 Ibid., pp. 164–7.

27 Desbonnet, *Les rois de la force*, pp. 380–87, 395, 397–8.

28 Jan Todd, 'The Legacy of Pudgy Stockton', *Iron Game History*, 11/2 (1992), pp. 5–6.

29 Jan Todd, 'Pudgy Stockton, the Belle of the Barbell', *Iron Game History*, X/1 (2007), p. 3.

30 Todd, 'The Legacy of Pudgy Stockton', p. 7.

31 See www.bodybuilding.com, 'Olympia 2013: Weekend Photos', accessed 12 October 2013. The different galleries feature the top competitors and winners in each class of the contest for both men and women. See www.wbffshows.com, 'Events', for the WBFF men's and women's categories.

32 *Fame* (1980), directed by Alan Parker and starring Irene Kara.

33 Kenneth Cooper, *Aerobics* (New York, 1968), pp. 9–15.

34 Ibid., p. 6.

35 Kenneth Cooper, *The New Aerobics* (New York, 1970), p. 128.

36 See www.jackisorensen.com, 'Biographies', accessed 23 October 2013.

37 Jane Fonda, *My Life So Far* (New York, 2005), pp. 386–400.

38 Ibid., pp. 399–400.

7 MACHO MAN

1 Michel Foucault, *History of Sexuality: The Will to Knowledge*, vol. I, trans. R. Hurley (London, 1998), 'The Repressive Hypothesis', pp. 15–50.

2 Eric Chaline, *Gay Planet: All Things for All Gay Men* (New York, 2000), pp. 36–9.

3 David Chapman, *Sandow the Magnificient: Eugen Sandow and the Beginnings of Bodybuilding* (Urbana, IL, 2006), pp. 202–3.

4 Erick Alvarez, *Muscle Boys: Gay Gym Culture* (London, 2008), pp. 48–9.

5 Valentine Hooven, *Beefcake: The Muscle Magazines of America, 1950–1970* (Cologne, 1995), pp. 14–15.

6 Ibid., pp. 24–33.

7 Ibid., pp. 50–51.

8 Ibid., pp. 46–7.

9 Ibid., pp. 42–3.

10 Alvarez, *Muscle Boys*, pp. 99–102.

11 Ibid., pp. 96–8.

12 *Jeffrey* (1995), directed by Chrisopher Ashley and starring Steven Webber and Michael T. Weiss.

13 See www.sohogyms.com, accessed 13 November 2013.

14 Chaline, *Gay Planet*, 'Hope', pp. 62–71.

15 Alvarez, *Muscle Boys*, pp. 139–44.

16 Ibid., p. 93.

17 Harrison Pope, Katherine Philips and Roberto Olivardia, *The Adonis Complex: The Secret Crisis of Male Body Obsession* (New York, 2000), p. 213.

18 Alvarez, *Muscle Boys*, pp. 140–44, 151.

19 Ibid., pp. 76–9.

20 Ibid., p. 90.

8 CONSUMING FITNESS

1 The relative proportions of body fat and lean muscle mass. For body fat, essential fat M: 2–5 per cent, W: 10–13 per cent; average fat M: 18–24 per cent, W: 25–31 per cent; obese M: 25 per cent+, W: 32 per cent+.

2 In the UK and U.S., shows such as *Ten Years Younger* use a mix of cosmetic and surgical procedures to transform subjects (www.channel4.com, 'Ten Years Younger', accessed 1 December 2014).

3 For a full discussion of these topics, see Anthony Giddens, *Modernity and Self-identity: Self and Society in the Late Modern Age* (Cambridge, 1991) and *Runaway World* (London, 1999).

4 Body Mass Index (BMI) rates are calculated by an individual's weight in kilograms divided by the square of their height in metres; a BMI of 18.5–25 is normal; 25–30 is overweight; 30–35 is moderately obese; 35–40 is severely obese; and 40+ is very severely obese.

5 See www.surgeongeneral.gov, 'Obesity – Facts at a Glance', accessed

3 November 2013; www.cornell.edu, 'Obesity Accounts for 21 Percent of u.s. Health Care Costs', accessed 21 September 2014.

6 See www.who.int, 'Factsheets – Obesity', accessed 6 November 2013.

7 See IHRSA, 'Fitness Industry Stands Strong Despite Downward Economic Trend', at www.theleisuredatebase.com, accessed 20 August 2013.

8 *The Men Who Made Us Thin*, www.bbc.co.uk.

9 *The Men Who Made Us Thin*, episode 2.

10 Suzie Dale, Sue Godinet, Natalie Kearse and Adrian Field, *The Future of Fitness* (Auckland, 2009), p. 8.

11 See www.cdc.gov, 'Genomics and Health', accessed 30 January 2014.

12 Dale et al., *The Future of Fitness*, p. 1.

13 Ibid., p. 6.

14 A round cast-iron weight with a handle that is used to perform dynamic weight-training exercises that develop a mix of strength, endurance and flexibility.

15 See www.ginmillerfitness.com, 'Gin Miller Biography', accessed 7 November 2013.

16 Eric Chaline, *Simple Path to Yoga* (London, 2001), pp. 102–3.

17 See www.crossfit.com and, for example, www.psyclefitness.com.

18 Exergaming is a combination of exercise and gaming; Dale et al., *The Future of Fitness*, p. 6.

19 See www.sohogyms.com, 'Gyms', accessed 20 December 2013.

20 See www.blinkfitness.com and www.easygym.co.uk.

21 See www.equinox.com and www.hardcandyfitness.com.

22 See www.tonyhortonsworld.com.

SELECT BIBLIOGRAPHY

Alvarez, Erick, *Muscle Boys: Gay Gym Culture* (London, 2008)

Amoros, Francisco, *Gymnase normal, militaire et civil: Idée et état de cette institution au commencement de l'année 1821* (Paris, 1821)

—, *Manuel de l'éducation physique, gymnastique et morale* (Paris, 1830)

Andrieu, Gilbert, *La gymnastique au XIXe siècle* (Paris, 1999)

Bentham, Jeremy, *Selected Writings on Utilitarianism* (Ware, MA, 2001)

Boddy, Kasia, *Boxing: A Cultural History* (London, 2008)

Budd, Michael, *The Sculpture Machine: Physical Culture and Body Politics in the Age of Empire* (Basingstoke, Hampshire, 1997)

Camp, John, *The Archaeology of Athens* (New Haven, CT, 2001)

—, and Elisabeth Fisher, *Exploring the World of the Ancient Greeks* (London, 2002)

Chaline, Eric, *Gay Planet: All Things for All Gay Men* (New York, 2000)

—, *Simple Path to Yoga* (London, 2001)

—, *Traveller's Guide to the Ancient World: Greece in the Year 415 BCE* (London, 2008)

Chapman, David, 'Hippolyte Triat. From: Edmond Desbonnet's *Les rois de la force*', *Iron Game History*, IV/I (1995), pp. 3–10

—, *Sandow the Magnificent: Eugen Sandow and the Beginnings of Bodybuilding* (Urbana, IL, 2006)

Cooper, Kenneth, *Aerobics* (New York, 1968)

Dale, Suzie, Sue Godinet, Natalie Kearse and Adrian Field, *The Future of Fitness* (Auckland, 2009)

Desbonnet, Edmond, *Les rois de la force* (Paris, 1911)

Flacelière, Robert, *Daily Life in Ancient Greece at the Time of Pericles*, trans. P. Green (London, 1965)

Fonda, Jane, *My Life So Far* (New York, 2005)

Foucault, Michel, *The History of Sexuality*, vol. III: *The Care of the Self*, trans. R. Hurley (London, 1990)

—, *The History of Sexuality*, vol. II: *The Use of Pleasure*, trans. R. Hurley (London, 1992)

—, *The History of Sexuality*, vol. I: *The Will to Knowledge*, trans R. Hurley (London, 1998)

Fukuyama, Francis, *The End of History and the Last Man* (New York, 1992)

Gay, Peter, *The Enlightenment: The Rise of Modern Paganism* (New York, 1995)

Gibbon, Edward, *The History of the Decline and Fall of the Roman Empire* (Ware, MA, 1998)

Giddens, Anthony, *Modernity and Self-Identity: Self and Society in the Late Modern Age* (Cambridge, 1991)

Glass, S. L., 'The Greek Gymnasium', in *The Archeology of the Olympics*, ed. W. J. Raschke (Madison, WI, 1988)

Golden, Mark, *Sport and Society in Ancient Greece* (Cambridge, 1998)

Greer, Germaine, *The Female Eunuch* (London, 1971)

Hallett, Christopher, *The Roman Nude: Heroic Portrait Statuary 200 BC–300 AD* (Oxford, 2005)

Hébert, Georges, *La Culture Virile et les Devoirs Physiques de l'Officier Combattant* (Paris, 1913)

Homer, *The Iliad* (Ware, MA, 1995)

Hooven III, Valentine F., *Beefcake: The Muscle Magazines of America 1950–1970* (Cologne, 1995)

Hubbard, Thomas K., ed., *Greek Love Reconsidered* (New York, 2000)

Jahn, Friedrich, *Die Deutsche Turnkunst* (Berlin, 1816)

—, *A Treatise on Gymnasticks*, trans. Charles Beck (Northampton, MA, 1828)

LaLanne, Jack, *The Jack LaLanne Way to Vibrant Good Health* (New York, 1970)

Le Coeur, Marc, 'Couvert, découvert, redécouvert . . . L'invention du gymnase scolaire en France (1818–1872)', *Histoire de l'éducation*, 104 (2004), published online on 27 May 2009, www.histoire-education.revues.org

Lewis, Peter, *The Martial Arts: Origins, Philosophy, Practice* (London, 2001)

Locke, John, *Some Thoughts Concerning Education* (Oxford, 1989)

Mélio, George, *Manual of Swedish Drill* (London, 1889)

Mercuriale, Girolamo, *De Arte Gymnastica*, trans. V. Nutton (Florence, 2008)

Mill, John Stuart, *On Liberty*, ed. Edward Alexander (Peterborough, ON, 1999)

Miller, Stephen, *Arete: Greek Sports from Ancient Sources* (Berkeley, CA, 2004)

Norwich, John Julius, *Byzantium: The Apogee* (London, 1993)

—, *Byzantium: The Decline and Fall* (London, 1996)

—, *Byzantium: The Early Centuries* (London, 1990)

Osborne, Robin, *The History Written on the Classical Greek Body* (Cambridge, 2011)

Pope, Harrison, Katherine Philips and Roberto Olivardia, *The Adonis Complex: The Secret Crisis of Male Body Obsession* (New York, 2000)

Porter, Roy, *The Greatest Benefit to Mankind* (London, 1997)

Rao, V. K., *Teaching of Physical Education* (New Delhi, 2008)

Rothstein, Hugo, and Pehr Ling, *The Gymnastic Exercises of P. H. Ling*, trans. M. Roth (London, 1853)

Rousseau, Jean-Jacques, *Emile, or, On Education*, trans. Allan Bloom (New York, 1979)

Salzmann, Christian, and Johann Guts Muths, *Gymnastics for Youth, Or, A Practical Guide to Healthful and Amusing Exercises for the Use of Schools: An Essay Toward the Necessary Improvement of Education, Chiefly as it Relates to the Body* (London, 1800)

Sandow, Eugen, *Strength and How to Obtain It* (Aldershot, Hampshire, 1897)

Swatmarama, *Hatha Yoga Pradipika* (Munger, India, 2005)

Sweet, Waldo, *Sport and Recreation in Ancient Greece* (Oxford, 1987)

Todd, Jan, 'The Classical Ideal and its Impact on the Search for Suitable Exercise: 1774–1830', *Iron Game History*, II/4 (1992), pp. 6–16

—, 'The History of Cardinal Farnese's "Weary Hercules"', *Iron Game History*, IX/1 (2005), pp. 29–34

—, 'The Legacy of Pudgy Stockton', *Iron Game History*, II/2 (1992), pp. 5–7

—, 'From Milo to Milo: A History of Barbells, Dumbbells, and Indian Clubs', *Iron Game History*, III/6 (1995), pp. 4–16

—, 'The Origins of Weight Training for Female Athletes in North America', *Iron Game History*, II/2 (1992), pp. 4–14

—, 'Pudgy Stockton, the Belle of the Barbell', *Iron Game History*, X/1 (2007), pp. 1–3

—, '"Strength is Health": George Barker Windship and the First American', *Iron Game History*, III/1 (1993), pp. 3–14

—, and Terry Todd, 'Steve Reeves: The Last Interview', *Iron Game History*, VI/4 (2000), pp. 2–14

Vitruvius, *On Architecture*, trans. R. Tavernor and R. Schofield (London, 2009)

Weeks, Jeffrey, *Making Sexual History* (Malden, MA, 2000)

—, *Sex, Politics and Society: The Regulation of Sexuality since 1800* (Harlow, 2012)

—, *Sexuality and Its Discontents: Meanings, Myths and Modern Sexualities* (London, 1985)

Yesalis, Charles, ed., *Anabolic Steroids in Sport and Exercise*, 2nd edn (Champaign, IL, 2000)

PHOTO ACKNOWLEDGEMENTS

The author and publishers wish to express their thanks to the below sources for illustrative material and/or permission to reproduce it.

Getty Images: pp. 143, 168, 201; Jubilee Hall: pp. 228, 231, 233; © Pavel L Photo and Video/Shutterstock: p. 212; © Shutterstock: pp. 229, 241; © B. Stefanov/ Shutterstock: p. 136; © Trustees of the British Museum, London: pp. 14, 20, 25; courtesy of the Wellcome Library, London: pp. 27, 29, 59, 65, 76, 97, 108, 119, 126, 133, 180; © Vladimir Wrangel/Shutterstock: p. 194.

INDEX

Italic page numbers indicate illustrations

Decifrando o Apocalipse

AS PROFECIAS DA BÍBLIA

Luiz Roberto Mattos

SUMÁRIO

Introdução

A palavra *profecia* vem do grego *prophetéia*, e do latim *prophetia*, e significa *predição do futuro, que se crê por inspiração divina, anúncio de acontecimentos futuros*, segundo o dicionário da língua portuguesa Houaiss.

O propósito desta obra é fazer uma análise sistemática e conjunta de profecias feitas pelos profetas judeus ao longo de mais de dois mil e setecentos anos, principalmente acerca daquilo que ficou conhecido como *O Juízo Final ou Juízo Universal.* E, ainda, juntar aos escritos sobre essas duas expressões por demais conhecidas as revelações contidas no *Apocalipse* de São João, último livro da Bíblia Católica, e mais as profecias de *Nostradamus* a respeito dos fatos antes previstos pelos profetas judeus, inclusive Jesus Cristo.

Ao longo deste livro, pretendo estabelecer uma relação clara, nítida e lógica entre O Fim dos Tempos de que falava Jesus, O Juízo Final já pregado antes dele pelos profetas de Israel, o Apocalipse escrito pelo apóstolo João, e ainda as profecias de Nostradamus.

Mas não é só.

Pretendo, ainda, demonstrar que muitos fatos futuros previstos por Jesus, Nostradamus e as revelações dadas ao apóstolo João e registradas no livro Apocalipse estão relacionados entre si, e que o sofrimento futuro e maior da humanidade, visualizada há mais de dois mil e quinhentos anos atrás, será causado não por uma guerra nuclear, como muitos intérpretes de Nostradamus têm entendido, mas pela colisão de um asteróide ou um cometa com a Terra, de forma semelhante ao que aconteceu há 65 milhões de anos atrás, e que causou a extinção de cerca de 75% das espécies animais do planeta, e levou à extinção os dinossauros, como hoje se acredita, mas não acabou por completo com a vida na Terra, tanto que aqui estamos escrevendo e lendo.

Para isso, após estudar profundamente os livros dos profetas no Antigo Testamento, os quatro Evangelhos do Novo Testamento, o livro Apocalipse, de São João e o livro As Centúrias, de Nostradamus, tive que recorrer também ao estudo das enciclopédias e sites atualizados de astronomia na internet, inclusive da NASA, para aprender um pouco mais a respeito de meteoróides, meteoros e meteoritos, com suas diferenças, bem como sobre asteróides e cometas, e sobre os riscos potenciais e reais de colisão de um deles com a Terra a qualquer momento.

O que viso demonstrar com a interpretação dos diversos livros da Bíblia e ainda dos escritos de Nostradamus é que todos eles previram uma grande catástrofe no mundo, não causada por guerras, pois elas representariam apenas o início das dores, como descrito nos livros, inclusive dito por Jesus, mas por uma catástrofe natural, causada, no entanto, por algo vindo do espaço, um ou vários objetos vindos do "céu".

Demonstrarei, também, a possibilidade concreta de estar próximo o evento, conclamando a humanidade a uma reflexão urgente, e a uma revisão e mudança de valores de forma concreta, pois o evento catastrófico nos pegará de surpresa, sem tempo para mudança de vida e de atitude.

Com a catástrofe, haverá a tão falada separação do joio e do trigo, ou, em outras palavras, dos bons e dos maus. E depois dela a Terra será herdada pelos bons, pelos pacíficos, e *"as nações não se adestrarão mais para a guerra"*, como escreveu o profeta Isaías e confirmou Jesus seiscentos anos depois.

As duas guerras mundiais vividas pela humanidade no século XX foram apenas parte do início das dores, mas não são nada em comparação com o que ainda está por vir.

Guerras outras ainda teremos, talvez uma grande guerra "santa" entre Oriente Médio e Ocidente. Mas isso não será o "fim dos tempos", nem o "fim do mundo", nem tampouco a catástrofe maior prevista no Apocalipse. Esta última será materializada com a chegada e colisão com a Terra de um grande asteróide ou um cometa, e há muitos corpos rochosos nos rondando no espaço. Apenas em nosso sistema solar existem mais de 70.000 asteróides, como indicam os astrônomos, e como descreveremos em detalhes no primeiro capítulo deste livro.

Mostraremos que ao longo de toda a história de nosso planeta fomos e continuamos sendo bombardeados por meteoros, asteróides e fragmentos de cometa, como o que caiu na Rússia em 1.908, do mesmo modo que a Lua, Marte, Júpiter e Vênus, planetas de nosso sistema solar, cujas crateras de impacto são os retratos vivos desses choques de corpos rochosos vindos do espaço.

Uma análise sistemática, e não isolada dos livros da Bíblia que contêm profecias e revelações nos mostra que a humanidade não desaparecerá da Terra, e que a vida não será extinta, mas que haverá grande dor e sofrimento, e muita destruição e morte, muito maior do que haveria em uma guerra nuclear moderna.

Mostrarei que vários corpos celestes como meteoros, asteróides e cometas passam próximo da Terra com relativa freqüência, e que recentemente grandes corpos celestes chegaram a ser mesmo considerados ameaça à nossa sobrevivência, mas que os astrônomos se equivocaram. E que a qualquer momento pode haver choques entre os milhares de asteróides do denominado "Cinturão de Asteróides", que fica entre as órbitas dos planetas Marte e Júpiter, com o deslocamento de um deles em nossa direção, com grande perigo para a humanidade, que não teria para onde fugir.

E o mais relevante é que a humanidade se lembre das palavras de Jesus, o qual não mentiria, e não aumentaria apenas para assustar, que disse que deveríamos estar preparados para não sermos pegos de surpresa, pois ninguém escaparia da catástrofe por ele prevista.

Estejamos, portanto, atentos, vigilantes, e em oração diária, pois a ninguém foi dado saber o dia e a hora em que isso acontecerá, como disse Jesus. Nem mesmo ele sabia a hora, como humildemente revelou. Somente Deus é conhecedor dessa hora dolorosa.

CAPÍTULO 1

Meteoros, Asteróides e Cometas.

METEORÓIDES, METEOROS E METEORITOS.

O que são, e qual a diferença entre os três?

Esses nomes são muito confundidos. Mas os astrônomos fazem distinção sutil entre eles, e apenas por uma questão didática, pois materialmente falando não há diferenças reais entre eles. São na verdade o mesmo corpo, apenas em fases distintas de aproximação da superfície da Terra.

Meteoróide é um corpo sólido, muito pequeno para ser classificado como asteróide ou como cometa, que gira ao redor do sol, no espaço interplanetário.

Meteoro é um meteoróide que entrou na atmosfera da Terra, e que, com o atrito com os gases da atmosfera se torna incandescente, ou seja, se incendeia, sendo visto da Terra como um raio de luz a cruzar o céu, a conhecida "estrela cadente". Assim, vemos que o meteoróide é chamado de meteoro quando entra na atmosfera da Terra. Muda de nome, mas é o mesmo corpo, apenas incandescente.

O termo meteoro vem do grego *meteoron*, que significa *fenômeno no céu*. Existem aproximadamente 2.000 asteróides com diâmetro maior do que 1 km, e que se aproximam da Terra, colidindo com ela a uma taxa de aproximadamente 1 a cada 1 milhão de anos. São descobertos por ano dois a três meteoros, e suas órbitas são muitas vezes instáveis, devido a interações gravitacionais com os vários corpos (planetas e asteróides).

Meteorito é um meteoro que sobrevive à passagem pela atmosfera de gases, ou seja, que não é totalmente destruído na atmosfera, e que cai na superfície da Terra, no solo.

Seguem adiante uma foto de um meteorito que caiu em região de gelo, e uma de meteorito que caiu sobre um automóvel (Fotos 1 e 2).

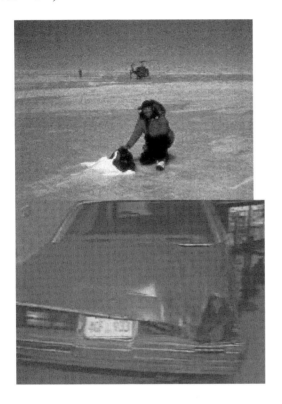

DE QUE SÃO FORMADOS OS METEORITOS?

Os meteoritos que caem na Terra são fragmentos de corpos sólidos como a Lua, Marte ou de um asteróide. Eles podem ser formados de rocha ou metal, ou por uma combinação de ambos.

ORIGEM DOS METEORITOS.

Os meteoritos têm sua origem na maioria das vezes em asteróides, podendo, também, se originar a partir de cometas.

Raros são os meteoritos que caem na Terra de origem marciana ou lunar.

CRATERA DE IMPACTO.

Uma cratera de impacto é uma formação no solo provocada pelo impacto de um meteorito, um asteróide ou um cometa.

Nosso planeta é bombardeado continuamente por meteoritos. Estima-se que diariamente a Terra receba mais de 10 mil quilos de material vindo do espaço, de diversos tamanhos, grande parte em forma de simples poeira estelar, face à desintegração dos meteoros devido ao atrito com o ar (gases) ao atravessarem a atmosfera terrestre.

Raros são os meteoritos de tamanho grande que chegam até a superfície de nosso planeta e formam uma cratera de impacto.

Um bom exemplo de cratera de impacto na Terra, formada pela queda de um meteorito, está no Estado do Arizona, nos Estados Unidos.

Ela foi formada entre 10 mil e 50 mil anos atrás (foto 3), com a queda de um meteorito de cerca de 30 a 50 metros de diâmetro, tendo a cratera 1.200 metros de diâmetro e 200 metros de profundidade.

Essa é a mais conservada de todas as crateras de impacto existentes na Terra, exatamente pelo pouco tempo de sua formação, já que a erosão do solo pela água das chuvas e pelo vento com o tempo destrói a formação circular característica das crateras de impacto.

Já foram identificadas mais de 150 crateras de impacto na Terra.

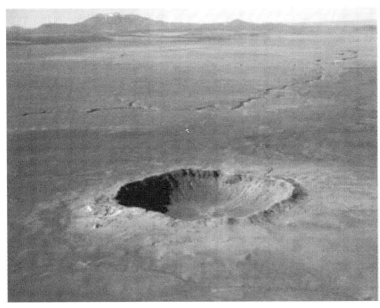 (Foto 3)

Os meteoros muito luminosos, quando vistos do solo, são descritos como "bolas de fogo", e a sua maior luminosidade está relacionada com o seu maior tamanho, que quando se incendeia ao entrar na atmosfera gera uma chama mais visível para quem está na Terra.

Anualmente são vistas da Terra as chamadas "chuvas de meteoros", provocadas pela entrada em grande quantidade de pequenos meteoros na atmosfera terrestre.

O maior meteorito já encontrado na Terra caiu em Hoba, Namíbia, e pesa 59 toneladas. Seu nome é "Hoba West" (Foto 4), e tem 2,7 metros de comprimento por 2,4 de largura.

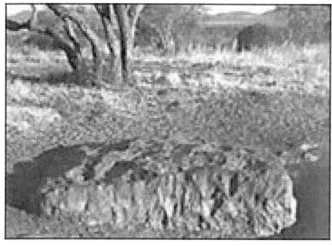

(Foto 4)

O maior meteorito em exibição em um museu é o Cabo York, que pesa aproximadamente 30 toneladas. Foi encontrado perto de Cabo York, Groelândia, em 1.897, pela expedição do Comandante Robert Peary, e está no Museu Americano de História Natural, Nova Iorque, Estados Unidos.

No Brasil, o maior meteorito encontrado é o chamado Pedra de Bedengó, que caiu no sertão da Bahia em 1.784 e está exposto no Museu Nacional, no Rio de Janeiro desde 1.888.

O meteorito "Willamette" (Foto 5), o maior já encontrado nos Estados Unidos da América, no Estado do Oregon, é o sexto maior encontrado no mundo inteiro.

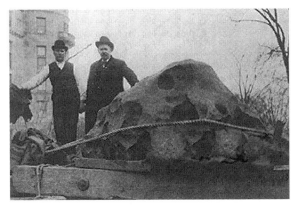

(Foto 5)

ASTERÓIDES.

Acredita-se que os asteróides são restos do processo de formação do Sistema Solar, gerados há 4,6 bilhões de anos atrás.

Os asteróides podem ser formados de rocha ou de metal, como os meteoritos conhecidos, e seus tamanhos podem variar de simples pedrinhas até 934 km de largura.

A maioria dos asteróides se comporta de forma ordenada, permanecendo em órbita regular ao redor de sol num cinturão de asteróides localizado entre as órbitas de Marte e Júpiter. No entanto, às vezes alguns escapam de sua órbita e terminam constituindo ameaça para nós na Terra.

Os astrônomos suspeitam que haja pelo menos 1.000 asteróides com diâmetro superior a 1 quilômetro. E um deles atinge a Terra pelo menos uma vez a cada milhão de anos, em média. Os maiores são menos numerosos, e seus impactos na Terra são menos freqüentes; mas, quando isso acontece, suas conseqüências são desastrosas.

A teoria científica mais aceita para explicar a extinção dos dinossauros envolve a queda de um grande asteróide na região costeira do México, há 65 milhões de anos atrás, tendo o objeto cerca de 10 quilômetros de diâmetro. Essa cratera, já não muito perceptível, tem cerca de 180 a 200 quilômetros de diâmetro, e está enterrada debaixo da selva perto de Chicxulub, na Península de Iucatã, México.

A energia desse impacto foi estimada em mais de 108 megatoneladas de TNT.

Adiante segue foto do asteróide denominado de Eros (Foto 6), fotografado em 12 de fevereiro de 2.000.

Pode-se ver que há crateras de impacto no asteróide, provavelmente causadas pelo choque de outros corpos que vagueiam pelo espaço.

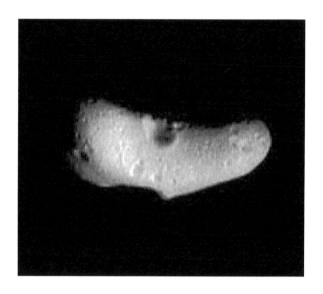

(Foto 6)

Além de cometas, meteoróides, e de uma fina e rala poeira interplanetária, o Sistema Solar é povoado também por milhares de corpos maiores, muitos deles com alguns quilômetros de diâmetro, que são os asteróides. Cerca de trinta deles têm diâmetro superior a 200 km, e o maior de todos, Ceres (o primeiro a ser descoberto, em 1.801 por Piazzi), tem 1.025 quilômetros de lado a lado. Ceres, sozinho, acumula aproximadamente metade da massa de todo o cinturão de asteróides. O cinturão inteiro possui apenas cerca de um centésimo da massa de Mercúrio, o menor planeta de nosso Sistema Solar.

Um outro cinturão de asteróide foi descoberto em 30 de agosto de 1.992 pelos astrônomos David Jewett e Jane Luu. Eles encontraram um objeto de mais de 200 quilômetros de diâmetro situado além das órbitas de Plutão e Netuno. Essa descoberta de um corpo tão grande além do que se imaginava ser os últimos planetas do Sistema Solar causou muita impressão. Posteriormente, vários outros cinturões de asteróides foram descobertos nos anos seguintes, em distâncias próximas, comprovando a existência de um novo cinturão de asteróides chamado Cinturão de Kuiper, nome dado em homenagem ao astrônomo holandês que previu sua existência em 1.951. Estima-se que haja pelo menos 70 mil corpos neste cinturão, situados entre 30 e 50 unidades astronômicas do Sol. Uma unidade astronômica é igual à distância média da Terra ao Sol; equivale a cerca de 149 milhões de quilômetros. Plutão está a 40 unidades astronômicas do Sol. A massa total do cinturão de Kuiper é muitas vezes maior que a massa do cinturão existente entre Marte e Júpiter. Há, no entanto, vários asteróides fora dos dois cinturões, muitos deles em trajetórias bastante ovaladas.

Hoje já são conhecidos cerca de duzentos asteróides cujas órbitas se aproximam da órbita da Terra. Mas a probabilidade de colisão, entretanto, é muito baixa, dizem os astrônomos. Mas não é improvável. Do contrário, a probabilidade seria zero.

O astrônomo norte-americano Carl Sagan, no livro **Pálido ponto azul**, estimou que a Terra é atingida por um objeto com cerca de 70 metros de diâmetro uma vez em alguns séculos. Uma queda dessas liberaria uma energia equivalente à das armas nucleares mais modernas. Já um corpo de 200 metros atinge a Terra em média a cada 10 mil anos, provocando uma colisão que poderia provocar alguns efeitos climáticos regionais muito graves.

Um asteróide é um corpo menor do sistema solar, geralmente da ordem de algumas centenas de quilômetros apenas. É também chamado de planetóide. O termo "asteróide" deriva do grego "astér", que significa estrela, e "óide", sufixo que indica semelhança. Assim, asteróide significa "semelhante a uma estrela".

Já foram catalogados mais de 3 mil asteróides, sendo que diversos deles ainda não possuem dados orbitais calculados. Provavelmente existem ainda milhares de outros asteróides a serem descobertos. Estima-se que mais de 400 mil possuam diâmetro superior a 1 quilômetro.

13

Ceres é o maior asteróide conhecido, possuindo diâmetro de aproximadamente 1.000 km. Desde 24 de agosto de 2.006, passou a ser considerado um planeta anão. Possui brilho variável, o que é explicado pela sua forma irregular, que reflete como um espelho a luz do Sol em diversas direções.

Existem alguns asteróides que descrevem órbitas muito excêntricas, aproximando-se periodicamente dos planetas Terra, Vênus e, provavelmente, Mercúrio. Os que podem chegar perto da Terra são chamados EGA (earth-grazers, ou earth-grazing asteroids). Um deles é o famoso Eros.

São conhecidas dezenas de milhares de asteróides, e estima-se que o seu número alcance os milhões. Cerca de 220 deles têm mais de 100 quilômetros de comprimento.

A grande quantidade de asteróides torna o cinturão um lugar muito dinâmico, e colisões entre asteróides ocorrem muitas vezes, em termos astronômicos. Uma colisão pode fragmentar um asteróide em inúmeros pequenos pedaços, formando-se assim uma nova família de asteróides, ou podem fazer com que se juntem dois asteróides, caso ocorram colisões em velocidades relativamente baixas. Após cinco milhões de anos, a população de asteróides dos dias de hoje é muito diferente da original.

Conhecidos pela sigla NEOs, de Near Earth Objects, asteróides e restos de velhos cometas constituem uma verdadeira ameaça à vida na Terra, e por isso se justifica que sejam permanentemente monitorados por diversos programas de observação astronômica, como o projecto LINEAR (Lincoln Near Earth Asteroid Research), do Instituto de Tecnologia de Massachussets, integralmente financiado pela Força Aérea norte-americana e pela NASA, o Spacewatch Program e o Jet Propulsion NEO Program, para além de outros desenvolvidos por alguns observatórios e centros de pesquisa.

A maioria dos asteróides é originária do cinturão de asteróides e desvia-se para "órbitas rasantes" por colisões entre si ou perturbações provocadas pelo planeta Júpiter.

Os asteróides se dividem em três grandes grupos:

1) grupo de Atenas, que permanece sempre dentro da órbita terrestre;

2) grupo de Apollo, que cruza a órbita do nosso planeta;

3) grupo de Amor, com um periélio um pouco exterior à órbita terrestre, entre 1 e 1,38 UA, e que podem se aproximar fortemente da Terra.

Esses asteróides potencialmente perigosos são relativamente raros, mas são seguidos com todo o cuidado.

Entre as recentes aproximações de asteróides com a Terra podemos mencionar o ocorrido em 14 de Junho de 2.002, quando um asteróide do tamanho de um campo de futebol, que levou a designação de 2.002 MN, passou a uma distância de 120 mil quilômetros da Terra, um terço da distância da Terra à Lua, e que se deslocava a 10 km/s.

O último a ser divulgado foi o Toutatis, com quase 5 km de diâmetro de comprimento e que em 19 de Setembro de 2.006 passou à tranqüila distância de pouco mais de 1,55 milhão de quilômetros da Terra, proximidade que não acontecia desde o ano 1.353, e só se repetirá no ano 2.652.

Apophis (nome astronômico 99942 Apophis, previamente catalogado como 2.004 MN4) é um asteróide descoberto por astrônomos em junho de 2004, tendo sido na época admitido estar ele em provável rota de colisão com a Terra prevista para 2.036.

Estas observações do asteróide, então ainda catalogado como 2.004 MN4, levaram às afirmações de que a órbita seguida por ele no espaço o levaria a um impacto direto com a Terra no ano de 2.029. Cálculos matemáticos mais refinados feitos nos meses seguintes acabaram eliminando a possibilidade de uma colisão nesse ano, mas mantiveram a previsão de que o asteróide passará pela Terra a pequena distância, num buraco gravitacional de cerca de 400m de largura, que o trará novamente ao planeta em 2036, com alguma possibilidade de um impacto direto, (1/43.000 em princípio, já rebaixada a até 1/37 por alguns cientistas) o que o colocou no nível 1 da Escala de Risco de Impacto de Turim.

Apophis está numa órbita em que completa uma volta em torno do Sol a cada 323 dias terrestres e o coloca duas vezes em cruzamento com a órbita da Terra a cada volta completa pelo Sol.

Baseado em estudos sobre o brilho do asteróide no vácuo, os astrônomos calcularam seu tamanho entre 320 e 415 m, e, no caso de colisão, o cálculo de sua massa, velocidade, composição e ângulo de entrada na atmosfera seriam suficientes para provocar uma explosão equivalente a 1480 megatons de TNT num impacto direto, o que representa 114.000 vezes a energia desprendida pela bomba atômica de Hiroshima e sete vezes mais energia que a desprendida pela explosão do vulcão Krakatoa, na Indonésia, em 1.883, capaz de volatilizar completamente uma extensão de terra do tamanho da ilha de Chipre e causar efeitos colaterais na geografia, no clima e no meio ambiente de 1/3 do planeta.

Os últimos estudos astronômicos indicam o dia 13 de abril de 2.036 como o da maior aproximação de Aphopis da Terra, numa distância de passagem de 35.000 km da superfície do planeta,.menor que a de alguns satélites geofísicos artificiais em órbita, mas como existem diversos estudos ainda divergentes, não se pode afirmar com absoluta certeza qual será realmente a distância de sua aproximação, nem eliminar completamente uma possibilidade de impacto. No momento atual, projeções mais precisas continuam sendo feitas e anunciadas regularmente e o Aphopis é hoje o corpo celeste mais vigiado no espaço pela comunidade científica.

Em 2.005, o ex-astronauta Russell Schweickart, tripulante da missão Apollo 15, que hoje dirige a Fundação B612 de estudos astronômicos, pediu em audiência ao congresso americano que fosse autorizada uma liberação de fundos a fim de ser enviada uma sonda ao asteróide, no intuito de depositar nele um rádio emissor, de modo que os astrônomos pudessem controlar sua posição correta e seus ângulos exatos de órbita em torno do Sol e da Terra até 2.070.

A preocupação de Schweickart, e da comunidade de astrofísicos, é a de que a primeira passagem pelo planeta em 2.029 deverá causar uma mudança angular na órbita do asteróide, colocando-o numa posição mais favorável a uma colisão na passagem de 2.036.

Segue abaixo um mapa com a localização das principais crateras de impacto já encontradas na Terra:

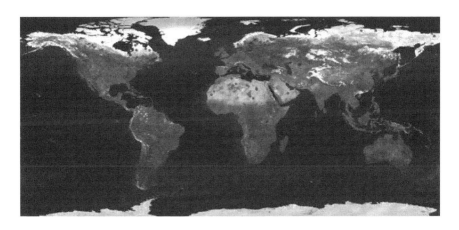

(Foto 7)

COMETAS.

O que são Cometas?
Basicamente, são "pedras de gelo sujo".
O gelo dessas pedras é formado principalmente por material volátil, que passa diretamente do estado sólido para o estado

17

gasoso, e essa "sujeira" é constituída principalmente por poeira e pedras de variados tamanhos.

Cometas são objetos do Sistema Solar que estão presos gravitacionalmente ao Sol. Ao contrário dos planetas, cujas órbitas são quase circulares, os cometas têm órbitas muito elípticas, o que realça o seu aproximar-afastar do Sol. Quanto mais distante for o afélio de um cometa (ponto de sua órbita mais distante do Sol) mais tempo o cometa levará para dar uma volta completa em torno do Sol, ou seja, para completar a sua órbita.

Como se formam os Cometas?

Em 1.950, a partir da análise das órbitas dos cometas, Jan Hendrik Oort (1.900-1.992) propôs o modelo atualmente aceito para a origem dos cometas de longo período. Segundo Oort, existe uma imensa "nuvem" de núcleos cometários orbitando o Sol, em órbitas aproximadamente circulares, a distâncias que variam de 30.000 UA a mais de 60.000 UA do Sol. Seriam mais de um trilhão de objetos, dos mais variados tamanhos. Essa "nuvem" é chamada de "Nuvem de Oort".

Cometas de curto período (menos de 200 anos) têm órbitas em planos próximos ao plano das órbitas dos planetas; cometas de longo período (de centenas a centenas de milhares de anos) têm órbitas em planos com as orientações as mais variadas, e parecem vir de todas as direções do céu. Seus aparecimentos são imprevisíveis.

Quando perturbados, esses objetos podem começar um movimento de "queda" para as regiões internas do Sistema Solar, adquirindo órbitas bastante elípticas, tornando-se, dessa forma, cometas de longo período.

Em 1.951, Gerard Peter Kuiper (1.905-1.973) sustentou serem os cometas de curto período oriundos de uma região plana, coincidente com o plano das órbitas dos planetas, com início logo após a órbita de Netuno (aproximadamente 30 UA do Sol) e se estendendo até aproximadamente 100 UA. Esse é o modelo atualmente aceito para a origem dos cometas de curto período. Essa "arruela" de núcleos cometários é hoje chamada de "Cinturão de Kuiper".

Estima-se que o Cinturão de Kuiper seja constituído de cerca de 10.000 objetos com mais de 300 quilômetros de diâmetro, sendo que 35.000 deles têm mais de 100 quilômetros, e 3.000.000 com mais de 30 quilômetros. Releva lembrar que o objeto que caiu na Terra há 65 milhões de anos e causou a extinção dos dinossauros tinha apenas 10 quilômetros de diâmetro, ou seja, era muito menor que todos esses corpos existentes ainda em nosso sistema solar, e que constituem uma ameaça potencial para a humanidade.

Abaixo, uma foto de um cometa, com sua cauda de milhares de quilômetros de extensão (Foto 8).

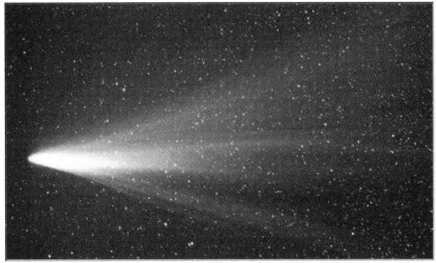

(Foto 8)

A seguir, outra foto de cometa, distanciando-se da Terra e da Lua (Foto 9).

19

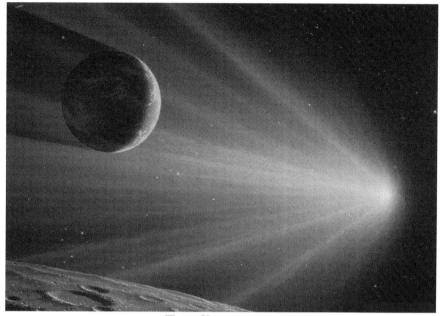

(Foto 9)

Mais Informações sobre os Cometas.

Diferentemente dos outros pequenos corpos do sistema solar, os cometas são conhecidos desde a antiguidade. Há registros chineses do Cometa Halley datados de pelo menos 240 a.C. A famosa tapeçaria Bayeux, que comemora a conquista normanda da Inglaterra em 1.066, retrata o aparecimento do Cometa Halley.

Até o presente, 878 cometas foram catalogados, e suas órbitas calculadas, pelo menos aproximadamente. Desses, 184 são cometas periódicos, que têm períodos orbitais inferiores a 200 anos; alguns dos cometas restantes são também periódicos, mas suas órbitas não foram determinadas com suficiente precisão para se ter certeza.

Os cometas são às vezes chamados de "bolas de neve suja" ou "pelotas de barro congelado". Eles são uma mistura de gelo (água e gases congelados) e poeira que, por alguma razão, não se transformaram em planetas quando o sistema solar foi formado. Por essa razão os cometas são uma importante amostra do passado de nosso sistema solar.

Quando os cometas estão próximos ao Sol, e ativos, têm várias partes distintas, que são:

1 – Núcleo – que é relativamente sólido e estável, formado principalmente de gelo e gás, com uma pequena quantidade de poeira e outros sólidos;

2 – Coma – que é uma densa nuvem de água, dióxido de carbono e outros gases neutros sublimados do núcleo;

3 - Nuvem de hidrogênio – que é um invólucro imenso, com milhões de km de diâmetro, mas bastante esparso, de hidrogênio neutro;

4 - Cauda de poeira – que tem até dez milhões de km de comprimento, composta de partículas de poeira, expelidas do núcleo pelos gases de escapamento. Esta é a parte mais visível de um cometa, e que pode ser vista a olho nu, tendo o nome vulgar "cauda do cometa";

5 - Cauda de íons – que tem até 100 milhões de km de comprimento, sendo composta de plasma e é enlaçada por raios e flâmulas causados pelas interações com o vento solar.

Os cometas são praticamente invisíveis para nós, exceto quando estão próximos do Sol. A maioria dos cometas tem órbita extremamente excêntrica, que o leva para além da órbita de Plutão; estes são vistos uma única vez e depois desaparecem por milênios. Somente os cometas de períodos curtos e intermediários como o Cometa Halley permanecem dentro da órbita de Plutão por uma parte considerável do trajeto de suas órbitas.

Com as repetidas passagens pelo Sol, a maior parte do gelo e gás do cometa se evapora, deixando um objeto rochoso semelhante a um asteróide. Um cometa cuja órbita o leve próximo do Sol poderia ou colidir com um dos planetas ou ser ejetado para fora do sistema solar em virtude de uma maior aproximação, especialmente com Júpiter.

O mais famoso cometa é o conhecido Cometa Halley, mas o cometa SL 9 foi o grande "astro" por uma semana no verão de 1.994.

Uma chuva de meteoros às vezes ocorre quando a Terra passa através da órbita de um cometa. Algumas ocorrem com grande regularidade. A chuva de meteoros Perseida ocorre todos os anos, entre os dias 9 e 13 de agosto, quando a Terra passa através da órbita do Cometa Swift-Tuttle. O Cometa Halley é a fonte da chuva Orionida de outubro.

Duas vezes no século XX grandes objetos colidiram com a Terra.

Em 30 de junho de 1.908 aconteceu um dos mais recentes impactos de fragmento de cometa na superfície terrestre, em Tunguska, na Sibéria, no norte da Rússia. O objeto tinha cerca de 60 metros de diâmetro, mas se desintegrou inteiramente antes de bater no solo, provocando, no entanto, mesmo assim, a derrubada das árvores num raio de 50 quilômetros (Foto 10), e o som do impacto foi ouvido em Londres. A força da explosão foi equivalente a 10 a 20 megatoneladas de TNT, com base nos registos microbarográficos. O fragmento de cometa tinha aproximadamente 100 mil toneladas e matou muitos animais com o impacto.

Não se formou cratera desse impacto, face à desintegração do fragmento de cometa antes de bater no solo. E não foi encontrado vestígio de rocha meteorítica ou metal oriundo de meteoro, o que reforça a teoria de que ele era formado basicamente de gelo. Ou seja, uma enorme bola de gelo (60 metros de diâmetro) caiu na Terra em 1.908 e causou a derrubada de árvores em um raio de 50 quilômetros, e o choque pôde ser escutado em Londres. Imaginem o estrago que teria feito um fragmento de cometa ou asteróide com alguns quilômetros de diâmetro caindo na Terra.

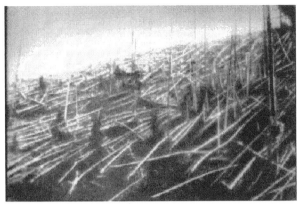
(Foto 10).

A foto acima foi tirada a 20 km do centro da explosão na região do Rio Tunguska, no centro-norte da Sibéria, em 1.927 (20 anos depois da explosão).

As duas fotos seguintes também são da floresta onde caiu o objeto do espaço (Fotos 11 e 12).

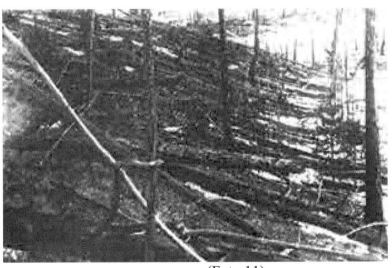
(Foto 11)

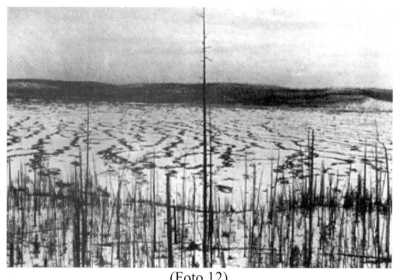

(Foto 12)

A primeira bomba de hidrogênio, chamada Bravo, foi testada em 1 de março de 1.954 pelos americanos, no Atol de Bikini, e tinha 15 Mton de TNT. A bomba de hidrogênio mais poderosa foi testada pelos russos e atingiu 50 Mton de TNT. A força da explosão do fragmento de cometa que caiu em Tunguska em 1.908 foi de 10 a 20 Mton de TNT, ou seja, mais ou menos igual à força da explosão da bomba de hidrogênio explodida pelos americanos em 1.954.

O segundo impacto do século XX ocorreu em 12 de fevereiro de 1.947, na cadeia de montanhas Sikhote-Alin, perto de Vladivostok, também na Sibéria. O impacto, causado por um asteróide de ferro-níquel de aproximadamente 100 toneladas que se rompeu no ar, foi visto por centenas de pessoas e deixou mais de 106 crateras, com tamanhos de até 28 m de diâmetro e 6 metros de profundidade.

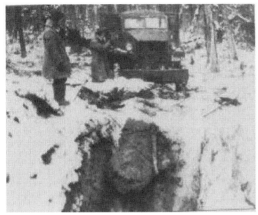
(Foto 13).

Essa foto mostra a recuperação do maior pedaço do meteorito de Sikhote-Alin, de 1.745 kg, sendo tirado de sua cratera por um caminhão. Mais de 9.000 pedaços, compondo 28 toneladas foram recuperados.

Em 18 de janeiro de 2.000, um meteoro explodiu sobre o território de Yukon, no Canadá, gerando uma bola de fogo brilhante detectada por satélites de defesa e também por sismógrafos. A energia liberada foi da ordem de 2 a 3 kton TNT. Denominado Tagish Lake, em referência ao local da queda, foi recuperado um pedaço de 850 g do meteoro que deve ter tido 200 toneladas e 5 m de diâmetro.

As Crateras da Lua

Impactos de grandes meteoritos deixam crateras, e se ele for de material muito denso e compacto pode se enterrar bem fundo. Quando o meteorito é formado por rocha, ao se chocar contra o solo na grande maioria das vezes se esfacela em milhões de partículas de poeira, misturando-se ao chão da região em que caiu.

Na explosão do impacto muito material do local também é lançado para fora da cratera. Assim, quando ocorrem impactos, o objeto que o provocou pode ou não ser destruído e partido em pequenos pedaços, que, por sua vez, podem formar uma série de crateras menores em torno da cratera principal.

Objetos como meteoróides, asteróides e cometas, que cruzam nossos céus, ainda que já não sejam hoje tão numerosos como no passado, ainda representam grande perigo para nós, devido à possibilidade de impacto com a Terra.

Como após cada impacto de meteoros, asteróides e cometas diminui a quantidade desses objetos no espaço, pode-se concluir que a taxa do número de impactos deveria ter sido muito mais alta num passado distante. De uma forma ou de outra, todos os corpos do Sistema Solar sofreram e ainda sofrem impactos, quer seja de meteoritos, cometas ou até mesmo de algum asteróide de maior tamanho, como no caso da Lua, como mostram as fotos a seguir:

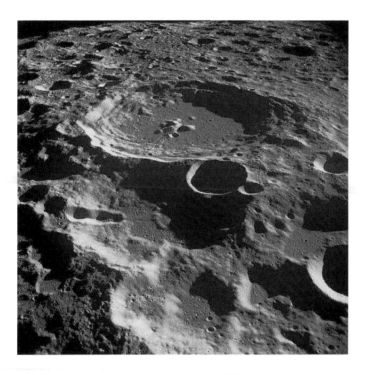

(Foto 14)

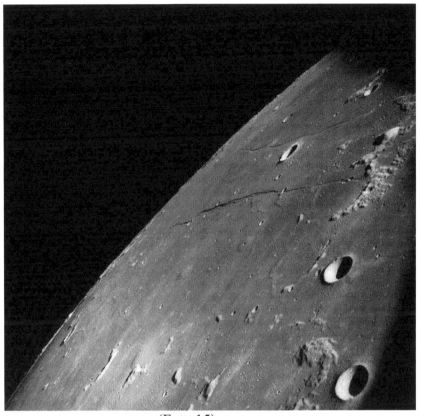
(Foto 15)

Qualquer imagem da Lua possibilita vermos centenas de crateras de variados tamanhos, que podem ser observadas através de lunetas e telescópios, e então veremos milhares delas espalhadas por toda a superfície da Lua. Existem cerca 30 mil crateras de impactos na Lua.

A Terra também já foi palco de muitas quedas de meteorito desde sua origem e durante a evolução de sua história geológica. Mas a Lua apresenta uma enormidade de crateras visíveis, diferentemente da Terra, porque a Lua não tem atmosfera para

27

queimar a maioria dos meteoróides que são atraídos por sua gravidade, nem alguns dos processos de erosão pelo vento, pela chuva e pela lava de vulcões, como acontece na Terra, e, por isso, todos os meteoróides que chegam muito próximos da Lua se chocam contra sua superfície, criando as crateras que lá se encontram.

Tanto na Lua como em outros corpos do Sistema Solar a maioria das crateras apresenta forma circular, têm uma depressão central, bordas elevadas e uma cobertura de material ejetado a rodeá-la, e outras ainda apresentam uma saliência, elevação ou pico central bastante pronunciada. Embora algumas raras crateras lunares apresentem formato oval alongada, a esmagadora maioria delas, que nós vemos na Lua, na Terra e nos outros corpos do Sistema Solar é totalmente ou quase circular. A razão disso é que uma explosão acontece no impacto, e as forças associadas a uma explosão sempre são esfericamente simétricas, ou seja, na explosão materiais são jogados do centro para fora de forma igual.

A vasta maioria das crateras lunares é formada através de impactos, e várias razões podem ser dadas para explicar esta afirmação.

O fato de as crateras apresentarem formas circulares é que a ejeção delas normalmente é radialmente simétrico, ou seja, apontam para a origem das crateras de uma fonte centralizada muito pequena. O material lançado de crateras grandes é significativo e indica que grandes quantidades de material foram deslocadas do local da cratera. Em alguns casos, o material ejetado como também pequenas crateras secundárias podem ser encontradas a milhares de quilômetros de seu ponto de origem. Isso mostra que eles foram lançados quase na velocidade de fuga lunar.

A energia exigida para causar este tipo de movimento de massa de uma zona central pequena só pode vir de impacto de objetos vindos do espaço.

A crosta lunar não é bastante forte para conter um grande impacto em um ponto pequeno sem lançar energia para criar grandes crateras lunares. Foi sugerida a idéia de que um colapso pudesse causar grandes crateras lunares, mas a idéia de colapso não pode explicar a maior parte das crateras marcianas que resistiram e que estão mais ou menos devastadas pela erosão. E muitas das crateras marcianas mais recentes têm uma morfologia que sugere que a superfície estava úmida quando ocorreu o impacto.

O chamado lado distante da Lua, não visível da Terra, até mesmo mais que a face visível da Lua voltada para a Terra, apresenta um largo registro do bombardeio sofrido pela Lua ao longo de sua história, o que exemplifica o ataque freqüente de objetos vindos do espaço, que se chocaram com a superfície lunar. As crateras nesta área da face não visível são encontradas em várias formas, tamanhos e graus de degradação que atestam uma grande variedade de processos formativos, energias de formação e idades. Cada cratera circular individual provavelmente foi produzida pelo impacto de um corpo do espaço interplanetário. Quanto maior for a cratera, maior energia de impacto foi necessária para provocá-la; quer dizer, um corpo maior despendeu uma maior velocidade e energia de impacto. Os impactos mais recentes que aconteceram na Lua apagaram as marcas das crateras mais antigas e produziram as crateras que hoje vemos em ambas as faces da Lua.

Há crateras na Lua com diâmetro de até 5.000 km, o que indica que foram criadas por um imenso asteróide ou cometa, tendo sido imensurável a sua força de impacto. E não podemos esquecer que a Lua é nosso satélite, nossa vizinha, muito próxima da Terra, e se ela foi atingida por esses grandes corpos celestes, também a Terra deve ter sido atingida muitas vezes no passado, e ainda poderá ser no futuro.

Crateras de Marte

No hemisfério Sul de Marte existe um velho planalto de lava basáltica semelhante aos "mares" da lua, e coberta por crateras do tipo lunar. No entanto, a paisagem marciana é diferente da paisagem da Lua, devido à existência de uma atmosfera no Planeta Marte.

O vento carregado de poeira foi produzindo ao longo do tempo um efeito de erosão que destruiu muitas crateras, apesar de ainda existir um número considerável delas em Marte. Assim, existem muito menos crateras em Marte do que na Lua, apesar de o planeta se situar mais perto do cinturão de asteróides.

Grande parte das crateras de Marte se localiza no seu hemisfério sul, onde fica a maior delas, chamada de Hellas Planitia, e que tem 6 km de profundidade e 2.000 km de diâmetro, estando coberta por areia alaranjada e é tratada como se fosse uma planície, tal como outras enormes crateras antigas e planas desse planeta.

A cratera Schiaparelli, em Marte, tem 450 Km de diâmetro. O impacto que a formou deve ter sido muito forte, e o corpo que ali caiu devia ser absurdamente grande.

Se Marte abrigasse vida na época dos impactos dos corpos celestes que formaram as crateras de Hellas Planitia e Schiaparelli, a primeira com 2.000 e a segunda com 450 Km de diâmetro, ela provavelmente teria sido extinta, a julgar pelo impacto na Terra do corpo de 10 Km de diâmetro que causou a extinção dos dinossauros, cuja cratera no México é de apenas 200 Km de diâmetro. E Marte é muito menor do que a Terra.

IMPACTOS EM JÚPITER.

Um episódio ocorrido em 1.994 nos fez lembrar a todos que a violência cósmica ainda é realidade no presente. O cometa Levy-Shoemaker 9, que girava ao redor do Sol há bilhões de anos, foi capturado pelo campo gravitacional de Júpiter há algumas décadas. No dia 7 de julho de 1.992, as fortes marés causadas no cometa pela gravidade do planeta gigante despedaçaram o seu núcleo.

Um grupo de astrônomos liderados por Eugene Shoemaker e David Levy viram o cometa pela primeira vez em 25 de março de 1.993, quando ele já se transformara em uma fileira de fragmentos rodopiando em direção ao Planeta Júpiter.

Seis espaçonaves da Nasa, espalhadas pelo Sistema Solar, e inúmeros astrônomos na Terra suspenderam suas tarefas para observar o que seria a colisão do milênio. Os fragmentos do cometa atingiram a atmosfera de Júpiter entre 16 e 22 de julho de 1.994, um após o outro, a 60 quilômetros por hora.

Foram observadas bolas de fogo se erguendo nos pontos de colisão (Foto 16), que em muitos casos se tornavam mais brilhantes que todo o resto de Júpiter considerado em seu conjunto. As explosões deram lugar a manchas escuras do tamanho do Planeta Terra. Imaginem a força de impacto. E as manchas vistas ficavam apenas na atmosfera. Não foi visto o estrago na superfície, se é que os fragmentos do cometa chegaram a atingir o solo daquele planeta.

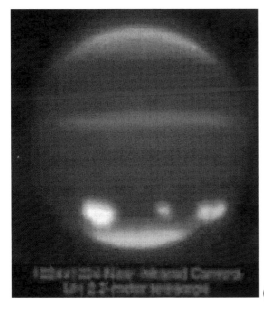

(Foto 16)

Calcula-se que um cometa desse porte atinja Júpiter em média uma vez a cada mil anos. Uma colisão dessas com a Terra poderia destruir nosso planeta.

31

Com tanta gente pensando que o livro Apocalipse e as profecias de Nostradamus falam de guerra nuclear, catástrofes ecológicas, etc., o cometa Levy-Shoemaker 9 nos fez lembrar que na verdade é a Natureza quem tem maior poder e dá a última palavra em matéria de destruição.

A queda na Terra de um asteróide como o que levou à extinção dos dinossauros há 65 milhões de anos atrás ou dos fragmentos de cometa que atingiram em 1.994 o Planeta Júpiter causaria imensa destruição na Terra, ainda que não extinguisse por completo a raça humana.

É essa possibilidade, juntamente com chuvas de meteoros e aproximação de cometas que estaremos analisando em capítulos seguintes, relacionando-os com diversas profecias e revelações.

Como já vimos antes, a maioria dos asteróides se comporta de forma ordenada, permanecendo em órbita regular ao redor de sol num cinturão de asteróides localizado entre as órbitas de Marte e Júpiter, e às vezes alguns escapam de sua órbita e terminam constituindo ameaça para nós na Terra.

Vejam os leitores que Marte fica muito perto da Terra, sendo o próximo planeta em direção ao sol.

Júpiter é um planeta gigante, comparado com a nossa pequenina Terra. E Júpiter é o maior planeta de nosso sistema solar.

O cinturão de asteróide está muito perto da Terra, e por isso a possibilidade de um asteróide se deslocar de lá até a Terra não é tão remota.

CAPÍTULO 2

BREVE HISTÓRICO DO POVO JUDEU.

Como nesta obra estaremos analisando basicamente as profecias feitas por profetas judeus, de Moisés a Jesus, e depois as revelações feitas ao apóstolo João, que constitui o livro Apocalipse, bem como Nostradamus, é importante conhecer um pouco, ou relembrar, a história desse povo ímpar, que existe já há 4.000 anos, para melhor entendermos seus momentos históricos e situar no tempo as profecias ao longo do tempo de sua existência.

O povo judeu teve sua origem com Abraão, que nasceu por volta do ano 2.000 a.C., e viveu na cidade de Ur, na Caldéia, no sul da Mesopotâmia. Vivia ele em uma tribo idólatra

Após receber uma revelação divina, segundo o livro Gêneses da Bíblia, Abraão deixou sua cidade e país de origem (cidade de Ur, na Mesopotâmia) acompanhado de sua esposa Sara e um sobrinho chamado Ló, com seus pertences, e se dirigiram para a terra denominada de Canaã, por indicação de Deus. Ali permaneceram até que um período de fome os fez migrarem para o Egito. Nesse país Abraão fez fortuna, e depois de algum tempo retornou para Canaã com sua família, fixando-se em Hebron, nas imediações do Mar Morto. Contudo, Ló e sua família não acompanharam Abraão, preferindo ir para a cidade de Sodoma.

Abraão e sua família, quando chegaram em Canaã, foram chamados de hebreus, palavra que deriva de "ivri", e que quer dizer "o que está do outro lado do rio", significando que eles eram imigrantes em Canaã, tendo vindo de além rio, que, no caso, era o Rio Eufrates, que ficava na Mesopotâmia, atual Iraque. Os hebreus foram os ancestrais dos judeus, e esse nome, hebreus, era dado aos israelitas por outros povos. Os parentes de Abraão não se autodenominavam de hebreus na época.

O idioma falado e escrito pelos hebreus era o hebraico, que pertence ao subgrupo lingüístico cananeu e está intimamente ligado ao fenício e ao moabita.

O hebraico era o idioma predominante na Palestina até o início do século III a.C., época em que foi suplantado pelo aramaico, idioma do povo chamado arameu, que vivia no norte da Mesopotâmia, e tem origem incerta. Contudo, apesar de ter deixado de ser o idioma falado pelos hebreus, o hebraico continuou a ser usado na liturgia e na literatura do povo hebreu.

O documento mais antigo escrito em hebraico, que se conhece, é o Canto de Débora, contido no livro Juizes, da Bíblia. Esse canto foi grafado em caracteres fenícios, e se acredita ter sido escrito antes do ano 1.000 a.C.

A destruição de Jerusalém e a partida dos hebreus para o cativeiro da Babilônia, no século IV a.c., marcaram o início do declínio do hebraico falado na Palestina. A língua, a partir dessa época, sofreu infiltrações das línguas canaanitas, bem como do acadiano e do aramaico. Assimilou também grande número de palavras sumérias, latinas e persas, uma vez que a região foi invadida e dominada por vários povos diferentes ao longo do tempo.

As três principais religiões monoteístas do mundo - Cristianismo, Islamismo e Judaísmo - reconhecem Abraão como sendo o primeiro dos patriarcas de Israel. Ele representa para todas essas religiões a transição da idolatria para a crença em um só Deus, que consideram verdadeiro.

Depois de Abraão, a personalidade mais importante para os hebreus foi Moisés. Nascido no Egito, filho de hebreus, no final do século XIII a.C., foi criado por uma filha do faraó. Ao ver, certa vez, um feitor maltratando um trabalhador hebreu, Moisés o matou, e teve que fugir. Soube já em idade adulta que era filho de hebreus, o que acabou por influenciá-lo a favor desse povo.

Após ter contato com Iavé, que era Deus para os hebreus, Moisés trabalhou incessantemente para tirar os hebreus do Egito, por orientação de Deus, cujos fatos são detalhadamente narrados na Bíblia no livro Êxodo.

O êxodo, ou saída dos hebreus do Egito, ocorreu no século XII a.C., tendo Moisés feito o povo hebreu andar pelo deserto do Sinai durante 40 anos, a fim de purificar a religião da influência egípcia, visto que os hebreus eram monoteístas, enquanto os egípcios eram politeístas.

Moisés é considerado pela tradição judaica o maior profeta hebreu. Foi ele quem criou propriamente a nação dos judeus.

Moisés morreu muito velho, com cem anos ou mais, entre o final do século XII e o início do século XI a.C.

Conforme lhe informara Iavé, não chegaria a pisar a Terra Prometida. E de fato Moisés morreu muito próximo, podendo vê-la de cima de um monte. Antes, porém, recebeu de Deus os Dez Mandamentos no Monte Sinai, e preparou um conjunto de leis baseadas nos mandamentos de Deus, e designou seu sucessor Josué, que levaria os hebreus até a Terra Prometida.

O primeiro profeta do povo hebreu após o êxodo comandado por Moisés, e já na Terra Prometida, foi Samuel, que viveu no século XI a.C., tendo sido contemporâneo de Josué, provavelmente. Foi ele quem garantiu a independência dos hebreus contra os filisteus, e foi o fundador da monarquia. Ungiu o primeiro rei dos hebreus, Saul, e depois ungiu também Davi.

Davi foi rei de Israel no século XI a.C., durante 40 anos, logo após Saul. A Bíblia relata a façanha de Davi ao derrotar um gigante filisteu com uma funda, em uma batalha. Foi Davi quem fixou a capital de Israel em Jerusalém, cidade que conquistou dos jebuseus, e para onde levou a Arca da Aliança. E foi sob o seu reinado que o Estado de Israel, na antiguidade, atingiu seu esplendor máximo.

Salomão foi o sucessor de Davi, e seu filho. Viveu em meados do século X a.C., e notabilizou-se por sua sabedoria. Foi o rei que conduziu Israel ao máximo poderio militar e comercial, e quem construiu o templo de Jerusalém, chamado depois de Templo de Salomão. Possuía um harém com 700 esposas e 300 concubinas.

Após a morte de Salomão, por volta do ano 930 a.C., o Estado hebreu foi dividido em dois, chamados de Israel e Judá, enfraquecendo com isso a nação, e permitindo que pouco tempo depois suas terras fossem invadidas e a nação conquistada respectivamente por assírios (722 a.C.) e babilônios (587 a.C.).

No século IX a.C. reinou Acab de Israel, de 874 a 854 a.C., que, influenciado por esposas estrangeiras que viviam no seu harém, introduziu no país o culto a Baal, o que implicou em retrocesso religioso, afastando o povo do monoteísmo e de Iavé para prendê-lo à idolatria. Nesse tempo vivia o profeta Elias, que tinha uma "língua de fogo", pois suas palavras "queimavam". E Acab entrou em choque com Elias por causa da idolatria. Elias nasceu para restaurar a fé dos judeus, e para reconduzir o povo desorientado e entregue à idolatria. Foi sucedido pelo profeta Eliseu que, segundo a tradição, viu seu mestre ser levado por uma carruagem de fogo.

Entre os séculos IX e VII a.C., viveram ainda os profetas Natã, Sofonias, Naum e Habacuque.

Isaías foi um dos maiores profetas de Israel, considerado o primeiro dos quatro profetas maiores. Viveu no século VIII a.C. e anunciou – profetizou - a ruína de Judá e Israel. Em 722 a.C. uma de suas profecias se confirmou, quando os assírios invadiram Israel, ao norte, e em 587 a.C. os babilônios invadiram Judá, ao sul, e destruíram Jerusalém, levando os sobreviventes como escravos para a Babilônia.

Isaías foi o primeiro profeta judeu a centrar o Reino Messiânico em Jerusalém. No capítulo 2 de seu livro ele escreveu que de Sião sairia a lei, e de Jerusalém a palavra do Senhor, que julgaria as nações e argüiria muitos povos; que das espadas dos povos seriam feitos arados, e das lanças foices; e que não mais levantariam a espada uma nação contra a outra, e nem se adestrariam mais para a guerra. Isto coincide em muitos aspectos com as palavras de Jesus. E Jesus deve ter sido mesmo a confirmação das profecias de Isaías.

Isaías foi o primeiro profeta a anunciar a vinda do Messias, conforme se vê no capítulo 7 de seu livro, ao dizer que o Senhor daria um sinal, dando luz uma virgem a um filho, que seria chamado Emanuel. Os evangelhos identificam Jesus com essa criança, e a virgem seria Maria, mãe de Jesus. Essas profecias foram feitas mais de setecentos anos antes de Jesus nascer. No capítulo 9, Isaías, referindo-se à Galiléia, escreveu que aquele povo, que andava em trevas, viu uma grande luz, e aos que habitavam na região da sombra da morte nasceu o dia. E que eles se alegrariam quando o Senhor lhes aparecesse.

Isaías escrevia como se as coisas fossem já presentes, pois via de fato os acontecimentos como sendo o presente, como se eles estivessem acontecendo. Ainda no capítulo 9, escreveu: *"porquanto já um pequeno se acha nascido para nós, e um filho nos foi dado a nós, e foi posto o principado sobre o seu ombro, e o nome com o qual se apelide será admirável, conselheiro, Deus forte, pai do futuro século, príncipe da paz. O seu império se estenderá cada vez mais, e a paz não terá fim. Assentar-se-á sobre o trono de Davi, e sobre o seu reino, para firmá-lo e fortalecer em juízo e justiça, desde então e para sempre"*.

Desde Isaías, no século VIII a.C., até Jesus, nenhum profeta ou homem comum de Israel ousou se identificar com o Messias, na forma anunciada por Isaías no texto acima transcrito. Somente Jesus o fez, e logo depois veio a destruição de Jerusalém e a diáspora, não tendo mais havido profetas em Israel até os dias atuais, neste início do terceiro milênio.

Isaías ainda escreveu sobre o reino universal e pacífico do Messias nos capítulos 11 e 12 de seu livro. Escreveu ele: *"Louvai ao Senhor, e invocai o seu nome. Façam notórios entre os povos os seus desígnios. Lembrai-vos que o seu nome é excelso"*. E *"Cantai ao Senhor, porque Ele fez coisas magníficas. Anunciai isto em toda a Terra"*. E ainda *"Exulta e louva, morada de Sião, porque o grande, o Santo de Israel está no teu meio"*. Isaías escrevia como se fosse presente, vendo os fatos acontecerem, como geralmente os profetas e grandes videntes vêem. Via Jesus, provavelmente, e suas obras, que chamou de coisas magníficas, e com razão, mais de setecentos anos antes de acontecerem.

No capítulo 13, Isaías escreveu coisas parecidas com as que Jesus falou acerca do juízo que haveria na sua volta, e com os escritos do Apocalipse, de João. E no capítulo 24, mais ainda, narra acontecimentos semelhantes aos preditos e narrados por Jesus a seus discípulos quando falou dos sinais dos tempos e da proximidade do juízo. Isaías também escreveu sobre o juízo universal.

Entre os séculos VIII e VII a.C. viveu o profeta Miquéias (740 a 687 a.C.), que também anunciou a vinda do Messias como futuro rei de Israel, e indicou o lugar de seu nascimento como sendo Belém. No capítulo 4, Miquéias escreveu coisas semelhantes às que escreveu Isaías, sobre o dia da vinda do Senhor. No capítulo 5, escreveu Miquéias: *"E tu, Belém Efrata, tu és pequenina entre as milhares de Judá! Mas de ti é que me há de sair aquele que há de reinar em Israel, e cuja geração é desde o princípio, desde os dias da eternidade. Por isso Deus os abandonará até o tempo em que parirá aquela que há de parir, e então as relíquias de seus irmãos se ajuntarão aos filhos de Israel. E ele estará firme, e apascentará o seu rebanho na fortaleza do Senhor, na sublimidade do nome do Senhor seu Deus, e eles se converterão, porque agora se engrandecerá ele até as extremidades da Terra. E ele será a paz"*.

Entre os séculos VIII e VII a.C., viveu o profeta Ezequiel. E ainda no século VII a.C., os profetas Sofonias e Naum.

Entre os séculos VII e VI a.C., viveu o profeta Jeremias (640 a 587 a.C.), que pregou por mais de 40 anos.

No século VI a.C., ainda, viveram os profetas Ezequiel, o segundo Isaías, Zacarias, que profetizou de 520 a 518 a.C. e celebrou o nascimento do Messias, e, entre o século VI e o século V a.C., viveram também os profetas Ageu, que defendeu a reconstrução do templo de Jerusalém, Daniel, Abdias, Malaquias, Joel e Jonas, que teria sido engolido por um grande peixe e expelido vivo três dias depois, citado por Jesus em uma passagem dos evangelhos ao se referir ao único prodígio que o povo veria, comparando sua ressurreição com o fenômeno ocorrido com Jonas.

Um denominador comum entre os profetas de Israel era a defesa de Iavé (Deus) e sua ética. Todos os profetas judeus eram profundamente éticos, religiosos, e criticavam os reis quando cometiam erros, chamando-os ao arrependimento.

O último profeta judeu a anunciar a vinda do Messias havia sido Zacarias, entre 520 e 518 a.C., até que apareceu João Batista, já contemporâneo de Jesus de Nazaré. Assim, havia já mais de 500 anos que os judeus esperavam a vinda do Messias, desde a última previsão profética, feita por Zacarias, e sem receberem nenhum outro profeta, como outrora era comum e freqüente. E esse tempo sem profetas se encaixa perfeitamente nos escritos do profeta Miquéias, ao dizer que Deus abandonaria os judeus até que parisse aquela mulher que haveria de parir, ou seja, até que Maria, mãe de Jesus, lhe trouxesse à luz.

Foram 500 anos sem profetas, até que surgiu João Batista. Se considerarmos que ele tinha mais ou menos a mesma idade de Jesus, ele nasceu quando Maria pariu Jesus, o que coincide com a profecia de Miquéias, ou seja, Deus abandonou o povo judeu em termos de enviados seus, os profetas, até que Maria pariu Jesus, e foi exatamente nesse tempo que também nasceu João Batista. Isso leva à conclusão de que a profecia de Miquéias estava correta, e de que João Batista era de fato também um enviado de Deus, para preparar o surgimento e a chegada iminente do Messias, Jesus de Nazaré, que já estava se preparando para começar a sua missão e se anunciar como o Messias esperado e anunciado pelos antigos profetas.

João Batista também foi um profeta, pois falava em nome de Deus, e defendia a sua ética, criticando o rei Herodes por seu comportamento imoral, dando um exemplo ruim para o povo. João dizia para as pessoas se arrependerem e fazerem penitência, porque o Reino de Deus estava próximo. E dizia que estava próxima a vinda do Messias.

Jesus se apresentou para ser batizado por João Batista quando tinha cerca de trinta anos, e então João o indicou aos seus discípulos como sendo o Messias esperado há tanto tempo, e de quem ele, João, não era digno nem de desatar as correias das sandálias. João se recusou a princípio a batizar Jesus, mas acabou cedendo à sua insistência, e o batizou, e depois disso Jesus começou sua pregação, e João foi preso e decapitado, tendo que minguar para que Jesus crescesse.

Jesus se apresentou aos judeus como o Messias, o Filho de Deus, tendo feito muitos milagres, principalmente curas, e fez algumas previsões para o futuro, mas somente para seus discípulos, que depois escreveram os chamados evangelhos.

Morreu Jesus entre os anos 32 e 34 da Era Cristã, como hoje acreditam os historiadores, sem que tenha conseguido convencer todo o povo judeu a não lutar contra os romanos, mas a amá-los. E pouco depois de sua morte o Sinédrio (centro do poder religioso de Israel) se transformou em Conselho de Guerra, e insuflou o povo à revolta contra os romanos, que dominavam Israel desde o ano 63 a.C. No ano 70 d.C. os romanos cercaram Jerusalém durante vários meses, impedindo a chegada de alimentos e água, enquanto atacavam a cidade. As tropas de Tito, que depois se tornaria imperador de Roma, não deram trégua, até invadirem a cidade e matarem à espada a maior parte da população. Jerusalém foi totalmente destruída, inclusive o Grande Templo. Os que sobreviveram foram vendidos como escravos para várias partes do Império Romano. E começou-se a diáspora, a dispersão dos judeus pelo mundo.

Depois da diáspora, nos séculos seguintes, a Palestina foi sucessivamente ocupada por bizantinos, persas, árabes, cruzados, mamelucos, otomanos e britânicos.

No final do século XIX começou-se a fixação de colonos judeus na Palestina, e já havia movimento na Europa e Estados Unidos para a criação do Estado judeu na Palestina.

Em 1.897 foi realizado o Primeiro Congresso Sionista na Suíça, tendo como objetivo a criação de um Estado judeu na Palestina.

Em 1.922 a Liga das Nações (criada em 1.920) outorgou o mandato sobre a Palestina ao Reino Unido, e os britânicos facilitaram então a imigração dos judeus para a Palestina, desrespeitando antiga limitação de imigrantes judeus. Mas protegeram os britânicos ao mesmo tempo os direitos dos habitantes árabes.

Em novembro de 1.947 a ONU (Organização das Nações Unidas - criada em 1.945) aprovou a partilha da Palestina, e em 14 de maio de 1.948 foi proclamado o Estado de Israel. Com isso, os britânicos declararam findo o seu mandato na Palestina e deixaram o país, que foi imediatamente invadido pelos árabes pelo leste e pelo sul, dando início à guerra da Palestina.

Israel esteve em guerra com o Egito e com outros vizinhos árabes. Conseguiu fazer a paz com o Egito graças ao presidente egípcio Sadat, e somente em 1.993 assinou acordo de paz com os palestinos, através de Arafat, líder da OLP (Organização para a Libertação da Palestina).

Até os dias atuais os conflitos entre judeus e palestinos acontecem, com mortes de parte a parte. Bombas colocadas em mercados, em shoppings, em pontos de ônibus, nas ruas, etc., não param de acontecer em Israel. Choques na fronteira com o Líbano, com mortes freqüentes, sempre acompanhados de bombardeios por parte da aviação israelense aos acampamentos dos guerrilheiros que ficam no sul do Líbano. E uma guerra civil começa a se instalar em territórios dentro de Israel, entre os próprios palestinos, por causa de divergências políticas entre as duas mais fortes organizações político-religiosas dos palestinos.

Durante a Guerra do Golfo, em 1.991, o Iraque lançou vários mísseis sobre o território de Israel, para provocar a sua entrada na guerra e fazer com que outros países muçulmanos se juntassem e também lutassem contra os Estados Unidos. Este país ajudou Israel a se defender dos mísseis iraquianos, conseguindo a muito custo impedir sua entrada na guerra, porque, se Israel entrasse, poderia ter chegado ao ponto de usar armas nucleares, como bombas atômicas, possuindo Israel pelo menos cem delas na época. O desastre teria sido muito grande naquela região.

Os palestinos prometeram declarar independentes alguns territórios dentro de Israel em maio de 1.999, o que não ocorreu graças a insistentes apelos de líderes políticos junto a Arafat. E Israel vive há tempo uma guerra civil não declarada, entre palestinos, que são muçulmanos, e judeus. A região continua ainda sendo um imenso barril de pólvora, sempre prestes a explodir, sempre à beira do limite do suportável de violência.

Este é apenas um ligeiro e muito sintético resumo da história de Israel e do povo judeu, importante para situarmos os profetas e Jesus no tempo e entendermos um pouco melhor o povo entre o qual ele viveu.

CAPÍTULO 3

A VIDA DE JESUS – UM POUCO DE HISTÓRIA

Hoje é certo e pacífico entre os historiadores que pesquisam a vida de Jesus Cristo que seu nascimento não se deu no ano que hoje é o marco para a contagem do tempo, ou seja, o ano zero da Era Cristã. Teria nascido Jesus, na verdade, entre os anos 8 e 6 a.C., ou seja, na verdade Jesus nasceu seis a oito anos antes da data que se fixou na Idade Média como sendo aquela de seu nascimento. E esse erro de datação do nascimento de Jesus se deveu ao monge Dionísio, o Pequeno (500-545 d.C.), que foi encarregado de organizar um calendário pelo Papa da Igreja Católica no século V d.C.

A afirmação dos historiadores se baseia na citação feita no Evangelho Segundo Lucas, quanto ao recenseamento feito pelos romanos, ocorrido na época do nascimento de Jesus, e que foi o primeiro feito na Palestina, destinando-se a regularizar a cobrança de impostos. Os historiadores situam esse acontecimento, o recenseamento, entre os anos 8 e 6 a.C.

O astrônomo alemão Johannes Kepler (1.571-1.630 d.C), pai da moderna astronomia, e profundo conhecedor da astrologia antiga, buscando explicação científica para o que poderia ter sido a "Estrela de Belém", mencionada nos Evangelhos da Bíblia, e vista na época e no dia em que Jesus nasceu, acabou por apresentar uma teoria. Segundo seus estudos, uma conjunção entre os planetas Saturno e Júpiter em Peixes seria vista na Terra com imensa luminosidade, semelhante ao que se denominou de "Estrela de Belém". E a última conjunção desses planetas ocorreu em 22 de agosto do ano 7 a.C. Note-se que, coincidentemente, esta data está em acordo com o recenseamento feito pelos romanos na Palestina (entre 8 e 6 a.C.). Procurou-se elaborar o mapa astral de uma pessoa nascida nessa data, e concluiu-se que ela seria uma pessoa destinada a mudar o mundo. Incrível coincidência. É possível que Jesus tenha nascido no dia 22 de agosto do ano 7 a.C.

No Evangelho segundo Mateus (capítulo 2), escreveu ele: *"Tendo, pois, nascido Jesus em Belém de Judá, em tempo do rei Herodes, eis que vieram do Oriente uns magos a Jerusalém, dizendo: Onde está o rei dos judeus, que é nascido? Porque nós vimos no Oriente a sua estrela: e viemos adorá-lo*". Nos outros evangelhos não há registro dessa passagem.

Note-se que Mateus não fala em reis, mas em magos. A Mesopotâmia, onde se situava o Império Babilônio naquela época, era a terra dos magos, e dos astrólogos. O berço da Astrologia foi a Mesopotâmia, como hoje se reconhece.

Alguns interpretam a "Estrela de Belém" como sendo um OVNI (objeto voador não identificado). Contudo, o texto de Mateus é claro ao mencionar uma estrela. Ademais, essa estrela foi vista também pelos magos no Oriente. Isto nos leva a crer que realmente se tratava de uma estrela, ou um planeta irradiando grande luminosidade, ou talvez mesmo uma conjunção de planetas, aumentando a luminosidade vista da Terra, conforme a teoria de Kepler. Ou, quem sabe, um cometa passando perto da Terra. Naquele tempo os conhecimentos de astronomia eram muito rudimentares, e não se distinguia muitas vezes planeta de estrela, e não se conheciam ainda os cometas. OVNI é pouco provável.

Ainda em Mateus (capítulo 7), está escrito: "*Então Herodes, tendo chamado secretamente os magos, inquiriu deles com todo o cuidado que tempo havia que lhes aparecera a estrela*". Isto demonstra que os reis naquele tempo tinham magos, ou astrólogos na corte, para aconselhá-los. Isto era comum, e até mesmo no império romano isso acontecia. E Herodes quis saber deles quanto tempo tinha que a estrela havia aparecido, para que pudesse encontrar a criança nascida.

Os maiores astrólogos daquele tempo estavam na Babilônia. Assim, é bem provável que astrólogos, que também eram magos, tivessem previsto o nascimento de alguém muito importante para a humanidade na data do aparecimento da chamada "Estrela de Belém", que pode ter sido mesmo a conjunção de Saturno com Júpiter em Peixes, ocorrida no dia 22 de agosto do ano 7 a.C. Do contrário, o que os levaria a sair de um país tão distante a cavalo ou camelo à procura da criança nascida?

É muito provável também que os magos (astrólogos) do oriente conhecessem as escrituras dos judeus, relativamente ao messias que havia de nascer. Pois eles perguntaram em Israel pelo rei que teria

43

nascido lá. Eles deveriam logicamente saber da profecia sobre um rei ou messias que havia de nascer, e ligaram a profecia à estrela que eles viram no oriente, em sua terra, e também em Israel.

Quanto ao ano em que morreu Jesus, está associado ao tempo em que Pôncio Pilatos era o Governador Romano da Palestina, que era uma província romana, tendo sido dada a sentença de morte a Jesus, por crucificação, entre os anos 34 e 32 da Era Cristã, como hoje acreditam os historiadores com base no período de governo de Pitalos na Palestina. Assim, Jesus viveu na verdade entre 39 e 41 anos, e não apenas 33 anos, como se pensava. Como Lucas em seu evangelho registrou que Jesus tinha mais ou menos 30 anos quando iniciou sua pregação, tem-se que ele pregou durante 9 a 11 anos, e não apenas por 3 anos. Esse tempo maior justifica o que escreveu João em seu evangelho, que *Jesus realizou tantas obras que se fossem todas registradas por escrito o mundo não conteria todos os livros* (João, cap.21, v.25).

Jesus nasceu em Belém, na Judéia, que hoje faz parte de Israel. Viveu em Nazaré após voltar do Egito, para onde sua família fugiu para livrá-lo da morte ordenada por Herodes. Só deixou a cidade Nazaré definitivamente quando iniciou sua missão, com cerca de trinta anos de idade.

A existência de fato de um homem chamado Jesus, que teria sido crucificado em Jerusalém, dando nascimento depois a uma religião com muitos seguidores hoje não pode ser contestada. E isto porque, além dos evangelhos reconhecidos pela Igreja Católica e pelos historiadores, que relatam sua vida, ensinamentos, milagres e profecias, há também documentos outros, históricos, de origem não-cristã, que mencionam Jesus, a exemplo dos escritos do historiador da corte romana de Domiciano, o judeu Flavio Josefo, que menciona a morte de João Batista em termos que coincidem substancialmente com os relatos evangélicos, dando-lhes com isso autenticidade, e ainda registrou o mesmo Flavio Josefo o martírio de Tiago, "irmão daquele Jesus que é chamado Cristo", segundo palavras suas. Josefo escreveu sobre a história do povo judeu por volta do ano 50 d.C., e menciona Jesus como "obrador de feitos extraordinários". Ele devia ser criança quando Jesus foi morto, e deve ter colhido muitos relatos acerca dos feitos de Jesus, que foi um homem muito famoso em seu tempo. A existência de Jesus e mesmo sua morte eram recentes para o historiador Flavio Josefo.

Há também o maior historiador romano, Tácito, que mencionou a figura de Cristo, ao referir-se ao incêndio de Roma. Nero, para desculpar-se, atribuiu o incêndio aos cristãos, cujo nome, afirma Tácito, *"lhes vem de Cristo, o qual, sob o principado de Tibério, o procurador Pôncio Pilatos entregara ao suplício..."*. E o Talmude de Jerusalém e também o da Babilônia confirmam a existência histórica de Jesus de Nazaré.

Em abril de 1.992, para alvoroço dos historiadores, e para maior confirmação da existência histórica de Jesus de Nazaré, descobriu-se em uma das grutas do sítio arqueológico de Qumran, às margens do Mar Morto, próximo à cidade de Jericó, na Palestina, território de Israel, um fragmento de papiro datado aproximadamente do ano 50 d.C. O texto está escrito em caracteres gregos, e trata-se de uma conhecida passagem da vida de Jesus descrita no Evangelho de Marcos. Até então, entre os famosos Manuscritos do Mar Morto, nada havia sido identificado como fazendo referência à existência de Jesus. Mas naquele ano de 1.992 as coisas mudaram de rumo, e os historiadores tiveram a certeza de que não só existira de fato um homem chamado Jesus naquela região, como também foram feitos registros a seu respeito desde pelo menos vinte anos após a sua morte, o que mudou a crença anterior de que os registros evangélicos somente tardiamente foram elaborados. Alguns historiadores sustentavam que os evangelhos somente tinham sido escritos cerca de cem anos após a morte de Jesus, o que hoje está ultrapassado.

Os Manuscritos do Mar Morto foram escondidos em gruta pelos essênios, membros de uma seita judaica dissidente e purista, que viviam em uma comunidade às margens do Mar Morto. A maior quantidade dos manuscritos foi encontrada logo após a Segunda Guerra Mundial por jovens pastores, mas somente recentemente traduzida, e só em 1.992 foi encontrado o fragmento que menciona Jesus. A sobrevivência desse fragmento pode ser considerada, em certo sentido, um verdadeiro milagre, encontrado já no final do milênio, e a confirmar a existência e importância de Jesus de Nazaré já bem pouco tempo depois de sua morte. Se Jesus tivesse sido um homem comum, sem maior importância, não teriam escrito sobre ele, e ainda mais em grego, quando os judeus falavam e escreviam em aramaico no seu tempo, e não teriam escondido os escritos na gruta. Jesus deve ter sido considerado muito importante por quem escreveu sobre ele em grego.

Arqueólogos encontraram em Cafarnaum, nas imediações da sinagoga do século I d.C., vestígios de uma casa com anzóis e jarros para peixe, onde se encontrou em escavações uma placa com a inscrição: *"Casa do Príncipe dos apóstolos"*. É mesmo possível que se tratasse da casa do apóstolo Pedro, pois os evangelhos indicam que Pedro vivia em Cafarnaum quando foi chamado por Jesus.

Em 2.002 foi divulgada a descoberta nos arredores de Jerusalém de uma urna funerária com uma inscrição em aramaico, a língua falada em Israel no tempo de Jesus, que diz: "Ya'akov bar yosef akhui di yeshua", que em português quer dizer *"Tiago, filho de José, irmão de Jesus"*. A Bíblia indica a existência de um irmão de Jesus chamado Tiago. Exames atestaram que a peça encontrada é mesmo da época de Jesus, ou seja, do século I d.C.

A palavra *cristianismo* deriva de Cristo, que na sua raiz grega significa *ungido*. Jesus se identificou com a figura do Messias esperado pelos judeus, e prometido por Deus desde os tempos dos profetas Miquéias, Isaías e Zacarias, por intermédio deles. O Messias, o Salvador, era esperado há mais de 500 anos quando nasceu Jesus.

Na época em que Jesus viveu a nação judaica estava sob domínio estrangeiro fazia muito tempo, e os sonhos de liberdade eram já muito antigos. A região ficava situada numa zona de tensão entre os grandes impérios do mundo oriental, e por isso a nação perdeu sua independência política desde o exílio da Babilônia, nos fins do século VI a.C. Depois vieram os persas, os gregos com Alexandre, o Grande, e por último os romanos, em 63 a.C.

Na época de nascimento de Jesus a Palestina era foco constante de revoltas e resistência contra Roma, e por isso muitos foram crucificados antes e depois de viver Jesus. E os judeus esperavam um Messias, um Salvador, que efetivamente os salvasse, mas do domínio dos romanos, o que dificultou a aceitação de Jesus quando ele se recusou a ser coroado rei dos judeus, pois eles queriam que Jesus liderasse a revolta armada contra os romanos, o que estava fora dos planos de Jesus. Dizia ele: *"meu reino não é deste mundo"*; *"quem com ferro fere, com ferro será ferido"*; *"amai vossos inimigos"*. Jesus não podia liderar um exército contra os romanos. Ele até curava romanos.

Jesus viveu num tempo de intensa agitação política na Palestina. As principais forças políticas de seu tempo eram compostas pelos *saduceus*, que negavam a imortalidade da alma, e foram os principais responsáveis pela condenação de Jesus; *escribas*, ou doutores da lei, que eram os intérpretes das escrituras; *fariseus,* puristas e nacionalistas, que esperavam do Messias a libertação do jugo romano, acreditavam na imortalidade da alma e na ressurreição do corpo; *zelotas,* dissidentes dos fariseus, ultranacionalistas, que pretendiam expulsar os romanos pagãos pelas armas, sendo por isso ferozmente perseguidos pelos romanos; e *essênios,* sacerdotes dissidentes e leigos exilados, que viviam em comunidades ultra fechadas em Qumran, considerando-se os únicos puros de Israel.

Pelo que indicam os evangelhos, Jesus era carpinteiro, profissão que deve ter exercido até iniciar sua vida missionária aos trinta anos de idade. Isto devia fazer dele um homem forte, do ponto de vista físico, devido ao trabalho braçal. Seguiu o mesmo ofício de José, seu pai, o que era comum naqueles tempos em Israel.

Na região onde Jesus viveu o povo era preponderantemente moreno, de cabelos escuros e olhos castanho-escuros, como são até hoje os árabes e os chamados palestinos que vivem em Israel, bem como os jordanianos, egípcios, iraquianos, iranianos, turcos e muitos outros povos vizinhos. Assim, seria naturalmente de se esperar, por ser o mais natural, e provável que Jesus fosse também moreno, de cabelos pretos ou castanho-escuros, o mesmo se dando com os olhos. O tipo louro e de olhos azuis não se coaduna com o tipo étnico da região nos tempos de Jesus. A imagem do Cristo louro e de olhos azuis foi criação dos cristãos europeus, estes sim, em grande parte louros e de olhos claros. Todavia, não se pode descartar totalmente a possibilidade de ter sido ele claro e de olhos azuis, visto que durante vários séculos Israel foi dominada pelos gregos e depois pelos romanos, que eram claros e tinham olhos claros. Quem sabe o sangue helênico ou romano não se misturou com os antepassados de Jesus...isso não é impossível. Além disso, não se pode descartar de forma absoluta a hipótese de realmente Jesus não ter sido gerado por José, seu pai, ou seja, que ele não tinha os mesmos traços dos judeus, já que os textos evangélicos lhe atribuem outra origem, divina, mesmo do ponto de vista físico, genético. Maria, segundo os evangelhos, ficou grávida sem contato físico com José, que era ainda seu noivo. Sua gravidez, se acreditarmos nos evangelistas, não teve origem humana. O relato envolve a presença de um anjo. Não é impossível que a genética de Jesus não fosse humana, e que fosse perfeita, sem a possibilidade de doenças congênitas, fraquezas, predisposições a doenças, e que lhe possibilitasse o desenvolvimento de poderes paranormais além da compreensão humana. Um dos milagres descritos na Bíblia. É questão de fé. Acredita-se ou não.

O Santo Sudário, em cuja veracidade acreditamos, como tivemos oportunidade de expressar em nosso livro "Os Milagres de Jesus Cristo", e objeto de um dos últimos capítulos desta obra, mostra que Jesus tinha 1,81 cm de altura, o que está muito acima da média dos judeus de seu tempo, e mesmo da média mundial no século XX. Jesus era um homem muito alto para os padrões gregos, romanos e judeus de seu tempo. Ele devia chamar atenção pela altura, pela fortaleza física, e pelo olhar firme e penetrante. Certamente por essa razão não foi rechaçado e impedido no ato de expulsão dos vendedores do templo em Jerusalém. Ninguém ousaria, estando desarmado, enfrentar Jesus sozinho.

Ao longo de sua missão na Terra, Jesus Cristo operou muitos dos chamados milagres, como curas, multiplicação de alimentos, levitação sobre as águas, ressuscitamento de mortos, etc. E também profetizou acontecimentos futuros, dos quais estaremos falando ao longo desta obra, principalmente as previsões relativas ao Juízo Final e aos Sinais dos tempos.

CAPÍTULO 4

OS PROFETAS JUDEUS ANTES DE JESUS

Todas as profecias analisadas nesta obra emanaram de judeus.

Coincidência ou não, os antigos profetas de Israel, como Isaías, Miquéias, Daniel, João Batista e o próprio Jesus eram todos judeus. Moisés, o primeiro profeta na seqüência bíblica, era hebreu, e não conheceu e não pisou na Terra Santa, a Terra Prometida. O profeta Nostradamus, que viveu no início do século XVI d.C., e é famoso até nossos dias, era igualmente judeu, convertido ao catolicismo apenas para sobreviver, em uma época de grande perseguição aos judeus na Europa, e no auge da Inquisição da Igreja Católica.

Não se tem conhecimento de profetas e profecias em larga escala, com detalhes sobre os acontecimentos futuros, e que não tivessem relação com o povo judeu.

Nesse contexto, pode-se mesmo dizer que os judeus foram escolhidos por Deus, seja para receberem os mais variados profetas ao longo de mais de dois mil e quinhentos anos, seja para receber em sua terra o maior de todos os profetas, Jesus de Nazaré, ou Jesus Cristo, em que pese muitos judeus não tê-lo reconhecido como o Messias por eles esperado.

Lembraremos neste capítulo algumas profecias dos antigos profetas de Israel, anteriores a Jesus, e de forma cronológica, tendo sido algumas já concretizadas e outras ainda aguardam concretização. E em seguida veremos as profecias de Jesus já concretizadas, e aquelas ainda também por se concretizarem, para depois analisarmos e compararmos essas profecias com as revelações do livro O Apocalipse e com as profecias de Nostradamus, e ver os pontos em comum entre todas elas.

Não podemos perder de vista, ao lermos as profecias contidas na Bíblia, do contexto da época em que foram escritas. Todos os profetas foram pessoas religiosas, e na época em que foram escritos os livros do Antigo Testamento a visão de Deus era a de um ser que ficava bravo, irado, que era vingativo, que manda matar até mesmo velhos e crianças, como podemos ver em diversas passagens dos primeiros livros do Antigo Testamento. Já Jesus trouxe uma nova e revolucionária visão de Deus, compassivo, clemente, que perdoa e que ama a todos, indistintamente. Assim, os escritos das palavras de Jesus não trazem o mesmo peso dos escritos dos profetas do Antigo Testamento, que falam muito na ira do Senhor, na vingança do Senhor, etc., o que não se observa mais nas palavras de Jesus. Mas isso não retira a essência de suas profecias, principalmente quando vemos muitas delas sendo cumpridas ao longo do tempo.

MOISÉS.

Moisés é considerado o primeiro profeta dos hebreus, antes mesmo, porém, de o povo ser chamado de judeu.

Viveu, segundo os historiadores, entre os séculos XIII e XII a.C., ou seja, entre 1.300 e 1.200 anos antes de cristo, e morreu com cem a cento e vinte anos de idade.

A tradição rabínica de Israel atribui a Moisés a autoria dos cinco primeiros livros da Bíblia, do Antigo Testamento, que são Gêneses, Êxodo, Levítico, Números e Deuteronômio.

Moisés, além de possuir, segundo os livros da Bíblia, poderes extraordinários, tinha também o dom de profetizar, ou seja, de prever o futuro. E ele o fez, como indicam algumas profecias adiante analisadas.

No capítulo 27 Moisés escreveu sobre maldições sobre os hebreus; no capítulo 28 continua prevendo maldições, além de doenças e derrotas, e também invasões e sofrimento infligido pelos inimigos.

No capítulo 28, a partir do versículo 49, Moisés fez profecias terríveis, que parecem ter sido cumpridas mais de 1.200 anos depois de sua morte. Escreveu ele:

"O Senhor mandará de longe, das extremidades da terra sobre ti uma nação, à semelhança da águia que voa impetuosamente, cuja língua tu não possas entender; nação atrevidíssima, que não terá respeito algum ao velho, nem se compadecerá do menino, e devorará tudo o que nascer dos teus gados, e os frutos da tua terra, até que pereças, e não te deixará nem pão, nem vinho, nem azeite, nem nanadas de bois, nem rebanhos de ovelhas, até que te haja destruído, e te haja aniquilado em todas as suas cidades, e até que em toda a tua terra sejam derrubados os teus fortes e altos muros

em que ponhas a tua segurança. Serás sitiado dentro das tuas portas em toda a tua terra, que o Senhor teu Deus te dará, e comerás o fruto do teu ventre, e as carnes de teus filhos e de tuas filhas que o Senhor teu Deus te houver dado na angústia e desolação, com que te oprimirá o teu inimigo. O homem mais delicado dos teus, e o mais entregue aos prazeres, será mesquinho com seu irmão, e com sua mulher, que dorme com ele, e não lhes dará das carnes de seus filhos, que ele comerá, por não ter nenhuma outra coisa no cerco e na penúria, a que te reduzirão os teus inimigos dentro de todas as tuas portas. A mulher tenra e mimosa, que não podia andar sobre a terra, nem firmar nela um pé por causa da sua demasiada brandura e delicadeza será mesquinha com seu marido, que dorme ao seu lado, das carnes de seu filho e de sua filha, e da asquerosa hediondez das páreas, que sairá do seu ventre, e dos filhos que no mesmo momento lhe nascerem, porque os comerão ocultamente pela falta de todas as coisas, no cerco e desolação, com que te oprimirá o teu inimigo dentro das tuas portas".

Profecia por demais chocante, mas que parece ter se cumprido.

Lembremo-nos que o sul de Israel, chamado no passado de Judá, foi invadido em 587 a.C. pelos babilônios, que levaram os sobreviventes como cativos para a Babilônia, onde permaneceram por cerca de 50 anos, e em 722 a.C o norte, chamado na época de Israel, foi invadido pelos assírios, como profetizado por Isaías.

Jerusalém foi totalmente destruída na época de sua invasão.

Todavia, se atentarmos bem para o texto de Moisés no Deuteronômio, como acima transcrito, veremos que as atrocidades dos assírios e babilônios não foram tão grandes quanto àquelas promovidas pelos romanos a partir do ano 70 d.C, quando, sob o comando do general Tito, as tropas romanas sitiaram Jerusalém, a Cidade Santa dos judeus, durante cerca de um ano, sem deixarem entrar comida alguma. Como teriam sobrevivido os sitiados por tão longo tempo? Não havia comida estocada suficiente para todos, e para tão longo período de tempo, bem como água abundante para tanta gente. Assim, não é mesmo impossível que tenham alguns judeus chegado a praticar realmente o canibalismo, matando crianças, e comendo inclusive bebês recém nascidos, e fetos abortados, como consta expressamente no texto de Moisés acima transcrito da Bíblia.

Se acreditarmos em Moisés, não devemos duvidar de que isso tenha realmente acontecido, por mais chocante que isso possa parecer agora, no início do século XXI.

Outra coisa intrigante é que os romanos tinham como símbolo a águia, que carregavam em seus porta-estandartes. E eles falavam uma língua totalmente nova, estranha e incompreensível para os judeus, o que está previsto no livro de Moisés, e confirma a sua profecia. Há coincidência entre a simbologia da águia, utilizada por Moisés, e o símbolo material da águia utilizada pelos romanos, que bem demonstra o seu espírito conquistador.

Os gregos antes dos romanos já haviam conquistado também a região da Palestina, no século IV a.C. Todavia, não há registro de atrocidades perpetradas pelos gregos como as que fizeram os romanos em Israel.

No mesmo capítulo 28, Moisés continua ainda fazendo profecias terríveis para os hebreus, como o advento de pragas, doenças, e a drástica redução da população, com a dispersão do povo pelo mundo.

Vejamos o que escreveu Moisés a partir do versículo 63 do capítulo 28 do livro Deuteronômio:

"E assim como antes se comprazia o Senhor em vos fazer bem, multiplicando-vos, assim se comprazerá em acabar-vos, e destruir-vos, para serdes exterminados da terra, em cuja posse estais a entrar. O Senhor te espalhará por todos os povos desde uma extremidade da terra até os seus fins, e lá servirás a deuses estranhos, que tu e teus pais ignoram, a paus e a pedras. Tampouco terás repouso entre esses povos, nem a planta do teu pé achará descanso. Porque o Senhor te dará ali um coração medroso, e uns olhos descaídos, e uma alma consumida de tristeza. E a tua vida estará como suspensa diante de ti. Temerás de dia e de noite, e não crerás na tua vida. Pela manhã dirás: Quem me dera chegar à tarde? E à tarde: Quem me dera ver a manhã? Por causa do temor com que serás aterrado em teu coração, e por causa daquelas coisas, que verás com os teus olhos. O Senhor vos fará tornar por mar ao Egito, donde ele vos tinha dito que não tornásseis mais a tomar o caminho. Lá sereis

vendidos aos teus inimigos para serdes escravos e escravas, e não haverá quem os compre".

Outra seqüência de profecias terríveis feita por Moisés aos hebreus, e que parece ter sido mesmo cumprida, quando eles já eram chamados de judeus.

Vemos nessas profecias que os judeus seriam exterminados em sua terra, o atual Estado de Israel, o que de fato aconteceu no tempo em que os romanos dominavam a Palestina, como eles chamavam a região naquele tempo. O cerco e a destruição de Jerusalém em 70 d.C. foi o marco inicial da matança dos judeus pelos romanos, motivada pela revolta dos judeus, que não aceitavam o domínio romano. O último reduto da resistência dos judeus foi Massada, que ficava em um monte próximo ao Mar Morto, onde pouco mais de mil judeus conseguiram resistir por cerca de um ano ao cerco romano, e ao final se suicidaram, antes da invasão romana que se seguiu à construção de uma imensa rampa de terra e cascalho para alcançar o alto do monte.

Ainda no século I da Era Cristã, os romanos venderam os judeus sobreviventes por todo o mundo romano, que não era pequeno, e passaram os judeus sobreviventes a ser escravos.

O profeta hebreu ainda escreveu que o povo seria obrigado a pau e pedra a adorar deuses de outros povos, e que eles viveriam com medo, de dia e de noite.

Observe-se que durante toda a Idade Média os judeus foram intensamente perseguidos e escorraçados em quase toda a Europa, principalmente na época da Inquisição da Igreja Católica, e muitos, para sobreviverem, tiveram que se converter ao cristianismo, como fez a família de Nostradamus, como vimos em capítulo anterior.

Os judeus, por causa da perseguição religiosa, não paravam em país algum, estando sempre a fugir e a migrar, o que o profeta chamou de *não descansar a planta do pé, nem encontrar repouso entre os povos.*

Moisés escreveu que os judeus teriam um *coração medroso, e uns olhos descaídos, e uma alma consumida de tristeza.* E de fato durante muitos séculos os judeus tiveram baixa auto-estima, viveram tristes, e com medo, principalmente na época em que o nazismo se implantou na Alemanha, com o surgimento de Hitler, o grande carrasco dos judeus da Europa, e um dos instrumentos do cumprimento das profecias de Moisés.

Nos anos de caçada aos judeus na Europa, na década de 1.940, por ordem de Hitler, os judeus se escondiam em sótãos, porões, casas abandonadas, florestas, sem saber se chegariam até a noite, ou até a próxima manhã, o que está em total acordo com as chocantes palavras de Moisés no texto antes transcrito.

A vida de um judeu na Europa, principalmente na Alemanha e Polônia, não valia nada na época do domínio nazista. Assim, os judeus não acreditavam na sua vida, ou seja, na sua sobrevivência, o que confirma as palavras de Moisés.

Por incrível que possa parecer, Moisés viu, 1.200 anos antes de Cristo, o que aconteceria nos anos de 1.939 a 1.945, ou seja, anteviu o futuro dos judeus mais de três mil anos antes. Essa distância no tempo entre a profecia e seu cumprimento não encontra similar em outro profeta, já que Moisés foi o primeiro e mais antigo profeta do povo judeu.

Moisés no século XII a.C. viu fatos e acontecimentos futuros que somente há pouco mais de 60 anos se cumpriram, e que estão relacionados com as profecias de Jesus e o Apocalipse, no que diz respeito à volta dos judeus à terra onde no passado viviam, a Terra Santa, a Terra Prometida.

ISAÍAS

Um dos quatro profetas maiores de Israel, que viveu no século VIII a.C., profetizou sobre a ruína de Israel e Judá, e em 722 a.C. ela começou a se concretizar, com a invasão dos assírios e a destruição de Israel ao norte e a invasão que seguiu pelo sul pelos babilônios, destruindo a cidade de Jerusalém, e levando os sobreviventes como escravos para a Babilônia.

Isaías foi o primeiro profeta judeu a centrar o Reino Messiânico em Jerusalém.

No capítulo 2 de seu livro, Isaías escreveu que de Sião sairia a Lei, e de Jerusalém a palavra do Senhor, que julgaria as nações e argüiria muitos povos; que das espadas dos povos seriam feitos arados, e das lanças foices; e que não mais levantariam a espada uma nação contra a outra, e nem se adestrariam mais para a guerra.

Jesus foi a confirmação parcial também das palavras e profecias de Isaías. Mas nem todas as profecias de Isaías já se cumpriram, posto que ainda existem muitas armas no mundo, e as nações ainda fazem guerra umas contra as outras, e ainda se preparam para a guerra. Essa profecia feita há 2.700 anos ainda está por se cumprir, o que mostra a longa distância no tempo entre a profecia de Isaías e a sua confirmação e concretização. Ele previu fatos que aconteceriam em breve, ainda no seu tempo, e que foram efetivamente confirmados, como a destruição de Jerusalém e a escravidão na Babilônia, e coisas que somente aconteceriam mais de 2.600 anos depois, e ainda não confirmados.

Os verdadeiros profetas, como Isaías, e como Jesus, anteviam fatos que somente após milênios se tornariam realidade. Eles viam o futuro como se fosse presente, mas sem fixar datas para os acontecimentos que previam, mesmo porque o calendário judeu de seu tempo não era igual ao adotado no mundo moderno. Além disso, as visões dos profetas não indicam época, nem datas, ou sequer os anos em que os fatos aconteceriam. Aliás, de um modo geral, os videntes de hoje também não datam os acontecimentos que prevêem. Apenas vêem as imagens, muitas vezes seqüenciadas. Até Nostradamus pouco indicou datas, e quando o fez errou, como veremos em capítulo adiante.

Os profetas vêem algo acontecendo, como um filme passando em sua mente, como se estivesse acontecendo naquele momento, e não têm idéia de quando o fato acontecerá.

Isaías no século VIII a.C. previu a chegada de Jesus, o que somente aconteceu mais de seiscentos anos depois dele. E nesse meio tempo ninguém em Israel ousou se identificar com o Messias previsto por Isaías.

Esse profeta falou dos Sinais dos Tempos, do Juízo Universal, da dispersão dos judeus pelo mundo (a Diáspora) e tantas outras coisas, sendo que algumas delas já aconteceram, e outras ainda aguardam a sua concretização.

Em seu livro Isaías escreveu (cap.11), falando do reinado pacífico do messias, que *"o lobo habitará com o cordeiro, e o leopardo se deitará ao pé do cabrito; o novilho, o leão e a ovelha viverão juntos, e um menino pequenino os conduzirá. O novilho e o urso irão comer nas mesmas pastagens, as suas crias descansarão umas com as outras, e o leão comerá palha com o boi. E se divertirá a criança de peito sobre a toca do áspide; e na caverna do basilisco meterá a sua mão a que estiver já desmamada. Eles não farão dano algum, nem*

55

matarão em todo o seu santo monte, porque a terra está cheia da ciência do Senhor, assim como as águas do mar que a cobre".

É evidente que esta profecia, se não for apenas uma figura retórica, ainda não se cumpriu, ainda que tenha meramente sentido figurado, dizendo respeito aos homens, e não aos animais.

No capítulo 13 Isaías inicia a profetizar a respeito do que ele chamou de Dia do Senhor, que assolaria a terra, causando debilitação das mãos e desânimo nos corações dos homens, que quebrantados ficarão, em dores, e atônitos.

Escreveu Isaías no mesmo capítulo que *o dia do Senhor seria cruel, e que poria a terra numa solidão, e que as estrelas do céu e o resplendor delas não espalhariam a sua luz, e o sol e a lua não dariam mais a sua luz, e a terra seria movida de lugar.*

Isaías mescla fatos futuros que aconteceram em breve tempo, a partir do tempo em que escreveu as profecias, com fatos naturais e catástrofes que somente muitos séculos depois aconteceriam, fatos estes também profetizados por Jesus, quase setecentos anos mais tarde, bem como por São João, no Apocalipse, e por Nostradamus mais de dois mil anos depois de Isaías.

O que poderia fazer com que o sol, a lua e as estrelas deixassem de irradiar luz para a Terra?

Um eclipse, seja lunar ou solar, não impediria a luz das estrelas de chegar até a Terra. E um eclipse não tem ligação com terremoto, ou alteração do eixo da Terra.

Vemos que Isaías fala em trevas em relação à luz do sol, da lua e das estrelas, ou seja, algo impediria por completo a chegada dessa luz à Terra.

E vemos também que ele fala que a terra seria movida de lugar. Terremoto ou inclinação do eixo da Terra?

Somente o impacto de um grande corpo vindo do espaço, como um grande asteróide ou um cometa, ou fragmento de cometa, seria capaz de alterar a inclinação do eixo da Terra, e levantaria uma grande nuvem de poeira que cobriria todo ou quase todo o planeta por um longo tempo, barrando a entrada dos raios solares, da luz da lua e impedindo a visualização das estrelas durante a noite, como aconteceu há 65 milhões de anos atrás causando a extinção dos dinossauros.

No capítulo 24, Isaías escreveu que *a Terra seria dissipada e ficaria nua, e seria afligida a sua face, e que os seus habitantes se espalhariam*.

Sustenta que todos seriam igualmente atingidos, independentemente de suas atividades, sexo ou profissões.

Acrescenta que *a Terra em total estrago será desolada, e pela rapina saqueada, e que seria descaído o orbe*.

Poucos homens seriam deixados na Terra, segundo Isaías. E depois de descrever um quadro de dor e sofrimento para a humanidade, no mesmo capítulo 24 ele escreveu que para os habitantes da Terra estava aparelhado o susto, a cova e o laço.

E afirmou Isaías: "*E acontecerá: que o que fugir da voz do susto cairá na cova, e o que se desembaraçou da cova ficará preso no laço, porque as cataratas lá das alturas foram abertas e serão abalados os fundamentos da Terra. Com a ruptura de suas partes, será a Terra feita em pedaços, com o choque delas será a Terra esmigalhada, com o seu abalo será a mesma terra desconjuntada, pelo balanço será agitada como um embriagado, e será tirada como uma tenda duma noite, e carregará sobre ela a sua iniqüidade, e cairá, e não tornará a levantar-se*".

Essa parte dos escritos de Isaías só confirma o início do capítulo 24 de seu livro, mostrando que o sofrimento será geral.

Afirma Isaías que os fundamentos da Terra serão abalados. Isso poderá acontecer com o choque de um asteróide ou cometa com a superfície da Terra, causando inclinação do seu eixo, o que levaria a mudanças climáticas radicais e rápidas, com enchentes em alguns lugares e secas em outros. Haveria deslocamento dos oceanos, com inundações e maremotos em várias partes do globo.

É possível, ainda, que haja, segundo as afirmações de Isaías, grande transformação na distribuição das terras, com deslocamento das placas tectônicas, gerando grandes e fortes terremotos. Isso seria o resultado do que ele chamou de *abalo aos fundamentos da Terra*.

Parece mesmo que o profeta Isaías, 2.700 anos atrás, previu uma catástrofe global gerada pelo impacto de um ou vários corpos rochosos vindos do espaço, que causaria mudança no eixo da Terra, provocando mudanças climáticas rápidas e terríveis, deslocamento brusco das placas tectônicas, com grandes e fortes terremotos, além de maremotos e outras coisas mais, com total desequilíbrio ecológico.

Não se pode interpretar da leitura do livro de Isaías na Bíblia que haverá guerra atômica de grandes proporções, pois nada parecido com os efeitos de uma guerra nuclear é descrito pelo profeta. É muito mais lógico interpretar que haverá choque de um corpo sólido vindo do espaço, cujos efeitos já foram demonstrados no primeiro capítulo.

JEREMIAS.

Este profeta viveu entre os séculos VII e VI a.C. (640 a 587 a.C.), e pregou por mais de 40 anos.

No capítulo 4, versículos 5 em diante, Jeremias escreveu:

"Anunciai em Judá e fazei ouvir em Jerusalém: falai e publicai ao som da trombeta na terra, gritai em alta voz e dizei: Ajuntai-vos todos e entremos nas cidades fortificadas, levantai o estandarte em Sião. Esforçai-vos, não estejais parados, porque eu faço vir do aquilão um mal e uma grande assolação. Saiu o leão do seu covil, e levantou-se o roubador das gentes: saiu do seu país, para reduzir a tua terra a um deserto: as tuas cidades serão destruídas, sem que nelas fique algum habitador".

Estava Jeremias prevendo a invasão que se deu próximo ao seu tempo, em Israel, ou a invasão romana, mais distante um pouco do seu tempo?

De uma forma ou de outra, Jeremias previu uma invasão que se concretizou, com grande destruição das cidades e com a retirada dos judeus de sua pátria e remoção para outras nações, na condição de escravos.

No versículo 23 do mesmo capítulo 4, Jeremias escreveu:

"Olhei para a terra, e eis que estava vazia, e era nada; e para o céu, e não havia nele luz. Vi os montes, e eis que se moviam; e todos os outeiros tremiam. Olhei, e não havia homem, e todas as aves do céu haviam se retirado. Olhei, e eis que estava deserto o Carmelo; e todas as suas cidades foram destruídas na presença do senhor, e na presença da ira do seu furor".

Essa passagem de Jeremias não parece se referir ao seu tempo, nem tampouco à época de qualquer invasão de Israel. Parece na verdade com as profecias feitas por Isaías, e também por Jesus, e depois no Apocalipse.

Jeremias viu a terra vazia; o céu sem luz, ou seja, o céu coberto por nuvens, e sem a visualização da luz do sol ou das estrelas; os montes se movendo, causado provavelmente por um grande terremoto; a fuga das aves, por causa do terremoto ou outra causa de grande impacto na terra; as cidades destruídas, pelo terremoto ou algum impacto.

Mais adiante, Jeremias escreveu no versículo 27 do capítulo4:

"Porque isto diz o Senhor: Deserta ficará toda a terra, porém, contudo, eu não a destruirei de todo. Chorará a terra, e entristecerão os céus de cima, porque falei, considerei e não me arrependi nem desisti disso".

Jeremias confirma a destruição de parte da terra, que ficará deserta, mas não a sua destruição total, o que coincide com outras profecias analisadas neste livro.

DANIEL.

Viveu no século VI a.C., e escreveu no capítulo 9 de seu livro que *"Desde a ordem para Jerusalém ser segunda vez edificada, até o Cristo capitão, passarão sete semanas e sessenta e duas semanas: e segunda vez serão edificadas as ruas, e os muros na angústia dos tempos. E depois de sessenta e duas semanas, será morto o Cristo: e o povo, que o há de negar, não será mais seu povo. E um povo com o seu capitão, que há de vir, destruirá a cidade e o santuário: e o seu fim será uma ruína total e a desolação, a que ela foi condenada, lhe virá depois no fim da guerra. Esse Cristo porém confirmará para muitos o seu pacto numa semana: no meio da semana faltará a hóstia e o sacrifício: e ver-se-á no Templo a abominação da desolação: e a desolação perseverará até a consumação e até o fim".*

Pelo que se vê, a contagem de tempo empregada pelo profeta não se assemelha em nada à nossa forma de contar o tempo. Ele escreveu sobre a vinda do Cristo, sua negação pelos judeus e a posterior destruição de Jerusalém, o que aconteceu no ano 70 d.C., portanto, 38 anos depois da morte de Jesus, que se deu entre 32 e 34 d.C.

Em razão da revolta dos judeus, que nunca aceitaram o domínio romano, que existia desde 63 a.c., Jerusalém foi cercada e sitiada pelas tropas romanas comandadas pelo general Tito em 70 d.C., e depois foi invadida e completamente destruída, inclusive o Templo de Salomão, ou Grande Templo, e quem não morreu nessa guerra foi vendido como escravo e espalhado pelo mundo romano. Isso foi o começo do fim do que outrora fora o Estado judeu em Canaã, ou na Palestina, denominação dada pelos romanos à sua província, quando conquistaram a região.

A *abominação da desolação* foi a completa destruição do Templo, a sua ruína, e o deserto que se tornou Jerusalém durante um bom tempo após a sua destruição.

A mesma expressão viria mais tarde a ser utilizada por Jesus em suas profecias, algumas coincidentes com os escritos de Daniel.

O Templo de Salomão, segundo os escritos de Daniel, permaneceria desolado até a consumação e até o fim. E ele de fato até hoje não foi reconstruído, existindo em seu lugar, 2.000 anos depois de sua destruição, apenas um grande e alto muro formado por enormes blocos de pedra, resto do que teria sido o fundo do Grande Templo, e que passou a ser chamado pelos judeus de "O Muro das Lamentações", principal local sagrado para eles hoje, e onde diariamente centenas de judeus de várias seitas e correntes judaicas vão fazer suas orações e colocar papéis com pedidos entre os blocos de pedra.

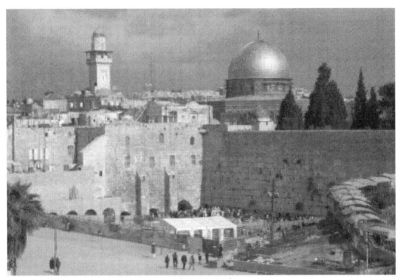
(Foto 17)

A desolação do templo de fato persevera até hoje. Quando será a consumação, e o fim a que refere o profeta? Será o do Dia do Juízo Universal? O dia do impacto do asteróide ou cometa?

Vemos também que o profeta acertou ao afirmar que o povo judeu negaria Jesus, o que de fato aconteceu, e por isso deixaria de ser o seu povo. Depois da morte de Jesus, nasceu o Cristianismo, e os judeus, que não reconheceram em Jesus o Messias previsto pelos profetas antigos, deixaram realmente de ser o seu povo, e aguardam até hoje a chegada do Messias, ao contrário dos cristãos que louvam Jesus como sendo o Salvador prometido muitos séculos antes por Deus.

MIQUÉIAS.
Viveu entre 740 e 687 a.C.

Em seu livro, no capítulo 1, escreveu Miquéias que *"Ele descerá, e pisará aos pés tudo o que há de grande na terra. E debaixo dele, os montes desaparecerão: e os vales se rasgarão como cera, diante do fogo, e como as águas, que se precipitam num abismo"*.

O cenário descrito pelo profeta nessa passagem também nos faz pensar na mesma catástrofe prevista por Isaías e Daniel, uma vez que também envolve montes desaparecendo, vales se rasgando, fogo, águas se precipitando. Isso parece ter a ver com o choque de um corpo vindo do espaço, que destruirá montes; o fogo de meteoros; terremotos e choques de placas tectônicas, abrindo o solo, e rios e mares descendo por aberturas na terra.

No capítulo 4 Miquéias também fala em julgamento e transformações dos povos, que não mais se baterão em lutas, fazendo de suas espadas arados, e de suas lanças enxadas, de forma semelhante aos outros profetas que igualmente fizeram essas previsões.

ZACARIAS.
Viveu no século VI a.C.
Profetizou de 520 a 518 a.C.
Vê-se logo no capítulo 1 de seu livro da Bíblia que suas visões, mostradas por um anjo, segundo o profeta, se assemelham muito em sua simbologia aos escritos de São João no Apocalipse.

Fala o profeta Zacarias em cavalos e cavaleiros, e em cornos, que com suas marradas (chifradas) fariam ir pelos ares Judá, Israel e Jerusalém.

No capítulo 2, Zacarias escreveu: *"Filha de Sião, entoa cânticos de louvor, e alegra-te: porque eis aí vou eu mesmo, e habitarei no meio de ti, diz o Senhor. E naquele dia se chegarão muitas gentes ao Senhor, e serão o meu povo, e eu habitarei no meio de ti"*.

Podemos ver nitidamente que o profeta escreveu sobre Jesus, que nasceu entre os judeus, e a ele muita gente procurou, tanto em Jerusalém quanto em outras cidades e aldeias da região.

No versículo 9 do capítulo 9 Zacarias escreveu: *"Salta de extremo prazer, ó filha de Sião, enche-se de júbilo, ó filha de Jerusalém! Eis aí, o teu rei virá a ti, justo e salvador! Ele é pobre, e vem montado sobre uma jumenta, e sobre o potrinho da jumenta"*.

Novamente Zacarias faz referência a Jesus, e sua entrada em Jerusalém montado em uma jumenta, conforme confirmado pelos escritos dos evangelhos da Bíblia.

O profeta anteviu a entrada de Jesus naquela em Jerusalém 500 anos antes disso acontecer.

No versículo 6 do capítulo 14, Zacarias escreveu que: "*acontecerá naquele dia: Não haverá luz, mas sim frio e gelo. E haverá um dia conhecido do Senhor que não será nem dia, nem noite, e na tarde desse dia aparecerá a luz*".

O Dia do Senhor, como os profetas escreviam, seria o Dia do Juízo Final, ou do Juízo Universal. E nesse tempo não haveria luz, mas apenas frio e gelo. Como isso se daria?

O impacto de um grande asteróide, ou de fragmentos grandes de um cometa criaria uma nuvem de poeira imensa, cobrindo a toda ou quase toda a atmosfera terrestre, impedindo assim a penetração da luz solar, e com isso teríamos um inverno prolongado, com muito frio e formação de gelo na Terra. E falta da luz solar tornaria dia e noite iguais (**não será nem dia, nem noite...**).

JOÃO BATISTA.

Foi contemporâneo de Jesus, tendo talvez alguns poucos meses ou poucos anos de diferença de idade em relação a ele.

João adotou a vida ascética, retirando-se para o deserto, onde pregava aos judeus, recomendando-lhes fazer penitência e se arrependerem, porque o reino dos céus estava próximo; mandava prepararem o caminho do Senhor; dizia que batizava com água, mas aquele estava para vir depois dele batizaria no Espírito Santo e com fogo, e que seria mais poderoso do que ele.

João falava da chegada do Messias como se o fato fosse extremamente iminente, e de fato Jesus logo apareceu para ser por ele batizado.

Logo em seguida João foi preso e decapitado, e Jesus cresceu em fama e fez maravilhas.

João sabia, intimamente, pois não devia conhecer Jesus, nem saber do seu destino, que Jesus era o Messias, o Prometido por Deus aos antigos profetas. E ele falava da chegada do Reino do Céu como uma coisa próxima. Mas isso de fato ainda não se concretizou, posto que ainda há guerras, fome, doenças, sofrimento e muitas coisas ruins no mundo. Assim, sua profecia sobre a chegada do Messias se confirmou ainda nos seus dias, e ele teve o privilégio de batizar Jesus, que humildemente a ele se apresentou para isso. E morreu na glória, depois de conhecer e olhar nos olhos o homem mais importante que já pisou a Terra até nossos dias. Contudo, o reino do céu, ou o reino de Deus ainda não se estabeleceu na Terra, mesmo dois mil anos depois da morte de João Batista. O seu sonho e a sua profecia ainda será confirmada no futuro.

CAPÍTULO 5

AS PROFECIAS DE JESUS CRISTO

Inicialmente, vale relembrar que Jesus tinha a faculdade de ver o futuro, ou de profetizar, que é um dom divino. E ele tanto via o futuro próximo como o mais distante. Tanto viu a destruição de Jerusalém, que aconteceria em breve tempo, no ano 70 d.C., quanto o Dia do Juízo Universal, o Dia do Senhor, como muito tempo antes dele já haviam profetizado outros profetas de Israel como Isaías e Daniel.

É importante e relevante também lembrar e chamar a atenção para o fato de que Jesus nada escreveu. Os quatro Evangelhos contidos na Bíblia foram escritos vários anos depois de sua morte, sendo dois deles por apóstolos, João e Mateus, e dois por pessoas que não o conheceram, Lucas e Marcos, que escreveram relatando fatos que ouviram de outras pessoas, talvez de pessoas que tenham convivido com Jesus, podendo ter ouvido os relatos sobre Jesus até mesmo de outros discípulos ou apóstolos dele.

Assim, se levarmos em consideração que Jesus na confusão que se formou no Templo de Salomão, ou depois dela, em um monte falou de várias coisas futuras a seus apóstolos, é razoável pensarmos que, sendo a memória humana falha, tenham os apóstolos misturado as profecias relativas a acontecimentos breves com fatos que somente muito tempo depois aconteceriam. Como exemplo disso, encontramos a destruição de Jerusalém e do templo no ano 70 d.C. e a catástrofe descrita que levaria à morte grande parte da humanidade, e que não aconteceu ainda, nem em Israel, nem em parte alguma do planeta, e que apontamos como causa a queda de asteróide ou cometa ainda por acontecer.

O primeiro Evangelho na seqüência bíblica é o de Mateus.

Mateus era cobrador de impostos. E um cobrador de impostos tinha que ser, necessariamente, uma pessoa com certa cultura, que sabia ler e escrever bem, que tinha que ter conhecimento básico de matemática, para fazer os registros dos tributos arrecadados, e certamente inteligente e esperto.

65

Mateus devia ter posses. Não era pobre. Tinha algo a perder, do ponto de vista material, quando tudo largou para seguir Jesus. Ele deve ter ficado muito impressionado com o novo Mestre que surgiu repentinamente na Galiléia.

Partindo do princípio, como fazemos em relação a todos os escritos dos Evangelhos da Bíblia, que os escritos de Mateus são verdadeiros, e que somente relatam o que de fato ele ouviu de Jesus, passamos a analisar o que Jesus falou do futuro, as suas profecias, já confirmadas ou ainda pendentes de confirmação.

No Sermão da Montanha, narrado por Mateus no capítulo 5 de seu Evangelho, Jesus falou das Bem-Aventuranças. Disse ele que os mansos possuiriam a Terra.

Assim, se a Terra fosse totalmente destruída no futuro, ninguém restaria, e nada haveria a ser possuído pelos homens, o que reforça a idéia de que, mesmo com as catástrofes que se abaterão sobre o planeta, ainda restarão pessoas nele, a Terra ainda será habitada, mas apenas pelos mansos.

No capítulo 10 Mateus relata que Jesus disse para eles se resguardarem dos homens, porque eles os fariam comparecer em seus juízos, açoitar nas sinagogas, levar diante dos governadores e dos reis, para lhes servir e também aos gentios de testemunho.

Após a morte de Jesus, de fato começou a perseguição dos cristãos em Israel, e depois por todo o Império Romano, e muitos foram presos, levados à presença de reis e governadores, que os julgaram, e foram açoitados, crucificados, queimados vivos ou comidos por leões nos circos romanos.

Com isso, essa profecia inicial de Jesus foi completamente cumprida, e pouco depois de sua morte.

No capítulo 23, Mateus fala do discurso de Jesus aos fariseus, e no versículo 34 reafirma as mesmas coisas expostas acima em relação à perseguição dos profetas e dos cristãos.

No versículo 36 Jesus fala: *"Em verdade vos digo, que todas estas coisas virão a cair sobre esta geração"*.

E teve razão Jesus. A perseguição aos cristãos começou ainda na geração de seus apóstolos e discípulos, tendo muitos deles sido presos e mortos de forma violenta.

Alguns evangelhos, descrevendo a fala de Jesus de forma e seqüência um pouco diferentes de Mateus, podem dar a entender que tudo o que ele falou, inclusive a morte de grande parte da população da Terra se daria ainda naquela geração. Mas não foi isso o que Jesus disse. Mateus escreveu de forma correta, e na seqüência certa, pois o pior do que Jesus falou está registrado por Mateus depois da fala inicial sobre a perseguição e morte dos profetas e sábios enviados por Jesus.

Nos versículos 37, 38 e 39 Jesus falou: *"Jerusalém, Jerusalém, que matas os profetas, e apedrejas os que te são enviados, quantas vezes eu quis juntar teus filhos, do modo como uma galinha recolhe debaixo das asas os seus pintos, e tu não quiseste? Eis aí vos ficará deserta a vossa casa. Porque eu vos declaro que desde agora não me tornareis a ver até que digais: Bendito seja o que vem em nome do Senhor"*.

Nessa passagem de Mateus, Jesus já profetiza que Jerusalém ficaria deserta. E que os judeus não mais o veriam até que dissessem "Bendito seja o que vem em nome do Senhor", o que ainda não aconteceu, pois os judeus não reconhecem até hoje Jesus como o Filho do Homem, como mencionado nas escrituras sagradas dos judeus, ou como o Salvador, o Messias que haveria de vir, previsto pelos profetas antigos dos judeus.

Depois de dizer essas coisas no Templo, ia Jesus dele se retirando, quando se aproximaram dele seus discípulos, desejando mostrar-lhe a fábrica do templo. E Jesus lhes disse: *"Não verdade vos digo, que não ficará aqui pedra sobre pedra que não seja derrubada"*.

De fato, como já dito antes, no ano 70 d.C., cerca de 38 anos depois da fala de Jesus, as tropas romanas comandadas por Tito cercaram Jerusalém e por fim a destruíram e mataram grande parte da população. E do Grante Templo, do Templo de Salomão, somente restou o muro do seu fundo. Ou seja, o templo foi de fato destruído, e até hoje não reconstruído.

Depois, logo em seguida, Jesus estava sentado no Monte das Oliveiras, quando seus discípulos o chamaram em particular e lhes perguntaram: *"Diga-nos, quando sucederão essas coisas?"*. E Jesus lhes respondeu dizendo: *"Vejam, que ninguém vos engane. Porque virão muitos em meu nome, dizendo: Eu sou cristo. E enganarão a muitos. Havereis, pois, de ouvir guerras, e rumores de guerras. Olhai, não vos turbeis, porque importa que assim aconteça, mas não é este ainda o fim, porque se levantará nação contra nação, e reino contra reino, e haverá pestilência, e fome, e terremotos em diversos lugares. E todas essas coisas são princípios das dores".*

Nos últimos dois mil anos muitos falsos cristos e falsos profetas já apareceram na Terra, e neste século XXI ainda há falsos profetas. Muitas guerras e rumores de guerras temos conhecimento, sendo as duas maiores guerras aquelas ocorridas no século XX, as Primeira e Segunda Guerras Mundiais, tendo esta última causado a morte de 60 milhões de pessoas, fora feridos, aleijados, inutilizados, órfãos, viúvos e viúvas e tanto sofrimento causado.

Terremotos, a antiguidade registra inúmeros. O Palácio de Cleópatra foi destruído por um, o mesmo se dando com o Farol de Alexandria. A Grécia registra tantos terremotos na antiguidade. Cidades várias no passado distante e no século XX foram parcialmente destruídas por terremotos. Lembramos dos terríveis terremotos da Turquia, do México, do Japão e o de Los Ângeles.

Fome, a Idade Média registra até demais; revoluções foram feitas pela fome. Pestes. Lembramos da peste bubônica, da gripe espanhola, e houve outras que mataram milhões de pessoas na Europa.

Esses fatos dolorosos seriam, segundo Jesus, apenas o princípio das dores. Este não seria o fim. Mas Jesus não falou em momento algum do fim da raça humana, ou do fim da Terra.

Nos versículos 9 a 14, Mateus escreveu que Jesus disse que então eles seriam entregues à tribulação, e seriam mortos, o que já falamos antes. E disse, ainda, que seria pregado o evangelho por todo o mundo, e então chegaria o fim.

Esse é um dos marcos para a percepção da proximidade do que Jesus chamou de "fim". Ou seja, *a pregação do evangelho por todo o mundo*. Logo, o "fim" mencionado por Jesus não poderia se dar naquela época, nem mesmo durante a vida do último apóstolo a morrer, que foi João, porque no século I da Era Cristã o evangelho ainda estava apenas começando a ser divulgado pelo Oriente Médio e parte da Europa.

Somente muitos séculos depois, cerca de 1.500 anos depois da morte de Jesus, é que o cristianismo e o evangelho chegaram até o Japão, a China e a vários países asiáticos e ao continente americano, pois as grandes navegações tiveram início apenas por volta do ano 1.500.

Assim, se o fim tivesse que chegar à época da geração dos apóstolos, a maior parte dos habitantes da Terra ainda não teria conhecido a mensagem de Jesus. Isso contrariaria as suas palavras.

Falando da vinda do Filho do Homem, Jesus, conforme o versículo 28 do capítulo 24 de Mateus disse: *"Em qualquer lugar onde estiver o corpo, aí se juntarão também as águias"*.

A meu ver, Jesus quis dizer que em toda a parte onde houver ser humano na Terra haveria morte, pois isso atrairia as águias. Ou seja, a catástrofe será mundial, e não apenas localizada, em Israel ou em outra qualquer região do planeta.

No versículo 29 do mesmo capítulo, Mateus relata que Jesus disse: *"E logo depois da aflição daqueles dias, escurecer-se-á o sol, e a lua não dará a sua claridade, e as estrelas cairão do céu, e as virtudes do céu se comoverão; e então aparecerá o sinal do Filho do Homem no céu, e então todos os povos da Terra chorarão"*.

Esta passagem lembra uma já transcrita anteriormente, prevista por um dos profetas antigos de Israel.

Jesus fala de aflições anteriores, que devem ser as guerras, fome, pestes, terremotos e maremotos em diversas partes. E então, depois disso tudo, o sol escureceria durante o dia, a lua não daria mais a sua claridade durante a noite, e as estrelas cairiam do céu.

Como já vimos anteriormente, somente o impacto de um asteróide grande ou um cometa ou fragmento de cometa faria "o sol escurecer", pois na verdade o sol nada sofreria diretamente com tal impacto, apenas nossa visão dele é que ficaria turvada por nuvens de poeira que se levantariam na atmosfera terrestre. E da mesma forma a lua, durante a noite, não seria também vista da Terra, por causa das nuvens espessas de poeira a cobrir a Terra.

Quanto a estrelas caindo do céu, temos que lembrar ao leitor que Jesus e os profetas tiveram visões muitos milênios antes do surgimento da ciência. Em suas épocas as pessoas não sabiam que as estrelas eram sóis, como o nosso sol, e que a Terra gira em torno do sol. As pessoas pensavam, inclusive os sábios da época, que a abóbada celeste era fixa, firme, e daí o nome firmamento. Aquilo que vemos e chamamos de céu não passa de uma camada de gases, que dão o efeito da cor azul que vemos da superfície da terra.

Os antigos acreditavam que as estrelas eram como lamparinas presas e penduradas no firmamento, nada mais do que isso. Ninguém sabia da existência de cometas, asteróides, meteoros, etc. Assim, como até hoje chamamos de "estrelas cadentes" os meteoros que entram em nossa atmosfera terrestre, porque desde a mais remota antiguidade se pensava que os hoje conhecidos meteoros eram estrelas que caíam do céu, não é difícil concluir que as estrelas caindo do céu de que falou Jesus diziam respeito à queda de meteoros na Terra.

Depois da queda das estrelas, na verdade queda de meteoros, apareceria no céu o "sinal do Filho do Homem". Que sinal seria esse? Um cometa, visível da Terra, com sua cauda comprida e visível de vários quilômetros?

No versículo 34, do mesmo capítulo 24, Mateus relata que Jesus disse que tudo isso aconteceria ainda naquela geração. Ora, se considerarmos geração da mesma forma como hoje a entendemos, só podemos atribuir a um equívoco de interpretação do evangelista, que depois de ouvir tantas coisas, relativas ao cerco de Jerusalém e sua destruição e também coisas relativas a um futuro distante de seu tempo, misturou todas as informações como se tudo o que foi anunciado por Jesus fosse acontecer naquela geração. É claro que os acontecimentos relativos ao escurecimento do sol, da lua e a queda das estrelas não aconteceram no tempo de vida dos apóstolos. Nem em nosso tempo ainda não aconteceram essas coisas. E devemos levar em conta, ainda, que Mateus não deve ter escrito o evangelho no mesmo dia em que ouviu tais coisas de Jesus, mas muitos anos depois. E a memória é falha. Mateus certamente misturou fatos que aconteceriam primeiro com outros posteriores, sem perceber a ordem, ou sem lembrar da ordem em que Jesus colocou as coisas e os acontecimentos profetizados.

Nos versículos 36 a 41, do capítulo 24, Mateus relata que Jesus disse: *"Mas daquele dia, nem daquela hora, ninguém sabe, nem os anjos dos céus, senão só o Pai. E assim como foi nos dias de Noé, assim será a vinda do Filho do homem. Porque assim como nos dias antes do dilúvio estavam comendo e bebendo, casando-se dando-se em casamento, até ao dia que Noé entrou na arca, e não o entenderam enquanto não veio o dilúvio e os levou a todos, assim será também a vinda do Filho do homem. Então de dois que estiverem no campo, um será tomado, e outro será deixado. De duas mulheres que estiverem moendo em um moinho, uma será tomada, e outra será deixada"*. E segundo o versículo 42, Jesus disse: *"Velai, pois, porque não sabeis a que hora há de vir vosso Senhor"*.

Jesus deixou claro que nem ele mesmo sabia o dia e a hora em que tudo o que ele descreveu aconteceria. Só Deus conhece essa hora. E por isso deveríamos estar vigilantes.

O Evangelho de São Marcos, que não conheceu e não ouviu os relatos diretamente de Jesus, praticamente repete no seu capítulo 13 as mesmas coisas e palavras de Mateus, com exceção do contido nos versículos 14 a 23, que dizem: *"Quando, porém, vós virdes estar a abominação da desolação onde não deve estar, o que lê entenda, então os que estiverem na Judéia fujam para os montes; os que estiverem sobre o telhado não desçam à sua casa nem entrem para levar dela coisa alguma. E os que se acharem no campo não voltem atrás para buscar os seus vestidos. Mas ai das que naquele tempo estiverem grávidas, e criarem. Rogai, pois, para que não sucedam estas coisas no inverno. Porque naqueles dias haverá tribulações tais como nunca houve desde o princípio das criaturas, que Deus fez até agora, nem haverá. De sorte que, se o senhor não abreviasse aqueles dias, nenhuma pessoa se salvaria. Mas ele o abreviou em atenção aos escolhidos, de que fez escolha. E se então vos disser alguém: Reparai, aqui está o Cristo, ou, ei-lo acolá está, não lhe dê crédito, porque se levantarão falsos Cristos, e falsos profetas, que farão prodígios, e portentos para enganarem, se possível fosse, até os mesmos escolhidos. Estejam vós, pois, de sobreaviso, e olhai que eu vos preveni de tudo"*.

Observemos que Jesus nesta passagem de São Marcos é taxativo ao afirmar que as tribulações que haveria naqueles dias nunca antes haviam acontecido da mesma forma, desde o princípio das criaturas, e nunca mais aconteceria. E disse que se Deus não abreviasse as tribulações, nenhuma pessoa se salvaria. Mas Deus abreviaria as tribulações, e pessoas escapariam da morte.

Mesmo se tomarmos como hipótese uma guerra nuclear entre grandes potências, não há como pensar que todas as coisas descritas nos evangelhos de Mateus e Marcos se encaixem perfeitamente nessa hipótese. Primeiro porque nem todos os países do mundo seriam atingidos com mísseis ou foguetes com ogivas nucleares.

Imaginem se as grandes potências iriam se preocupar em mandar armas nucleares para destruírem o Brasil e os demais países da América do Sul, que não incomodam as grandes potências, ou mesmo certos países asiáticos pequenos, a Austrália, a África, e tantos outros países. A guerra não atingiria diretamente a todos no planeta. Somente a radiação se espalharia, e a depender da quantidade e da potência das bombas utilizadas. Mas jamais uma guerra nuclear chegaria a obscurecer o sol e a lua, nem tampouco faria caírem as estrelas do céu.

Somente a queda na Terra, na forma já antes descritas, de um asteróide ou fragmentos de cometa levaria a humanidade a um sofrimento tão grande quanto o descrito pelos evangelistas, e que precisaria ser abreviado para que uma parte da humanidade escapasse da morte.

Jesus previu uma tão grande destruição que quase levaria a humanidade à total destruição. Mas, apesar de muitas mortes, nem todos seriam levados deste mundo. Em sua maneira de falar, Jesus disse que de cada dois, um seria levado, e um deixado, o que significa metade, 50%. Ou seja, se tomado ao pé da letra, Jesus disse que metade da humanidade seria morta na catástrofe por ele profetizada.

No Evangelho de São Marcos, terceiro na seqüência do Novo Testamento da Bíblia, ele repete muitas coisas contidas nos dois primeiros, que não repetiremos, por não haver necessidade, mas no versículo 11 do capítulo 21 ele acrescenta um detalhe não contido nos evangelhos de Mateus e Marcos.

Disse Jesus, segundo esse versículo, depois de falar nas guerras, terremotos, pestes e fome, que antecederiam a grande destruição, que *"aparecerão coisas espantosas, e grandes sinais no céu"*.

Mais uma vez, tomando como hipótese uma guerra nuclear, não podemos visualizar que ela nos mostrará grandes sinais no céu. As explosões se dão na terra, ou próximo do solo, não no céu. E uma explosão atômica já é hoje uma coisa de certo modo "banal", em face de tantos filmes mostrando esse tipo de explosão, inclusive as explosões reais de Hiroshima e Nagasaki. Isso não seria novidade, nem tão espantoso assim.

Já a aproximação da Terra de um grande asteróide ou de um cometa, coisa nunca antes vista pelos habitantes da Terra, seria sim uma coisa espantosa, talvez até mesmo para Jesus, que também nunca viu nada igual em seu tempo.

São Lucas coloca, segundo as palavras de Jesus, que antes disso tudo (guerras, terremotos, pestes, coisas espantosas e sinais do céu) haveria a perseguição e morte dos cristãos, o que de fato aconteceu, estando a seqüência de Lucas mais correta do que algumas outras, que deixam dúvidas, que misturam fatos mais recentes com os mais distantes no tempo.

Lucas narra nos versículos 20 a 24 do capítulo 21 a destruição de Jerusalém numa seqüência impecável, conforme adiante transcrito: *"Quando virdes, pois, que Jerusalém é sitiada de um exército, então sabei que está próxima a sua desolação. Os que nesse tempo se acharem na Judéia, fujam para os montes, os que estiverem dentro da cidade, retirem-se, e os que estiverem nos campos, não entrem nela, porque estes são dias de vingança, para que se cumpram todas as coisas que estão escritas. Mas ai das que estiverem prenhes, e das que então criarem naqueles dias! Porque haverá grande aperto sobre a terra, e ira contra este povo. E cairão ao fio da espada, e serão levados cativos a todas as nações, e Jerusalém será pisada dos gentios até se completarem os tempos das nações"*.

Essa passagem é ainda mais clara do que as mesmas descrições em Mateus e Marcos. Trata-se do cerco de Jerusalém pelos romanos em 70 d.C., liderados por Tito, que seria depois um dos imperadores de Roma.

Depois de um ano de cerco, sem entrar comida na cidade, ela foi finalmente invadida, destruída, mortos seus habitantes, em grande parte pela espada, e os sobreviventes foram de fato vendidos como escravos para várias províncias do Império Romano.

A recomendação de Jesus de que não voltassem à cidade quem fora dela estivesse era correta, e procedente, e o mesmo se dava para quem estivesse dentro da cidade, e que deveria dela sair. Será que na época alguém levou a sério as palavras de Jesus e escapou do cerco e da morte?

Após a destruição de Jerusalém e a dispersão dos judeus pelo mundo como escravos, de fato a cidade, e toda a Palestina, passou a ser morada de gentios, palavra utilizada pelos judeus para se referirem a quem não era judeu. E somente na primeira metade do século XX os judeus começaram a retornar para a região em larga escala.

Observemos que Jesus disse que Jerusalém seria morada dos gentios até que se completassem os tempos das nações.

Jerusalém efetivamente foi pisada dos gentios até 1.948, quando foi criado o Estado de Israel. Aí, então, deve ser considerado o marco final do que Jesus chamou de *tempos das nações*. Ou no máximo no início do século XX, a partir do ano 1.922, quando, ainda estando a Palestina sob controle e administração do Reino Unido, por outorga da Liga das Nações, os judeus começaram a migrar para lá em grande quantidade, ainda que sem autonomia política, e sem ser um Estado independente.

O que seriam os "tempos das nações"?

Certamente um tempo para alguma coisa. Mas para quê?

Jesus quis dizer que as nações teriam um tempo até a volta dos judeus à sua antiga terra, hoje Israel. E depois desse tempo, segundo a seqüência de Lucas (versículos 25 e 26), seriam vistos os *"sinais no sol, e na lua, e nas estrelas, e na terra consternação de gentes pela confusão em que as porá o bramido do mar, e das ondas, mirrando-se os homens de susto, e na expectativa do que virá sobre todo o mundo, porque as virtudes dos céus se abalarão"*.

Novamente somos forçados a afastar a hipótese de guerra nuclear para caracterizar o chamado Dia do Senhor, ou dia do Filho do homem, ou Dia do Juízo Universal, porque Jesus claramente falou de sinais no sol, na lua e nas estrelas, medo por causa da agitação do mar e das ondas que causariam grande susto nos homens, e medo do que estava ainda por vir depois disso tudo.

Os terremotos já acontecidos na Terra desde a antiguidade, os maremotos, as pestes, as guerras, os eclipses, não indicam o cumprimento das palavras de Jesus. Nem mesmo o recente Tsunami de 2.004, que matou mais de 220 mil pessoas nos leva a esse convencimento, porque foi apenas localizado, em pequenas regiões do globo.

As ondas do mar e a sua agitação de modo a matar de susto as pessoas devem ser provocadas pela queda de um asteróide, cometa ou fragmento de cometa no mar, criando ondas gigantescas a se espalharem por grande parte das regiões costeiras do planeta, causando inundações com destruição de cidades inteiras, matando

74

toda ou quase toda a sua população. Isso pode ser visto no filme Impacto Profundo.

O impacto do asteróide ou cometa em terra causará destruição pela onda de choque, com deslocamento de ar em velocidade muitíssimo maior do que o que se dá quando surgem ciclones e tornados, derrubando casas e edifícios.

Certamente, o asteróide ou cometa virá acompanhado de muitos meteoros, que chegarão até a Terra com uma imensa velocidade, em forma de rochas em chamas, com um impacto altamente destrutivo, criando a chamada "chuva de meteoros", ou bolas de fogo caindo do céu, ou ainda estrelas caindo do céu, nas palavras de Jesus e outros profetas antigos dos judeus.

Considero que a volta dos judeus à sua terra natal é o marco do *fim dos tempos das nações,* nas palavras de Jesus. E é a partir desse marco que se pode considerar que está chegando o tempo das catástrofes previstas pelos profetas de Israel, inclusive Jesus, e também no livro Apocalipse.

A concretização dos sofrimentos descritos por Jesus indica a proximidade do Reino de Deus, conforme indica o versículo 31 do capítulo 21 do Evangelho de Lucas.

Jesus disse (versículo 35, capítulo 21, Lucas): *"Porque ele, assim como um laço, prenderá a todos os que habitam sobre a face de toda a terra".* E disse, ainda: *"Vigiai, pois, orando em todo o tempo, a fim de que vos façais dignos de evitar todos estes males, que têm de suceder".*

Nessa passagem, Jesus reafirma que a catástrofe não será local, limitada, mas global, geral. E diz que deveríamos orar para sermos dignos de escapar do sofrimento, e que deveríamos nos preparar para o Reino de Deus, que viria em seguida, reino este de paz, sem guerra, sem fome, sem destruição causada por corpos vindos do espaço, etc.

João é o único dos apóstolos que não escreveu no seu Evangelho sobre as profecias de Jesus acerca das catástrofes que se abateriam sobre a Terra. Talvez por isso mais tarde ele recebeu as *revelações*, contidas no seu livro O Apocalipse.

CAPÍTULO 6

O APOCALIPSE DE SÃO JOÃO

João foi um dos doze apóstolos de Jesus, e o mais novo em idade.

Jesus começou sua pregação logo após ter sido batizado por João Batista, tendo Jesus na época cerca de 30 anos de idade, segundo registra um dos Evangelhos.

Se considerarmos, por hipótese, que João, o apóstolo, tinha cerca de 20 anos quando se juntou a Jesus, ele era cerca de 10 anos mais moço que o mestre.

Conforme já exposto no início desta obra, os historiadores hoje acreditam que Jesus nasceu entre os anos 8 e 6 a.C. Assim, João teria nascido, em nossa hipótese, entre os anos 2 e 4 d.C.

A tradição cristã sustenta que João viveu cerca de 100 anos ou mais. Se ele viveu 100 anos, morreu entre os anos 102 e 104 d.C., portanto, no início do século II d.C.

Jesus foi crucificado entre os anos 32 e 34 d.C. Assim, João viveu ainda cerca de 70 anos depois da morte do mestre na cruz.

João, no fim de sua vida, estava preso na Ilha de Patmos, que fica na costa da atual Turquia, sendo na época domínio romano, como quase toda a região do Mediterrâneo. E sua prisão fazia parte da perseguição aos cristãos, perpetrada pelos romanos, e como havia previsto Jesus.

Vivia João em seus últimos anos de vida em uma gruta na Ilha de Patmos, onde estive no mês de março de 2.007, em viagem à Grécia e Turquia.

Hoje existe uma pequena igreja cobrindo a gruta, a Igreja de São João.

O livro Apocalipse foi escrito por João na Ilha de Patmos na gruta onde vivia já próximo do fim da vida, e em idade bastante avançada.

A palavra *Apocalipse* é grega, e quer dizer *Revelação.*

Conta João, logo no início do livro, que em um dia de domingo foi *arrebatado em espírito*, e que ouviu uma voz parecendo de trombeta atrás dele mandando que ele escrevesse em um livro o que veria. E antes disso escreveu que a revelação lhe foi dada por um anjo que lhe foi enviado.

A descrição de João quanto a ter sido *arrebatado em espírito* em muito se assemelha ao que modernamente se denomina projeção astral, ou projeção da consciência, que é a saída do corpo, ou seja, o espírito deixa temporariamente o corpo, tem uma experiência, e depois a ele retorna. E isso é diferente de uma visão com a pessoa acordada, como Jesus costumava ter, e também os profetas antigos de Israel.

João não era profeta. Ele não via o futuro enquanto estava acordado, como Isaías, Zacarias, Daniel ou Nostradamus. João teve a revelação (apocalipse) fora do corpo, e quando a ele retornou escreveu tudo em um livro, o Apocalipse, que é o último livro que compõe a Bíblia Católica.

O livro Apocalipse é extremamente complexo, e está cheio de simbolismos de difícil interpretação. Em muito se assemelha às quadras de Nostradamus, contidas em seu livro As Centúrias.

Tentar interpretar e decifrar totalmente o Apocalipse é tarefa quase impossível, tanto quanto tentar interpretar e decifrar todas as previsões de Nostradamus.

Nesta obra não ousarei tentar interpretar complemente as visões de João quando arrebatado em espírito. Limitar-me-ei principalmente a mostrar as passagens, palavras e previsões do Apocalipse que se casam perfeitamente com as profecias anteriores dos profetas judeus, principalmente Isaías, Daniel e Jesus, dentro da linha geral seguida por esta obra, de modo a mostrar que as revelações feitas a João na Ilha de Patmos apenas confirmam aquilo que Jesus já havia afirmado, e profetizado, e também outros profetas antes dele.

Há detalhes que considero sem maior relevância no livro Apocalipse, e por isso não tentarei adivinhar ou afirmar com exatidão, por exemplo, o que ou quem viriam a ser os quatro cavaleiros do apocalipse, ou se a besta que sairia do mar seria humana, animal ou espírito, ou apenas uma alegoria, um simbolismo que pode ser interpretado de formas variadas, o que de fato acontece, da mesma forma como intérpretes fazem com as quadras de Nostradamus, e muitas vezes erram, como, por exemplo, quando apontaram o ano 1.999 como sendo o do início da Terceira Guerra Mundial. Muitos intérpretes de Nostradamus erraram ao apontar esse ano, porque nenhuma guerra de grandes proporções teve início em 1.999. E até a presente data, 9 de junho de 2.007, nenhuma guerra de grande porte teve início depois da Segunda Guerra, que se encerrou em 1.945.

Nosso objetivo neste livro não nos permite desviar a atenção do leitor e o foco de nossa análise para detalhes menores. O que importa é a mensagem principal do Apocalipse.

Passamos, assim, à análise do Apocalipse de São João.

Vemos logo nos versículos 12 a 17, do capítulo 1, o simbolismo apresentado a João, tendo ele visto sete candeeiros de ouro, e no meio deles alguém parecido com o Filho do homem, expressão usada por Jesus para indicar a si próprio, porque era uma expressão já empregada anteriormente em livros dos profetas.

João viu sete estrelas na direita do Filho do homem, e de sua boca saía uma espada aguda de dois fios, o que é difícil de interpretar, e não considero relevante.

As sete estrelas são os setes anjos das sete igrejas, e os sete candeeiros as sete igrejas, como explicado no próprio livro.

As mensagens iniciais do Apocalipse foram dadas para as sete igrejas cristãs primitivas, já existentes no tempo de João, e na forma de epístolas, o que diz respeito à época anterior ao nascimento da Igreja Católica Apostólica Romana.

No capítulo 4, que trata da visão preliminar, do Supremo Juiz, João foi novamente arrebatado, dessa vez para uma porta que se abriu no céu, e viu tronos e anciãos neles sentados, e viu no meio dos tronos animais variados que descreveu.

João viu um livro escrito por dentro e por fora, selado com sete selos.

Provavelmente João foi arrebatado mais de uma vez, em dias diferentes, até completar o texto do livro Apocalipse, que é muito grande e complexo.

Ao abrir o Cordeiro (Jesus) o primeiro selo, viu João sair um cavalo branco, e o que estava montado nele tinha um arco, e lhe foi dada uma coroa, e saiu vitorioso para vencer.

Seria o cavaleiro do cavalo branco um dos guerreiros conquistadores, como Átila, rei dos Hunos, chamado de "o flagelo dos deuses"? Ele levou o terror e o sofrimento a muita gente na Ásia e parte da Europa. Ou Gengis Khan? Ou seria uma alusão à Primeira Guerra Mundial? Impossível saber com precisão e exatidão se o cavaleiro era um homem, ou uma nação, ou outra coisa qualquer. E não adianta ficar fazendo adivinhações. Este não é o nosso propósito. Só dá para ter certeza de que o primeiro cavaleiro está relacionado efetivamente a guerra.

Aberto o segundo selo, viu João sair um cavalo vermelho, e foi dado poder ao que estava montado sobre ele, para que tirasse a paz de cima da terra, e que se matassem uns aos outros, e foi-lhe dada uma grande espada. Esse cavaleiro, pelo que se vê no texto, causará mais mortes do que o primeiro.

Seria o cavaleiro do cavalo vermelho também um guerreiro conquistador, como Gengis Khan? Ele matou muita gente na Ásia e Europa, e criou um vasto império a ferro e fogo. Ou seria uma alusão ao comunismo e ao império por ele também construído pela força das armas? A bandeira vermelha do comunismo pode estar relacionada à cor do cavalo. Ou seria uma alusão à Segunda Guerra Mundial, e aos nazistas, que também empunhavam bandeiras vermelhas? Ou pode ser uma coisa que nem nos passa pela cabeça. É impossível ter certeza, salvo quanto ao fato de que o segundo cavaleiro também está relacionado com guerra.

Como Jesus também havia falado de guerras antes dos acontecimentos e catástrofes naturais que causariam grande sofrimento à humanidade, é bem provável mesmo que esses dois cavaleiros primeiros sejam agentes de guerra, na forma de nações ou líderes guerreiros.

O terceiro cavalo do Apocalipse era negro, e sobre ele estava montado alguém com uma balança, símbolo da justiça, e que simboliza julgamento, mas que também pode significar comércio, pois os comerciantes utilizam também balanças para pesarem os alimentos, e na antiguidade não havia balanças digitais, como hoje, sendo elas balanças de pratos laterais, para equilibrar os pesos, exatamente como a balança do símbolo da justiça. E foi dito que *"Meia oitava de trigo valerá um dinheiro, e três oitavas de cevada, um dinheiro; mas não façais dano ao vinho, nem ao azeite"*.

Parece que o terceiro cavalo, o negro, está relacionado à fome, a falta de alimento, como trigo e cevada, seja pela sua falta, seja pelo alto preço, por isso diz o texto que meia oitava de trigo valerá um dinheiro, e três oitavas de cevada valerá também um dinheiro, o que significa que o trigo estará seis vezes mais caro que a cevada. Ou seja, com o mesmo valor (um dinheiro) serão compradas três oitavas de cevada, mas somente meia oitava de trigo.

Claramente a alusão aos alimentos e diferenças de preço diz respeito à falta de alimento, talvez por inflação alta em relação a alguns produtos alimentícios, à seca, ou alguma outra causa natural ou provocada por algo externo à Terra, como destruição de plantações pela queda de meteoros, asteróide ou cometa, ou ainda inundação provada pelo choque desses corpos com a superfície da Terra ou no mar.

O vinho e o azeite seriam poupados da destruição, o que pode significar terras de plantações de olivas (azeitonas) e uvas menos atingidas pela destruição causada pelo "cavaleiro do cavalo negro", sendo este apenas um símbolo, e não uma pessoa ou grupo de pessoas, como no caso dos dois primeiros cavaleiros.

O quarto cavalo é o amarelo, e seu cavaleiro tinha por nome Morte, e foi-lhe dado poder sobre as quatro partes da Terra para que matasse à espada, pela fome, pela mortandade, e pelas alimárias da terra.

Também o quarto cavaleiro não parece ser uma pessoa, mas talvez um povo, que levaria a morte através de guerra, bem como representa fome e doenças, que poderiam se seguir à guerra, ou ser provocada por uma guerra bacteriológica.

Lembremo-nos da febre amarela. E há outras doenças que deixam o doente com a cor amarelada.

Mas o quarto cavaleiro também está associado à espada, e isso representa arma, exército, guerra.

Os quatro cavaleiros juntos representam, pois, guerras, conquistas, carestia e falta de alimentos, fome e doenças.

O quinto selo aberto em seguida dá a entender que ainda haveria martírio de religiosos, tudo indicando que será de cristãos, antes do terremoto que viria com a abertura do sexto selo.

Quando se abriu o sexto selo, João viu o que descreveu assim: *"E eis que sobreveio um grande terremoto e se tornou o sol negro, como um saco de cilício, e a lua se tornou toda como sangue, e as estrelas caíram do céu sobre a terra, como quando a figueira, sendo agitada dum grande vento, deixa cair os seus figos verdes, e o céu se recolheu como um livro, que se enrola, e todos os montes e ilhas se moveram de seus lugares, e os reis da terra, e os príncipes, e os tribunos, e os ricos e os poderosos, e todo o servo e livre se esconderam nas cavernas e entre os penhascos dos montes. E disseram aos montes: Cai sobre nós e escondei-nos de diante da face do que está assentado ao trono e da ira do Cordeiro, porque chegou o grande dia da ira deles, e quem poderá subsistir?".*

Terremoto já havia sido previsto por Jesus antes da revelação dada a João mais tarde e escrita no seu livro Apocalipse. Só que no Apocalipse João viu um "grande terremoto", e em seguida viu o sol se tornar negro, o que parece indicar que o sol se tornaria negro *por causa* e *em seguida* ao grande terremoto. Tal coisa nunca aconteceu na Terra, que tenha sido registrado na história.

Nenhum dos terremotos havidos nos últimos dois mil anos fez o sol ficar negro, ou o escondeu de nossa visão. O que poderia tornar o sol negro?

Como já vimos anteriormente, o impacto de um grande asteróide ou cometa ou fragmento de cometa no solo terrestre faria levantar da superfície da Terra uma tão grande nuvem de poeira que obscureceria o sol e seus raios solares por alguns anos, a depender do tamanho do corpo que caísse na Terra. E essa nuvem de poeira escura daria a impressão de que o sol se tornara negro, escuro. A lua também seria vista de forma diferente, de outra cor, devido à mesma nuvem de poeira, e igualmente não daria a sua luz, assim como o sol, como já antes previsto por um antigo profeta de Israel, como vimos em capítulo anterior.

Quanto à queda das estrelas do céu sobre a terra, já foi amplamente explicado que se trataria da queda na Terra de inúmeros meteoros, verdadeiras bolas de fogo, em uma seqüenciada "chuva de meteoros", já conhecida pelos astrônomos.

A seqüência vista por João parece indicar que primeiro haveria um grande terremoto, generalizado, o que pode ser causado por uma grande movimentação das placas tectônicas em várias partes do planeta, talvez acompanhada por inúmeras erupções vulcânicas, que lançariam na atmosfera muita fumaça escura, pó, gases, podendo ser esta, também, talvez, a causa do escurecimento do sol e da lua, e em seguida viria a queda dos meteoros, que seria a chamada "queda das estrelas do céu sobre a terra". Mas também pode ser que a queda de um cometa ou asteróide provoque o grande terremoto, face ao grande impacto da queda na Terra, que seria capaz até mesmo de abalar os fundamentos (as entranhas) do planeta.

O grande terremoto moveria montes e também ilhas de seus lugares, tamanha a potência da movimentação das placas tectônicas.

João viu as pessoas, de reis e ricos a pessoas comuns se escondendo em cavernas e penhascos, para tentarem escapar da fúria do terremoto e da chuva de meteoros. Isso pode significar pessoas se escondendo em abrigos subterrâneos, escavados em montanhas, construídos com o propósito mesmo de se proteger da catástrofe iminente, que pode ser talvez prevista com um ano de antecedência pelos astrônomos, ou pensando em guerra nuclear. O filme Impacto Profundo mostra a utilização desse tipo de abrigo.

O que João escreveu sobre o sexto selo coincide em grande parte com as palavras de Jesus e Isaías. É bom rever a transcrição e análise das previsões dos profetas que antecederam Jesus e as dele próprio, em capítulos anteriores, para verificar a coincidência das informações dadas por eles.

Em seguida, no capítulo 7 do Apocalipse, João escreveu que viu quatro anjos, que estavam sobre os quatro ângulos da Terra, retendo os ventos, para que não soprassem sobre a terra, e um outro anjo disse em alta voz a eles para não fazerem mal à terra, ao mar, nem às árvores, até que fossem marcados os servos de Deus. Depois, João viu uma grande multidão, de todas as nações, e que não se podia contar, de gente com palmas nas mãos entoando cânticos religiosos.

Então, foi aberto o sétimo selo, e se fez silêncio no céu por quase meia hora.

Parece um tempo de trégua, para recomposição da humanidade, e para se prepararem para o que ainda havia de acontecer.

João então viu depois sete anjos diante de Deus, com trombetas, e um que tomou um turíbulo e o encheu de fogo no altar e o lançou sobre a terra, e logo se fizeram trovões, estrondos e relâmpagos, e um grande terremoto. E então os sete anjos se prepararam para fazer soarem suas trombetas.

Quando o primeiro anjo tocou a sua trombeta, formou-se uma chuva de pedra e de fogo, misturados com sangue, que caiu sobre a terra, e foi abrasada a terça parte da terra, e foi queimada a terceira parte das árvores, e queimada toda a erva verde.

Nessa passagem, vemos uma clara alusão a chuva de meteoros, em grande quantidade, que são verdadeiras bolas de fogo, do ponto de vista de quem está na terra. E eles queimaram a terça parte das árvores e da terra, e toda erva verde.

Um terço da terra e da vegetação queimada. E as ervas verdes queimadas por inteiro, é o que diz o texto, se considerado literalmente. Somente uma grande chuva de meteoros, e de tamanho razoável, poderia produzir tal quadro de destruição da vegetação terrestre.

Então, João viu o segundo anjo tocar a sua trombeta e foi lançado no mar um grande monte ardendo em fogo, ou seja, fala claramente de um asteróide ou cometa, ou fragmento de cometa, visto que isso daria a impressão de ser um monte, uma grande rocha, envolta em chamas, o que é causada na travessia das camadas de gases da atmosfera terrestre.

A queda no mar do asteróide ou cometa se seguirá à chuva de meteoros.

João escreveu que a terça parte do mar se tornará em sangue, e a terça parte das criaturas que habitarem o mar morrerão, e a terça parte das embarcações perecerão, ou seja, serão destruídas.

João viu a queda no mar de um corpo rochoso ardendo em chamas e que causará a morte de um terço dos animais marinhos e a destruição de um terço das embarcações.

O terceiro anjo tocou a trombeta, e João viu cair do céu uma grande estrela ardente, atingindo a terça parte dos rios e fontes de água, e muitos homens morrerão ao beber da água amarga.

A grande estrela ardente parece mais um cometa do que um asteróide. Pode ser que os elementos que constituem o cometa sejam venenosos para o homem, que morrerão ao beber as águas poluídas pelo material cometário vindo do espaço.

O quarto anjo tocou também a sua trombeta, e foi ferida a terça parte do sol, a terça parte da lua e a terça parte das estrelas, de modo que foi obscurecida a terça parte deles, que teriam sua luminosidade prejudica em um terço.

Vemos aí a confirmação de outras profecias anteriores relativamente ao obscurecimento do sol, da lua e das estrelas, o que seria causado pela nuvem de poeira levantada com o impacto de grandes corpos rochosos vindos do espaço com o solo terrestre, com a parte sólida da Terra.

João em seguida ouviu uma voz dizer: *"Ai, ai, ai dos habitantes da terra, por causa das outras vozes dos três anjos que haviam de tocar a trombeta"*.

A voz ouvida se compadecia da humanidade, que já havia sofrido muito, mas que ainda continuaria a sofrer após o toque das trombetas dos outros anjos. Mais infortúnios viriam pela frente.

O quinto anjo então tocou sua trombeta, e caiu na terra uma estrela, o que significa mais um meteoro, asteróide ou cometa, e após a sua queda se abriu um poço de abismo, o que significa uma fenda na terra, que pode ser causada pelo forte impacto, e da fenda ou poço subiu fumo, quer dizer, fumaça, gases, como se saindo de uma grande fornalha, o que pode significar que a fenda deixará exposto o magma incandescente, e a fumaça que subirá ao céu obscurecerá o sol e o ar.

Ao toque da trombeta do sexto anjo, foram soltos quatro anjos que estavam presos no riu Eufrates, e eles levariam à morte a terça parte dos homens. E João em seu escrito relaciona a morte de um terço da humanidade ao fogo, ao fumo e ao enxofre, que antes tinham sido relacionados com a abertura de uma fenda na terra, que seria um poço. Isso quer dizer que o que sairá das entranhas da Terra levará à morte a terça parte das pessoas na superfície do planeta, seja pelo calor, pelos gases tóxicos, pelo ar sufocante e sem condição de ser respirado, como também pelo fogo.

Foi anunciado em seguida que não haveria mais tempo, e que com o soar da trombeta do sétimo anjo se cumpriria o mistério de Deus.

Quando foi tocada finalmente a sétima trombeta, João ouviu vozes dizendo: *"O reino deste mundo passou a ser de nosso Senhor, e do seu Cristo, e ele reinará pelos séculos dos séculos. Amém"*.

Em seguida, João torna a descrever relâmpagos, terremoto e chuva de pedra. E descreve um grande sinal no céu, que consistiria no que ele chamou de "uma mulher vestida de sol". Um cometa, que próximo da Terra se assemelharia ao sol? E ela teria a lua debaixo de seus pés e doze estrelas sobre a sua cabeça. Meteoros acompanhando o cometa?

João fala ainda de um outro sinal que seria visto no céu. Um dragão vermelho, cuja cauda arrastava a terça parte das estrelas do céu e as fez cair sobre a Terra.

O dragão vermelho com cauda só pode ser um cometa, pois somente os cometas possuem caudas, como já vimos no primeiro capítulo desta obra ao estudarmos os cometas, os asteróides e os meteoros.

As estrelas arrastadas pelo dragão são meteoros que acompanham o cometa, pois quando os meteoros entram na atmosfera da Terra, são vistos como se fossem estrelas caindo, as chamadas "estrelas cadentes".

Nessa passagem, João viu, então, a chegada e a aproximação de um cometa acompanhado de meteoros, e a queda dos meteoros e depois também do próprio cometa na Terra, o que causará grande impacto, e grande destruição, tanto na terra quanto no mar.

João menciona depois um mar de vidro envolto em fogo, no capítulo 15, o que pode ser uma região gelada (Antártida ou Pólo Norte) em chamas, pois uma região com água congelada parece um mar de vidro, visto que o gelo se assemelha ao vidro. É possível que um asteróide ou cometa venha a cair em uma das regiões geladas do planeta.

João em seguida fala dos sete cálices derramados por sete anjos na Terra, e parece repetir as coisas como sendo coisas novas, como pragas, sendo na verdade coisas já antes descritas no seu livro, como a morte dos seres marinhos, o envenenamento das fontes de água potável, calor e fogo, e ainda fonte de água secando, causando grande sede, terremoto e relâmpago. Repetição de coisas já antes descrita.

João, no entanto, ao tornar a falar em terremoto, escreveu que ele seria tão grande, e causaria tamanho temor, nunca antes tendo havido um terremoto igual desde que o homem existe na Terra. Ou seja, não se trata de um terremoto simples, localizado, mas de um grande e devastador terremoto que poderá acontecer com a grande movimentação das placas tectônicas, ou provocado pelo grande impacto de um asteróide ou cometa na Terra.

A intensa chuva de pedras e de fogo de que trata João é a queda de grande quantidade de meteoros na Terra.

Fala João, também, no capítulo 16, da queda das cidades das nações, e da grande cidade. Nova Iorque, hoje a cidade mais importante do mundo, seu coração financeiro?

João fala da condenação da "grande prostituta", que está assentada sobre as águas. Isso mostra que se trata de um país ou cidade existente em uma ilha. Cidade ou nação de grande poder. Nova Iorque tem o seu centro econômico, Manhatan, em uma ilha.

João ao final do livro fala de um céu novo e uma nova terra, porque o primeiro céu e a primeira terra se foram, e o mar anterior já não existia mais.

Parece dizer respeito a uma mudança radical na formação da Terra. Uma possível inclinação do eixo do planeta, causada pelos impactos de cometa ou asteróide, e pela movimentação das placas tectônicas levaria à invasão de lugares secos pela água do mar, e tornaria descoberto o fundo de mares e oceanos.

Resumindo, o Apocalipse nos dá informações sobre uma seqüência de acontecimentos na Terra, sem dizer quando eles ocorreriam, nem se eles se sucederiam imediatamente, ou com intervalos de tempo, salvo no caso do intervalo que foi chamado de "quase meia hora", com silêncio no céu.

A seqüência, incluindo as repetições contidas no livro, seria: guerras; fome; doenças; martírio de cristãos; grande terremoto com o escurecimento do sol, da lua e das estrelas; queda de meteoros; montes e ilhas mudando de lugar (que parece mais associado ao grande terremoto); intervalo de "quase meia hora" (trégua); trovões, relâmpagos, estrondos e terremoto; chuva de pedra e fogo (chuva de meteoros), com destruição de um terço da vegetação; queda de asteróide ou cometa no mar, com morte de um terço dos seres marinhos e destruição de um terço das embarcações; queda de meteoros ou cometas em rios e fontes de água, com morte de um terço dos homens que beberem as águas amargas; queda de outro asteróide ou cometa abrindo uma fenda na terra, de onde sairiam gases, enxofre e fumaça, causando o escurecimento do sol e da lua, causando a morte pelo fumo, pela fumaça, pelo calor e pelo enxofre; relâmpagos (parece repetição); terremoto (parece repetição); chuva de pedra (parece repetição); grande sinal no céu (mulher vestida de sol – cometa); outro sinal no céu, consistente em um cometa (dragão vermelho) arrastando meteoros (estrelas) que cairiam na Terra.

O livro Apocalipse, de São João, da mesma forma que Jesus e os profetas mais antigos de Israel, não fixa datas, nem indica com precisão a época em que os fatos aconteceriam. Assim, não se pode indicar com exatidão o tempo em que as catástrofes acontecerão na Terra. No máximo podemos nos arriscar a tomar certos indicadores de épocas fornecidos nos livros analisados nesta obra para tentar pelo menos aproximar o tempo de sofrimento previsto para a humanidade. E um dos indicadores, como já expusemos antes, é a volta dos judeus à sua terra natal, Israel, o que aconteceu em 1.948, isto se considerarmos o retorno em maior número, com a criação do Estado de Israel, porque desde o início do século XX os judeus já estavam migrando para aquela área.

Jesus designou o que seria a volta dos judeus à "Terra Santa" como sendo o marco do fim dos tempos das nações. Isso mostra que há nítida relação entre esse marco do fim dos tempos das nações com o início das catástrofes.

Se considerarmos o retorno dos judeus à Palestina, em meados do século XX, com a criação de Israel em 1.948, como sendo o marco do fim dos tempos das nações, duas grandes guerras existiram, com grande sofrimento para a humanidade, uma de 1.914 a 1.918 e outra de 1.939 a 1.945.

Essas duas grandes guerras podem estar associadas com os dois primeiros cavaleiros do Apocalipse, o do cavalo branco e o do cavalo vermelho. Assim, na seqüência, viriam fome, pestes e doenças.

O século XX é um retrato muito perfeito de fome, na África (Somália e Etiópia, principalmente), em Bangladesh, Índia, isto só tomando em conta os grandes exemplos de fome.

Doenças, o século XX viu o surgimento da gripe espanhola, da varíola, dos vírus ebola e AIDS, e outros mais secundários, sem falar no aparecimento de vírus e bactérias super-resistentes aos mais modernos antibióticos, como as bactérias que causam a tuberculose e a pneumonia, doenças já praticamente extintas no mundo.

A humanidade vive hoje com medo de inúmeros vírus e bactérias resistentes aos mais potentes antibióticos modernos. Até doenças já erradicadas como a pneumonia retornaram, e matam pessoas.

Viroses são rotuladas muitas vezes sem que os médicos saibam exatamente com que vírus estão lidando.

Podemos considerar, pois há elementos suficientes em apoio a essa hipótese, que o século XX já demonstrou o fim dos tempos das nações, e que nele já houve duas grandes guerras com imenso sofrimento para nós humanos, como nunca houve antes, em toda a história da humanidade, bem como ao longo do século já tivemos bastante fome, doenças e pestes. Assim, podemos dizer que em seguida virá o martírio de cristãos, para depois vir o grande terremoto.

Os conflitos religiosos que retornaram no século XX, a ameaça de uma nova guerra santa, uma nova cruzada entre islamitas (muçulmanos) e cristãos, devido à invasão de ocidentais (cristãos) a países do Oriente Médio (islamitas), hoje não parece ser algo impossível, nem tão distante.

Tivemos duas guerras envolvendo muçulmanos e cristãos, com a invasão dos americanos e seus aliados ao Iraque, a primeira no final do século XX (1.991) e a segunda logo no início do século XXI (2.003). E a luta e a matança lenta por lá ainda perduram, e não há indicativos de terminar tão cedo.

O Irã ainda representa uma ameaça de guerra para os "ocidentais", inclusive com seu polêmico programa nuclear, que tantas discussões já geraram nas Nações Unidas.

Israel, centro dos problemas no Oriente Médio, desde a sua criação em 1.948, já se envolveu em três guerras com seus vizinhos muçulmanos, e o ódio dos muçulmanos aos judeus na região não terá fim tão cedo. Por isso a região continua sendo um verdadeiro barril de pólvora, sempre à beira da explosão. Aliás, Israel vive praticamente uma guerra civil não declarada, e já faz algum tempo.

Todas as profecias contidas nos livros da Bíblia, e até agora analisadas, têm como epicentro os judeus, que já foi o povo de Jesus, e não é mais, desde que esse povo o negou, e o entregou ao martírio, como escrito por um dos profetas, e já transcrito anteriormente em capítulo que tratou dos antigos profetas. E parece mesmo que Jesus vinculou os tempos das nações e o marco para o início dos acontecimentos por ele previstos, o mesmo se dando com o Apocalipse, à volta dos judeus à Terra Santa, Israel, o que já aconteceu na primeira metade do século XX. Dessa forma, atingido o marco, já começaram a se desencadear os acontecimentos apocalípticos.

CAPÍTULO 7

AS PROFECIAS DE NOSTRADAMUS – RELAÇÃO COM O APOCALIPSE.

Analisaremos a seguir as profecias de Nostradamus que têm relação com as profecias de Isaías, Zacarias, Miquéias, Daniel, Jesus e com o Apocalipse de São João, e após faremos um resumo mais objetivo e claro das profecias e seu cumprimento, já que estaremos de posse de todo o conjunto de profecias oriundas de profetas do povo judeu, que outrora fora o "povo de Jesus", e que segundo um dos profetas deixou de ser o seu povo por tê-lo negado e entregado para a morte pelas mãos dos incrédulos, os romanos. Esse profeta último se chama Nostradamus.

Michel de Nostradamus nasceu em 1.503, em Saint-Rémy, na França. Foi médico, astrólogo e astrônomo.

Aos 22 anos de idade, mesmo antes de ter concluído o curso de medicina, Nostradamus teve participação ativa e decisiva no tratamento de peste bubônica em epidemia de seu tempo, na França.

Quando a epidemia terminou, Nostradamus já era conhecido em todo o sul da França, mesmo antes de se formar.

Foi em sua peregrinação pela Itália que as visões de Nostradamus tiveram início.

Em 1.555 saiu a primeira publicação do seu livro Centúrias, que logo se espalharia pela Europa, levando Nostradamus à fama rápida. Mas as quadras de seu livro foram embaralhadas propositalmente para confundir os leitores, e a terminologia utilizada pelo vidente era a mais confusa possível, por causa do medo da Inquisição, que ainda era muito forte naquela época. E isso até hoje prejudica a sua correta compreensão e interpretação.

Somente analisaremos as quadras escritas por Nostradamus no livro Centúrias que consideramos relevantes e que indiquem clara ligação lógica e confirmem as profecias anteriores e já analisadas nesta obra.

Na quadra VIII, 98, escreveu Nostradamus:

> "O sangue de gente da Igreja será derramado
> com tanta abundância como a água que corre
> e por muito tempo não será estancado
> pois haverá ruína e dor no clero"

Trata-se de uma quadra de texto literal, sem qualquer alegoria ou simbolismo. Nostradamus viu o derramamento de sangue de gente da Igreja, querendo se referir logicamente à Igreja Católica, pois naquela época ainda não existiam outras igrejas cristãs. E deixou claro que seria sangue de sacerdotes, de gente do clero, não de fiéis.

Escreveu que o sangue, ou seja, a morte dos sacerdotes seria algo duradouro, não de curta duração, ao se referir ao fato de que o sangue não seria estancado por longo tempo, havendo muita dor e ruína no clero.

Isso lembra o próximo passo antes mencionado, no capítulo anterior, relativo ao martírio de cristãos, previsto tanto por Jesus quanto no Apocalipse, que acontecerá antes do grande terremoto, já que duas grandes guerras, muita fome e pestes já aconteceram no século XX, como vimos no final do capítulo anterior.

A quadra I, 44, segue a mesma linha da anterior, aqui transcrita.

> "Em breve voltarão os sacrifícios
> contraventores sofrerão o sacrifício
> já não haverá monges, nem abades, nem noviços
> o mel será muito mais caro do que a cera".

Nostradamus fala em retorno dos sacrifícios, fazendo clara alusão a tempo em que houve perseguição e sacrifício de muitos cristãos, muito tempo antes de sua época. E menciona contraventores, o que pode significar que sacerdotes farão coisas erradas e isso levará à sua perseguição e morte. E, ainda, que ninguém mais buscará o caminho do sacerdócio, e por isso a vela (cera) ficará barata, pois já não se acenderão tantas velas nas igrejas.

Temos visto freqüentes escândalos de pedofilia envolvendo padres da Igreja Católica, sobretudo nos Estados Unidos, o que levou nestes últimos dias (julho de 2.007) a Igreja a celebrar acordo de bilhões de dólares com vítimas dos sacerdotes católicos naquela país. Seria esse o tipo de contravenção a ser merecer o sacrifício descrito na quadra acima transcrita?

A revista brasileira ÉPOCA, número 473, de 11 de junho de 2.007, apresentou reportagem intitulada Os Cristãos Esquecidos, nas páginas 92 e 93, na qual informa que no Iraque havia cerca de 2 milhões de cristãos antes da invasão americana de 2.003, e eles hoje estão reduzidos a cerca de 500 mil apenas.

A matéria da revista mostra que radicais muçulmanos estão promovendo atentados a igrejas cristãs no Iraque, e seqüestrando e matando padres. Além disso, obrigam a retirada das cruzes do alto das igrejas cristãs.

Isso não acontecia com cristãos há muitos e muitos séculos. E traduzem a situação de intolerância religiosa, e a existência de uma certa guerra religiosa, com grande fanatismo e sectarismo no Iraque.

Aliás, o país está prestes a ser dividido entre Sunitas e Xiitas, e ainda entre curdos e árabes, não havendo lugar para os cristãos na nova ordem social que se antevê naquele país em guerra civil não declarada.

É possível que a intolerância religiosa contra cristãos no Oriente Médio se espalhe, com uma guerra de religião como foram as antigas Cruzadas no século XII d.C.

A matéria da revista nos faz lembrar as quadras de Nostradamus acima transcritas.

Na quadra I, 63, Nostradamus escreveu:

"Os açoites passados que pioraram o mundo
longo tempo de paz, terras desabitadas,
irmã irá por céu, terra e onda,
e logo novamente as guerras suscitadas".

Parece haver indicação na primeira linha da quadra de que *os açoites passados que pioraram o mundo* tenham sido guerras, quem sabe as primeira e segunda guerras mundiais do século XX.

Então haveria longo tempo de paz. De fato desde 1.945 nenhuma guerra de grandes proporções aconteceu no mundo até agora (2.007).

Quem ou o quê seria a "irmã", que iria por céu, terra e onda? Seria um ataque de país irmão a outro? Seria a irmã algo vindo do espaço, caindo na terra e no mar, causando ondas? Não dá para se ter certeza.

Na quadra I, 16, escreveu o vidente:

"A foice no tanque olha para Sagitário
em seu mais alto grau de exaltação,
peste, fome, morte por mão militar,
o século se aproxima de sua renovação".

Nostradamus viu peste, fome, guerra, coisas profetizadas por Jesus e contidas também no Apocalipse. E a aproximação da renovação do século parece indicar o final de um século, que pode ser o final do século XX.

Nostradamus não colocou suas quadras em seqüência cronológica. Assim, o que faremos é pegar algumas quadras que possuem informações que lembrem ou confirmem as profecias anteriormente analisadas, para mostrar ao leitor que ele viu de fato as mesmas coisas, apenas tendo embaralhado as informações para confundir seus leitores.

Na quadra II, 46, novamente o vidente menciona fome e peste, somando a isso chuva, sangue, leite e fogo no céu, correndo grande centelha.

Não indica claramente se tratar de uma guerra ao falar em fogo no céu. Pode ser meteoro entrando em nossa atmosfera, que também se parece a uma centelha correndo.

Já na quadra II, 62, o profeta é mais claro:

"Mabus então morrerá logo, virá
de pessoas e animais terrível tragédia.
Logo, subitamente, se verá vingança
cem, mão, sede, fome, quando corra o cometa."

Não sabemos quem é Mabus, nem se há alguma relação entre ele e as outras coisas descritas na mesma quadra.

A quadra indica claramente que surgiriam doenças transmitidas por pessoas e por animais, o que nos faz lembrar de doenças como AIDS e a gripe aviária, bem como a vaca louca, todas no século XX. E menciona novamente a fome, e acrescenta a sede, quando corra o cometa.

Aqui temos que fazer um parênteses.

No tempo de Nostradamus já se sabia o que eram os cometas, e ele era astrônomo e astrólogo. Assim, não incluiria a palavra cometa na quadra para simbolizar outra coisa, nem para confundir o leitor. Cometa, aqui, é cometa mesmo.

Nostradamus viu um cometa correndo no céu, e relacionou a ele fome e sede, da mesma forma como encontramos no Apocalipse.

Na quadra I, 80, escreveu o vidente:

"Da sexta claro resplendor celeste
virá trovejar muito forte em Borgonha.
Depois nascerá um monstro de besta muito odiosa,
março, abril, maio, junho, grande esqueleto e ronha."

Nostradamus aqui fala em trovões e resplendor celeste, o que lembra os trovões, relâmpagos e estrondos descritos no Apocalipse. E em seguida dá clara indicação que durará vários meses o sofrimento com a tempestade. E indica que nascerá um monstro de besta muito odiosa, o que pode ser uma pessoa a nascer na mesma época da tempestade, e haverá muitas mortes (esqueletos).

Na quadra II, 41, escreveu o profeta:

"A grande estrela arderá durante sete dias
nublado fará com que dois sóis apareçam,
o grande mastim latirá durante toda a noite
quando o grande pontífice mude de lugar."

Nostradamus viu uma "grande estrela", e isso seria visto como dois sóis pelos habitantes da Terra.

A grande estrela não deve de forma alguma ser considerada um novo sol que se aproximará da Terra, porque isso é

95

praticamente impossível de acontecer, pelos conhecimentos astronômicos atuais. Devemos lembrar que um cometa iluminado se aproximando da Terra será visto como se fosse um outro sol. Por isso o vidente escreveu que a grande estrela faria com que houvesse dois sóis.

Se a segunda parte da quadra estiver ligada à primeira, pode significar que o Papa (o grande pontífice) mudará de lugar quando o cometa estiver chegando, pois poderá o cometa se dirigir para a cidade de Roma, ou a Itália. Ou seja, se o cometa for detectado com antecedência razoável, o que certamente acontecerá, pelos conhecimentos atuais, e pelos organismos internacionais de pesquisas sobre corpos estelares, o Papa poderá ser evacuado de Roma e até mesmo da Itália, se houver perigo para ele, o que também seria feito com autoridades governamentais.

Na quadra I, 62, Nostradamus escreveu:

"A grande perda que sofrerão as letras
antes que o céu de Latrona seja perfeito
houve grande dilúvio por ignaros cetros
que por um longo século não se reconstituirá."

Nostradamus parece indicar grande perda de intelectuais, e também que haveria um grande dilúvio, com efeitos duradouros e longos.

Isso nos lembra que a queda de um cometa ou asteróide no mar causará grandes deslocamentos de água através de grandes ondas, que invadirão terras, criando um verdadeiro dilúvio, e que seus efeitos seriam prolongados, o que indica que muita água avançará sobre as terras, com grande destruição de cidades e plantações.

Nostradamus na quadra I, 67 fala em grande fome, que rondaria com freqüência e se faria universal, e que levaria as pessoas a arrancarem as raízes dos bosques e a tirarem os meninos do peito de sua mãe. Grande fome mesmo. O que também nos lembra Jesus e o Apocalipse.

A quadra I, 17, diz:

"Durante quarenta anos o arco-íris não surgirá

durante quarenta anos todos os dias se poderá
ver:
    a terra seca em aridez aumentará
    e haverá um grande dilúvio quando se o veja".

Nostradamus parece querer dizer que algo fará com que não vejamos arco-íris durante quarenta anos, e que durante esse tempo haverá grande seca.

Nos lugares desertos, como nos estados americanos de Arizona, Novo México, em desertos como o Saara, no norte da África, e o Atacama, no Chile, e em muitas outras regiões secas da Terra, como o Raso da Catarina no Nordeste brasileiro, não se vêem arco-íris, pelo simples fato de não haver nuvens, muito menos carregadas, que possibilitem a formação dos conhecidos arco-íris. Sem nuvens carregadas não há arco-íris.

Assim, indica o profeta que haverá grande seca no mundo, mesmo que não seja geral, com duração de quarenta anos. E que depois desse período de seca, haverá inundações, o que ele chamou de dilúvio. Ou seja, mudanças climáticas, que poderão estar associadas a queda de asteróides ou cometa, ou a fatores climáticos simples, provocados pela poluição, desmatamento e descongelamento das calotas polares.

Na quadra II, 43, Nostradamus escreveu:

    "Do tremor tão forte do mês de maio
    Saturno em Capricórnio, Júpiter e Mercúrio em Touro
    Vênus, também em Câncer, Marte em Nonnay,
    cairá granizo maior do que um ovo.

    Durante a passagem da estrela de cabeleira aparente...
    Feridas do céu, paz, terra fremente..."

Nostradamus também nesta quadra faz referência a um grande terremoto, e a chuva de granizo maior do que um ovo. E parece relacionar isso à passagem de um cometa, visto que "estrela de cabeleira aparente" não pode ser outra coisa a não ser um cometa realmente. A cabeleira aparente é a cauda do cometa, hoje por demais conhecida.

Feridas do céu, paz, terra fremente nos lembra uma seqüência de corpos caindo do céu, como asteróides ou meteoros (feridas do céu), seguido de um período de trégua, de paz, que lembra o silêncio de quase meia hora no céu, conforme vimos no Apocalipse, e depois terremoto (terra fremente).

A escritora A. galloti, autora do livro **As Profecias do Futuro**, fazendo cálculos a partir dos dados fornecidos por Nostradamus nesta quadra, sugere que a passagem desse cometa se dará entre os anos 2.096 e 2.156.

Na quadra IX, 83, o vidente escreveu:

"Sol a vinte graus de Touro, terremoto na Terra
o grande teatro repleto afundará
ar, céu e terra escurecerão e tremerão
quando Deus com seus santos envolva os infiéis."

Nostradamus viu um terremoto, e um grande teatro cheio de gente afundando. E também viu que o terremoto causaria o escurecimento do céu, do ar e da terra, causando grande medo.

Essa quadra nos faz lembrar do Apocalipse, que descreve os efeitos do grande terremoto, de forma muito semelhante ao que escreveu Nostradamus, com o escurecimento do sol, da lua e das estrelas. Além disso, Nostradamus relaciona o acontecimento ao Juízo Final, ao escrever "quando Deus com seus santos envolva os infiéis". Vale rever e conferir em capítulo anterior.

Na quadra V, 32, o vidente escreveu:

"Onde tudo está bem, todo o bem do sol e da lua
é abundante, se aproxima sua ruína.
Do céu avança para jogar fora tua sorte,
No mesmo estado que a sétima rocha."

Nostradamus previu que repentinamente do céu viria alguma coisa para jogar fora a sorte, e que isso seria igual à sétima rocha. O que isso quer dizer?

98

A sétima rocha é uma referência à rocha mencionada no livro Apocalipse, que seria lançada (cairia) no mar.

É clara a afirmação que o que arruinaria o sol e a lua viria do céu, o que somente pode ser um cometa ou asteróide, devido à dimensão da destruição prevista pelo vidente.

Na curta quadra I, 56, ele prevê que:

"Vereis, mais cedo ou mais tarde, produzir-se uma grande mudança.
Horrores extremos e vinganças..."

Essa passagem parece indicar que grandes mudanças sofreria a Terra, o que pode significar a inclinação do seu eixo, com alterações climáticas grandes, gerando inundações em alguns lugares e congelamento em outros, passando a fazer calor onde antes era frio e vice-versa.

Na quadra III, 42, está escrito:

"O menino nascerá com dois dentes na garganta
em Tuscia choverá e pedras cairão
muito em breve não haverá comida na panela
para salvar aqueles que de fome morrerão."

Nostradamus nesta quadra fala de chuva e queda de pedras, o que parece indicar chuva de meteoritos (nome dos meteoros quando caem no solo), posto que se fosse granizo (pedra de gelo) ele o teria dito expressamente, como em outra quadra já analisada. E menciona uma grande fome, que mataria a muitos. Isso tudo também lembra o Apocalipse, e as palavras de Jesus já analisadas.

A quadra II, 18, descreve:

"Uma nova e súbita chuva, de modo impetuoso,
irá parar dois exércitos inteiros;
rochas, céu e fogo tornam o mar pedregoso;
apressam a morte de sete terras e marinheiros."

Nostradamus faz referência, aqui, a uma chuva muito forte, e também a rochas incendiadas caindo do céu no mar, destruindo terras e navios com seus marinheiros. Isso também está no Apocalipse. Não se trata de fogo de batalha, de tiros ou bombas, mas fogo do céu, o que somente pode representar meteoros caindo no mar.

Na quadra V, 98, nova referência do profeta a enorme estiagem de verão, ou seja, seca, rios e mares ardendo pelo fogo que cairá do céu (meteoros ou cometas).

Na carta a seu filho César, escrita em 1º de março de 1.555, Nostradamus escreveu:

"E antes de 177 anos, 3 meses e 11 dias a contar da data em que escrevo isto, por pestilência, longa onda de fome e guerras e mais ainda por inundações que se repetirão muitas vezes, antes e depois do término que fixei, o mundo se encontrará tão diminuído e a população ficará tão pequena que não se encontrará quem queira trabalhar nos campos que ficarão vazios por tanto tempo quanto passaram em serviço. Eis o que aparece do estudo do céu visível".

Nostradamus na carta, neste trecho, fala abertamente, sem rodeios, sem simbolismos, sem metáforas, descrevendo coisas que em muito se assemelham ao que foi dito por Jesus e por João no Apocalipse. Só que Nostradamus, fugindo à regra geral adotada no seu livro, fez cálculos astrológicos e datou alguns desses acontecimentos por ele vistos, e terminou por cometer um grande erro.

Somando-se 1.555 com 177, chegamos ao ano 1.732, no qual de forma alguma o mundo ficou grandemente diminuído e a população tão pequena que não se encontraria quem quisesse trabalhar, ficando os campos vazios. Nada de tão terrível e especial ocorreu nesse ano de 1.732.

Isso mostra, como dito por Jesus, que *daquele dia e daquela hora nem ele nem os anjos do céu sabiam dizer, mas só Deus.* Tentar adivinhar o dia e a hora é cair no erro, e nisso Nostradamus acabou se traindo, e por isso errou. O mesmo se deu com vários de seus intérpretes que tentam datar os acontecimentos por ele previstos. Tantos quantos buscam fazer isso erram, como errou o seu mestre, o próprio Michel de Nostradamus.

Ninguém sabe mesmo quando tudo acontecerá. Pode começar a qualquer momento, e pode já ter realmente começado aquela fase que Jesus chamou de "o início das dores", mas não a queda de asteróides, cometas ou meteoros na Terra, nem tampouco o grande terremoto, a inclinação do eixo da Terra com movimentos violentos das placas tectônicas de forma altamente destrutiva para as cidades.

No próximo capítulo estaremos resumindo a marcha humana de sua origem até o século XIX.

CAPÍTULO 8

A marcha Humana até o século XIX

Segundo estudiosos da Bíblia que levam ao pé da letra e literalmente tudo o que nela está escrito, a humanidade existe há apenas cerca de seis mil anos. Já para a ciência, os primeiros humanóides surgiram há mais de um milhão de anos, e os homens modernos, chamados de homo sapiens-sapiens, saíram da África há 100 mil anos, e se espalharam pelo mundo.

Mais de 100 mil anos antes do homem moderno, o homem de Neandertal já havia deixado a África e se espalhado por boa parte do mundo, sobretudo na Europa, e chegando até a China.

Ao contrário do homem moderno, que sobrevive até hoje, o homem de Neandertal desapareceu há 50 mil anos atrás.

Não há certeza sobre as causas de sua extinção, mas alguns estudiosos sustentam que houve lutas entre as duas espécies humanas, podendo ter havido disputas por territórios de caça, já que ambas as espécies eram caçadores nômades. A espécie mais nova provavelmente se adaptou melhor às condições climáticas da época, tendo já dominado o fogo, e tinha armas mais eficientes, talvez técnicas de defesa melhores, e com isso venceu a luta, levando à extinção a espécie que já habitava a Terra há mais de 100 mil anos.

Hoje se sabe que o homem moderno chegou na Austrália há cerca de 40 mil anos atrás, e na América há cerca de 12 a 14 mil anos.

Como todos os chamados nativos do continente americano já usavam o arco e flecha quando desapareceu o Estreito de Bering, por onde devem ter entrado no continente, vindos da Ásia, e também como os aborígines da Austrália também utilizavam o arco e flecha, conclui-se que o homem moderno já utilizava esse tipo de arma antes de 40 mil anos atrás, o que mostra que a invenção (não descoberta) do arco e flecha é muito antiga, mas posterior ao uso da lança, que é uma arma bem mais simples. O arco e a flecha permitem atingir o inimigo ou a caça de uma distância muito maior e mais segura, o que faz uma grande diferença tanto na caçada quanto na guerra.

É mais provável que a invenção do arco e flecha seja de autoria do homem moderno, o que lhe deu uma grande vantagem nas caçadas e nas guerras tribais.

O homem moderno foi basicamente caçador e coletor durante o período pré-histórico, e vivia em cabanas, feitas com material da região, como paus e palhas, ou de peles de animais ou couro.

A última glaciação (Era do Gelo) terminou há 10 mil anos. Entre 9.000 e 8.000 anos atrás se iniciou o período Neolítico, que sucedeu o Paleolítico. Nele surgiu a agricultura e a domesticação de animais, o que levou o homem a uma grande mudança de comportamento.

Grande parte dos humanos modernos deixou então de ser caçador nômade e passou a plantar cereais, fixando-se ao solo, a uma região geográfica, o que levava a construção de moradas fixas, cabanas mais resistentes e duradouras, e isso levou, com o passar do tempo, ao surgimento de vilas, aldeias, e, por fim, das cidades.

Também a criação de animais, sobretudo de bois e cabras, levou a uma maior fixação do homem a regiões de melhores pastos, e com isso também à construção de vilas, aldeias e cidades.

A civilização, segundo os historiadores modernos, surgiu por volta de 4.000 anos a.C. Esse início se deu no Egito e na Mesopotâmia, estando divididos os estudiosos quanto a qual delas surgiu primeiro, e em seguida se alastrou pela Índia, e depois Creta, Grécia, Itália e outras localidades.

Coincidentemente, o início da chamada civilização, ou início da construção das cidades, se deu mais ou menos na mesma época em que alguns estudiosos da Bíblia atribuem ao início do homem, com Adão e Eva. Esse início teria também cerca de 6 mil anos.

Nas cidades surgiram várias profissões, várias atividades, e necessidades, com especializações diversas, e a necessidade fez surgir a matemática, e depois a escrita, inicialmente cuneiforme, e depois em estilo gráfico, como os hieróglifos do Egito. Posteriormente foi inventado o alfabeto, promovendo uma grande revolução na escrita, facilitando a sua transmissão e popularização, e isso se espalhou pelo mundo mediterrâneo.

Hoje atribui-se a invenção do alfabeto aos fenícios, e o seu aperfeiçoamento aos gregos. A escrita tem cerca de 4 mil anos.

Outra revolução humana, considerada a primeira revolução industrial, foi a metalurgia, bem mais recente.

Iniciou-se a metalurgia do cobre, do ferro, do ouro, etc. E isso afetou o mundo, pois aqueles que iniciaram a fabricação de armas de metal venciam as guerras contra os que ainda lutavam com lanças e arco e flecha.

Povos oriundos do norte da Europa, que iniciaram mais cedo a metalurgia do ferro, e a fabricação de espadas pesadas de ferro desceram a conquistar o sul do continente. Aqueles que se defendiam com espadas de cobre sucumbiam. Aqueles que ainda usavam armas de pau não tinham qualquer chance de vitória, e foram destruídos ou dominados.

A Idade do Ferro, seguida da Idade do Aço, mostra a conquista por parte daqueles que já usavam eficazmente armas mais avançadas, e tecnologia mais avançada e mais moderna. E isso se repete até nossos dias, com armas muito mais avanças.

Logo, em curto espaço de tempo, as armas de ferro e depois as de aço se espalhariam pelo mundo antigo.

Quando os Hititas avançaram sobre o Oriente Médio com seus carros de guerra rápidos, carroças de duas rodas puxadas por um ou dois cavalos, fizeram tremer os que estavam no seu caminho, porque ninguém conhecia esse tipo de arma e meio de transporte. Mas em pouco tempo os egípcios adotaram também o carro de guerra, que depois se tornou comum entre gregos e romanos. A chamada "biga".

No último milênio anterior à Era Cristã, grandes avanços ocorreram no mundo, e não apenas no campo militar. A agricultura se desenvolveu muito, o comércio cresceu entre os povos do Mediterrâneo, a escrita alfabética se popularizou, as cidades cresceram e se desenvolveram, com água encanada em muitas delas, como se vê no Palácio de Cnossos, na ilha de Creta, em Cartago, em Roma, e nas cidades Indianas, como Harapo, no vale do Rio Hindu.

O crescimento das cidades e do comércio, o enriquecimento de algumas delas e o domínio de rotas de comércio levaram os povos a inúmeras guerras na antiguidade, a exemplo da famosa e lendária guerra entre os gregos e os troianos, os romanos e os cartagineses, e as guerras internas na Grécia, com a grande rivalidade entre as duas maiores potências, econômica e militar, Atenas e Esparta.

Invasões de países por outros também tiveram motivações econômicas, ou simplesmente por vontade de dominar o mundo, como buscaram fazer os persas, que depois de conquistarem grande parte do Oriente Médio partiram para invadir a Grécia, sendo, no entanto, rechaçados pelos valentes atenienses na primeira invasão na batalha de Maratona, e pelos espartanos na segunda invasão, nas Termópilas, ambas no século V a.C.

A antiguidade está recheada de histórias de guerras de conquista. E não se tratava de tomar um território apenas porque ele tinha esse ou aquele minério, ou por se tratar de melhor solo para plantar, ou melhor pasto para os animais. Era a conquista pela conquista. Questão de vaidade, de domínio, de enriquecimento com os espólios de guerra, com os saques das cidades ricas, e domínio territorial. Além, é claro, da cobrança de impostos, o que os romanos melhor do que quaisquer outros sabiam fazer eficientemente, chegando a fazer recenseamento apenas para controlar a cobrança de tributos, como feito na Palestina na época do nascimento de Jesus, o que levou os pais de Jesus a Belém.

A humanidade teria uma história muito comum em seus diversos povos se não fosse algumas revoluções culturais e religiosas ocorridas em algumas regiões do planeta.

Os primeiros surtos civilizatórios se deram na Mesopotâmia e no Egito, logo seguidos pela Índia, Creta e Grécia. Depois eles foram seguidos por outros povos.

O Egito desenvolveu a matemática, a engenharia, a medicina, o cultivo de cereais, a astronomia antiga, a cosmética, e muitas outras coisas. A Mesopotâmia desenvolveu a astronomia, a engenharia, a irrigação, a agricultura e outras coisas.

Creta desenvolveu o encanamento de água, tendo uma cultura bastante avançada. E a Grécia, além de aprender com os Cretenses e os Egípcios muito do que eles já sabiam, avançou em técnicas militares, sobretudo os espartanos, maiores guerreiros de seu tempo, e o mais importante de tudo, iniciou a filosofia e a ciência, contribuição sem igual para a humanidade.

Os séculos VI a IV a.C. foram os séculos de ouro do mundo antigo. Nele viveram Buda na Índia, Zoroastro na Mesopotâmia, Confúcio e Lao-Tsé na China, e Tales de Mileto, Pitágoras, Heráclito, Parmênides, Demócrito, Sócrates, Platão, Aristóteles, Epicuro e muitos outros filósofos na Grécia.

É incrível a coincidência de época de nascimento de tantos luminares e pensadores ao mesmo. Nunca mais isso se repetiria.

Não se trata de um surto civilizatório regional apenas. Na Grécia nasceram dezenas de homens muito inteligentes que influenciaram a humanidade para sempre, sobretudo Sócrates, Platão, Aristóteles e Epicuro, mas na Índia, muito distante, e sem qualquer contato com a Grécia, havia Buda, e na China, também sem nenhum contato, havia Confúcio. Isso é uma incrível coincidência, que nos leva a pensar no planejamento do "Alto", para fazer crescer e evoluir a humanidade.

As guerras de conquista no passado tinham um certo efeito globalizante, diferente de hoje, pois não havia imprensa, na forma de jornais, rádios, televisão, internet, etc.

Quando Alexandre, o Grande, saiu da Macedônia, no norte da Grécia, a conquistar o mundo por ele conhecido, começando pela invasão do Império Persa, acabou levando com ele a civilização grega, que ele adorava e admirava, tendo sido, ele próprio, educado por um grego, e um dos maiores filósofos de sua época, Aristóteles.

O que se denominou de helenismo foi a fusão das culturas grega e persa, com predominância grega, a se espalhar pelo novo Império Grego de Alexandre.

No Egito, depois da morte de Alexandre, o general Ptolomeu reinou como faraó, e construiu uma das maiores bibliotecas do mundo antigo, a Biblioteca de Alexandria. Nesse país houve uma grande fusão de culturas.

Traços da cultura grega nunca mais foram extirpados de muitos países conquistados pelos exércitos de Alexandre.

Depois, os romanos conquistaram a Grécia, já decadente, depois da morte de Alexandre, tendo seu império sido dividido entre os cinco generais macedônios. E um império dividido é um império enfraquecido, e à mercê de invasores mais fortes e unidos.

Apesar de terem os romanos conquistado a Grécia, a cultura e civilização gregas lhes eram superiores, e na verdade a cultura grega conquistou mais do que foi conquistada pelos romanos.

Teatro, literatura, arquitetura, técnicas militares, escultura, filosofia, tudo foi copiado pelos romanos dos gregos. Até hoje se vê em Roma os estilos gregos de construção.

Os romanos também conquistaram muitas terras, formando um vasto império, sendo os dominantes de Israel (Palestina) no tempo em que lá viveu Jesus.

A cultura romana também se espalhou pelo mundo antigo, e ainda sentimos os seus reflexos até hoje, seja nas línguas de origem latina, na ciência, sobretudo na química, com a utilização do latim nos nomes dos elementos, nas construções, no Direito, na literatura, na escultura e em muitos outros campos.

Com a queda do Império Romano, povos menos civilizados invadiram a Itália e vários outros países europeus, pois já não havia mais a proteção dos exércitos romanos, como no passado. Com isso, iniciou-se o chamado período feudal, com grande retrocesso, e predomínio da lei do mais forte, com senhores feudais dominando de forma absoluta suas terras e seus vassalos. Reis reinavam sobre pequenas porções de terra.

A Europa foi imensamente dividida em territórios pequenos. E isso possibilitou a invasão e o ataque de povos chamados bárbaros, menos civilizados, vindos do leste, da Ásia, como os hunos com Átila e os mongóis com Gengis Khan.

A China, que vivia fechada em sua cultura isolacionista, também foi conquistada pelos exércitos poderosos de Gengis Khan.

A história humana é uma sucessão de guerras, de lutas, de matanças muitas vezes inteiramente desnecessárias, motivadas por interesses mesquinhos e fúteis. Ego e vaidade, levando sofrimento a milhares de pessoas inocentes que vivem suas vidas pacíficas a trabalharem para viver.

Em muitas épocas e lugares famílias tiveram suas propriedades invadidas e saqueadas por dois ou três exércitos diferentes, de nações diferentes, em uma só existência.

Império sucedendo a império. Conquistador sucedendo a conquistador. Morte e sofrimento constante...

O denominado Renascimento, movimento que teve início na Itália, no início do século XVI, buscando redescobrir e reviver os áureos tempos da Grécia e Roma antigas, teve profundo impacto na civilização européia. A Religião perdeu um pouco da sua força, naquilo em que era negativo, como a Santa Inquisição, e abriu espaço para novos vôos filosóficos e científicos. A Igreja que calou Galileu quando ele afirmou que a Terra girava em torno do sol, e não o contrário, perdia um pouco desse autoritarismo, e isso permitiu que os gênios aflorassem, como Newton e Leonardo Da Vinte.

Bússola, astrolábio e outros instrumentos de navegação foram inventados no Renascimento, e permitiram as viagens aos mares desconhecidos do Oceano Atlântico, levando à descoberta da América e muitas outras terras novas para os europeus, possibilitando a disseminação do conhecimento pelo vasto planeta, inclusive levando o cristianismo a todas as partes do globo terrestre, em cumprimento ao mandamento de Jesus.

Os filósofos gregos foram redescobertos, e reinterpretados. O Direito romano foi despertado novamente, e logo viria a fase do Iluminismo, com Voltaire e Russeau, e tantos outros a buscar e pregar a democracia, que depois viria a ser finalmente implantada.

O Renascimento abriu as portas para o Iluminismo e para a Revolução Francesa, que espalharia o ideal de liberdade, igualdade e fraternidade por todo o mundo ocidental.

O Oriente ficou imune às idéias democráticas, e por isso continuou a abrigar inúmeros déspotas hereditários até nossos dias.

Do Renascimento até o final do século XIX, a humanidade fez inúmeras descobertas e fez grandes invenções.

A mais importante, no entanto, foi a invenção da máquina a vapor. Ela gerou a Revolução Industrial.

No século XIX, a máquina a vapor fez surgir a locomotiva a vapor, verdadeira revolução no transporte de passageiros e cargas. Logo esse meio de transporte se espalharia por toda a Europa, América, Japão, Ásia, e todas as partes do mundo.

O trem levaria também tropas, canhões, armas e munição para as guerras, que se tornaram cada vez mais devastadoras e sangrentas, sem precedentes na história.

Trajes, armas, jóias, transportes, meios de comunicação, imprensa e muitas outras coisas foram ao longo dos séculos mudando a face da humanidade.

O telégrafo levava mensagens rápidas a grandes distâncias antes percorridas por homens montados em cavalos, agilizando em muito as comunicações urgentes.

A medicina avançou muito até o final do século XIX. Também a engenharia, a arquitetura, a música com seus novos instrumentos musicais, e também as armas foram ficando cada vez mais potentes, com canhões que podiam agora atingir longas distâncias sem que o inimigo sequer suspeitasse que seria bombardeado, sendo pegos de surpresa, com vantagem para o atacante.

Quem tivesse melhores e mais potentes armas dominaria o mundo. E isso levou os países no último século a uma corrida armamentista sem precedentes, com armas muitos mais potentes e letais, que seriam inventadas no século XX, com poder de destruição em massa jamais imaginado pela humanidade, e colocando em risco a sua própria existência, o que antes não acontecia.

Ao final do século XIX, a escravidão estava extinta no planeta, de um modo geral e aberta; o trem a vapor estava disseminado; todos os povos usavam canhões e armas automáticas em seus exércitos; mesmo os países antes isolados, como o Japão, já estavam se modernizando. A cultura estava se universalizando. A globalização estava sendo exercitada cada vez mais. E os mais fortes dominavam o comércio. Não havia uma nação muito mais forte do que as outras no final do século XIX, do ponto de vista estritamente militar.

A grande mudança, e grande revolução, viria no século seguinte, o século XX, que veremos adiante.

CAPÍTULO 9

SÉCULO XX

Ano 2.007, dia 12 de julho. Se Jesus de fato tiver nascido na data sugerida pelo astrônomo alemão Johannes Kepler (1.571-1.630 d.C.), pai da moderna astronomia, que seria o dia 22 de agosto do ano 7 a.C., como narrado em um capítulo anterior, estará completando neste ano exatamente 2 mil anos de seu nascimento na Terra.

Desde o ano 7 a.C até nossos dias, muitas coisas mudaram no mundo.

O Império Romano se desfez, apesar de ter um dia parecido eterno, e após durar mais de mil anos. Mas em sua duração serviu de alavanca para a divulgação da mensagem de Jesus, a Boa Nova (Evangelho) por todo o planeta.

A Igreja Católica nasceu exatamente dentro do Império Romano, no século IV d.C., e com o aval do imperador romano Constantino, que deu novo nome a Bizâncio, que passou a se chamar Constantinopla.

A nova igreja, cristã, totalmente diferente da religião pagã antiga de Roma, que era semelhante à religião da Grécia antiga, tinha como centro de sua doutrina os quatro evangelhos escritos ao longo do século I d.C. E essa igreja, iniciada por São Pedro, apóstolo de Cristo, e São Paulo, perseguidor dos cristãos e posteriormente convertido ao cristianismo, inicialmente clandestina, e depois chancelada pelo Estado, cresceu rapidamente, se expandiu, e se espalhou pelo mundo afora.

A Igreja Católica neste início de século (XXI) busca a retomada de seu rumo, após ter passado por tantas mudanças, tantos desvios, tantos desatinos. E deve mesmo rever antigas posições, mas deve também bater pé firme diante de certas "modernidades", mesmo que venha a ser taxada de retrógrada e ultrapassada por alguns.

Não se pode aceitar tudo, aceitar qualquer nova idéia só para agradar, para ficar bem com alguns fiéis, principalmente quando as

110

idéias contenham imoralidade, prejuízo para a vida física e moral das pessoas, e risco para a saúde e para a alma.

O século XX foi um século ímpar, sem precedentes na história humana.

Nunca a humanidade antes havia se desenvolvido tanto em ciência, tecnologia, arte, armamento, economia, produção, educação, diplomacia, controle da natureza, da vida, e também destruído tanto o meio-ambiente, o planeta.

O século XX viu cientistas e inventores colocarem em prática e em atividade nas cidades a luz elétrica, que iluminou o mundo; o automóvel, e veículos maiores como caminhões e ônibus, tornando os deslocamentos mais rápidos, encurtando o tempo de percurso da transmissão de bens de consumo, e transportes de passageiros; o telefone fixo, e depois o móvel, permitindo a comunicação mais rápida e completa entre as pessoas e as nações; o rádio, que facilitou em muito a difusão de informações, notícias e idéias no mundo; a televisão, meio de comunicação audiovisual mais completo que o rádio, com transmissão de som e imagem em tempo real pelo mundo; o computador e a internet, que incrementaram e aumentaram a velocidade de processamento, armazenagem e transmissão digital de dados; o avião, que encurtou as distâncias, acelerando o processo de troca de bens e cultura entre os povos; o cinema, que espalhou pelo mundo idéias, lazer e cultura; a geladeira, que possibilitou o armazenamento por mais tempo dos alimentos perecíveis; o gramofone, e depois a vitrola (toca-discos) e o toca CD, o DVD, o MP3, e várias outras formas de arquivo digital de som e imagem, de música e filme; o foguete, o avião (ônibus) espacial, a estação espacial; a câmera fotográfica digital, a câmera filmadora digital; a energia nuclear para fins pacíficos; o satélite de comunicação, que facilitou e agilizou a troca de informações através do mundo; as técnicas cirúrgicas, com utilização em cirurgias plásticas reparadoras e estéticas, devolvendo a beleza perdida em acidentes ou aumentando a beleza com a correção de defeitos congênitos; as cirurgias de ponte de safena, que tantas vidas têm salvado; as cirurgias de colocação de próteses, como braços e pernas mecânicas, para aqueles que tiveram membros amputados após acidentes ou doenças; cirurgias de olhos, dentárias, implantes de cabelo e próteses de silicone nos seios; os trens elétricos rápidos e seguros, permitindo viagens mais rápidas, econômicas e seguras; a indústria química, petroquímica, cosmética, têxtil, etc.; as gráficas rápidas e impressoras de computador caseiro; o scanner, a reciclagem de lixo, diminuindo a poluição ambiental; o radar, o sonar, o raio X, a ressonância magnética, o ultra-som, a tomografia computadorizada, o PET (tomografia por emissão de pósitrons); a engenharia genética, as sondas espaciais para estudar os planetas do sistema solar; o infravermelho; e muitas outras coisas que encheriam páginas e mais páginas.

O século XX se iniciou com as pessoas andando a pé ou a cavalo, de carroça ou carruagem, trem a vapor, ou viajando de navio, e terminou com as pessoas circulando em carros rápidos, trens elétricos velozes, que atingem até 300 Km/h, aviões ligeiros com mais de 300 passageiros, ida ao espaço em avião espacial, envio rápido de mensagens através da internet (correio eletrônico), comunicação de qualquer lugar através de telefones celulares (móvel), rastreamento de veículos e pessoas por satélite (GPS), pesquisa e compra pela internet, sem sair de casa, pagando com cartões de crédito, envio de declarações de imposto de renda pela internet, fiscalização dos gastos públicos pela internet, vida mais longa com um número cada vez maior de pessoas passando dos 100 anos de idade.

As mudanças foram muitas.

Começamos o século XX sem cinema, sem rádio e sem TV. E logo nas primeiras décadas chegou o cinema preto e branco e mudo. Antes mesmo da metade do século, já tínhamos o cinema com som e a cores. E bem antes do encerramento do século já existia o cinema em 3D (três dimensões).

O cinema holográfico já está sendo desenvolvido, e não demorará muito a chegar às salas de cinema.

A televisão de plasma, a televisão digital, o DVD Player e o Home Theater trouxeram o cinema para casa.

O radar permitiu um grande número de vôos ao mesmo tempo, com pequena possibilidade de choques entre as aeronaves no ar.

A penicilina e os modernos antibióticos descobertos ao longo do século XX já salvaram milhões de vidas, em tempo de paz e nas guerras.

Os medicamentos para dor, como morfina, trouxeram alívio para muita gente, como feridos em combate, acidentados e doentes terminais. Hoje quem vive em um país relativamente avançado não morre em hospital com dor.

A diplomacia teve grande avanço no século XX.

Nos séculos anteriores, normalmente as guerras eram travadas entre duas nações, entre dois povos. Não era comum a formação de alianças para as guerras. E o mais forte normalmente vencia, e nenhuma outra nação se envolvia no conflito para impedi-lo.

No início do século XX tivemos uma guerra terrível, que envolveu muitos países, com alguns milhões de mortos de saldo, entre os anos 1.914 e 1.918. A Primeira Guerra Mundial.

Após a guerra, formou-se a Liga das Nações, que buscou resolver algumas questões territoriais. Não resolveu tudo, tanto que não demorou a eclodir a Segunda Guerra, logo depois, em 1.939. Mas a experiência adquirida com a Liga das Nações não foi de todo perdida, e após o término da Segunda Guerra nasceu a ONU (Organização das Nações Unidas), órgão até hoje existente, e que, a despeito de estar longe da perfeição e do ideal, tem conseguido evitar muitos conflitos bélicos entre as nações. Ou seja, a ONU, mesmo não sendo perfeita, tem cumprido um papel bastante eficaz mantendo o mundo em relativa paz.

A Segunda Guerra, de 1.939 a 1.945, teve como saldo um total de 60 milhões de mortos. Se colocarmos também os feridos, os órfãos, as viúvas e viúvos, sem dúvida chegaremos a mais de 100 milhões de vítimas diretas da guerra. O prejuízo material é incalculável. Os traumas da guerra até hoje são sentidos. Muitos judeus que sobreviveram ao Holocausto nazista ainda estão vivos, com a clara lembrança dos horrores dos campos de concentração. Soldados ainda lembram dos combates na terra, no ar ou no mar. Aleijados em decorrência de explosões de bombas, minas terrestres ou tiros ainda vivem suas agonias e ainda têm pesadelos.

A lembrança da terrível Segunda Guerra Mundial ainda não teve tempo de ser totalmente apagada.

A humanidade vive hoje há 62 anos em paz, se considerarmos apenas a guerra de larga proporção, ou guerra mundial, envolvendo várias nações. Tivemos vários conflitos menores e localizados depois do fim da Segunda Guerra, como a guerra da Coréia, no início dos anos 1.950, a guerra do Vietnã, nos anos 1.965 a 1.975, a guerra das Malvinas, entre Argentina e Inglaterra, a guerra entre Irã e Iraque, na década de 1.980, a guerra do Golfo, com a invasão do

Iraque em 1.991 por forças internacionais lideradas pelos Estados Unidos, e várias guerras civis dentro de países, como a de Angola e a da Bósnia, com processos vergonhosos de "limpeza étnica".

Estamos livres de conflitos de grandes proporções desde 1.945. E apesar de haver no mundo centenas ou talvez milhares de bombas atômicas, e também bombas de hidrogênio, nunca mais, desde 1.945, outra bomba nuclear foi lançada no mundo, o que já demonstra uma maturidade política na humanidade, e o predomínio da razão, pois sabem os políticos o que poderia acontecer em uma guerra nuclear de grandes proporções.

No século XX tivemos a experiência do Mercado Comum Europeu, que depois amadureceu para a Comunidade Européia, que levou à criação de uma moeda única em sua região de atuação bem grande, além da livre circulação de produtos, com grande ganho para todos os países que integram a comunidade, tanto que hoje o Euro, moeda criada pela Comunidade Européia, está mais valorizado e forte do que o Dólar americano. É a união vencendo.

Essa experiência certamente ao longo do século XXI deverá influenciar outras regiões do planeta.

Tenta-se já no sul do continente americano a implantação do Mercosul, mas ainda sem sucesso, face à imaturidade das nações da região. O mesmo se dá com a Alca, na parte norte do continente americano.

No século XX tivemos muitas demonstrações de solidariedade entre os povos, principalmente em momentos de dificuldades e catástrofes naturais, como terremotos, enchentes e maremotos, ou em razão de desastres e epidemias.

Nações mais ricas muitas vezes enviaram equipes especializadas em resgates para ajudar a socorrer vítimas de terremotos na Turquia, no México e no Paquistão, além de ajuda com medicamentos, alimentos e roupas. Países africanos vários foram ajudados para conter epidemias, como a AIDS e o vírus Ebola.

Em momentos de calamidades de grandes proporções, as nações têm se mobilizado para enviar ajuda aos necessitados, muitas vezes esquecendo até mesmo divergências políticas antigas. Isso demonstra um avanço na capacidade de sensibilização humana com a dor alheia.

O combate ao narcotráfico se tornou internacional. Todas as nações entraram nessa guerra, ao perceberem a sua importância. Há troca não só de informações, mas também de presos. Há mais extradições de criminosos, de uma forma nunca antes vista no mundo.

Há mais cooperação entre as polícias das nações, com benefício geral, para todas.

Há mais trocas de informações científicas pela internet, e entre os centros de pesquisas. O egoísmo tem diminuído no mundo científico. A difusão das vacinas que salvam vidas está acima do mero desejo de lucro. Ou seja, o ser humano está valendo mais.

Nossa percepção é de avanço e melhoria do mundo como um todo. Mas ainda há muitos aspectos negativos a serem corrigidos, e aberrações a serem extirpadas da humanidade.

Fechamos o século XX com a volta das guerras de religião, um retrocesso ao tempo das cruzadas do século XII, travada entre cristãos e muçulmanos.

Hindus e muçulmanos disputam áreas montanhosas na fronteira entre a Índia e o Paquistão; judeus e muçulmanos brigam em Israel; católicos e protestantes lutaram durante várias décadas na Irlanda; cristãos ocidentais lutam pelo domínio do Iraque com muçulmanos de várias correntes.

O clima é tenso entre cristãos ocidentais e muçulmanos desde a segunda metade do século XX, tendo se iniciado com a instalação do Estado de Israel na Palestina em 1.948, depois de quase dois mil anos de predomínio muçulmano na região, o que parece que jamais será aceito pelos palestinos. E por isso a região é um imenso barril de pólvora, sempre com possibilidade de explosão, a qualquer momento, e levando vários países a uma guerra de larga proporção.

No século XX assistimos muitas cenas de pessoas protestando na rua e se incendiando com gasolina; cenas de criança correndo nua e quase sem pele no Vietnã em decorrência da utilização da bomba conhecida como napalm; notícias de canibalismo em centros urbanos de países ricos, como os EUA; pais abusando sexualmente de filhos menores; estupros de criança de até dois anos pelo próprio pai; terrorismo fanático com utilização até mesmo de crianças de 12 anos para explodirem seus corpos envolvidos com dinamite ou outros explosivos para matarem pessoas inocentes.

São tantas as aberrações que vimos ao longo do século XX que muitas vezes chegamos a dizer que estava próximo o fim do mundo, ou que o mundo deveria acabar.

O século XX, por outro lado, viu também o maior progresso material da humanidade, de forma nunca antes vista. Todavia, apesar de o dinheiro circulante ter aumentado enormemente no mundo, houve também uma maior concentração de renda, ou seja, mais dinheiro no mundo, mas nas mãos de um número menor de pessoas.

A globalização da economia, iniciada logo após o fim da União Soviética, no início dos anos 1.990, levou progresso material a regiões antes muito pobres, como a Índia e a China.

As empresas sem bandeiras, multinacionais ou transnacionais, procuram se estabelecer onde há razoável nível de educação (instrução) e possibilidade de pagar salários menores, para que então possam lucrar mais do que lucravam em seus países de origem. Assim, a China hoje produz quase tudo, sendo o país que mais cresce, pois não há muitos direitos trabalhistas, e os salários são baixos. Mas no fim todos ganham, pois a China está crescendo, sua população está melhorando a qualidade de vida, que o regime comunista não conseguiu dar, podendo em futuro próximo se tornar a grande potência econômica do século XXI.

A Índia segue a mesma estrada da China, só que com liberdade, uma vez que a China ainda adota o regime comunista, sem liberdade de expressão e de crítica ao governo.

O século XX viu o nascimento do comunismo na prática, uma vez que Carl Marx lançou o manifesto comunista no meado do século XIX.

A Rússia passou pela revolução bolchevista em 1.917, tornando-se a primeira nação comunista do mundo, arrastando com ela muitas nações e povos vizinhos, e depois da Segunda Guerra ainda levou outras mais, como parte da Alemanha, que se tornou também comunista (Alemanha Oriental).

Na Rússia, somente nos primeiros anos de comunismo, o governo matou de fome cerca de 10 milhões de camponeses, que não aceitavam o novo regime imposto à força e que por isso tiveram confiscadas suas colheitas. E ao longo de seus mais de 70 anos de comunismo, a União Soviética trancafiou milhões de pessoas em campos de "reeducação", na verdade prisões políticas, porque elas representavam "ameaça" ao regime, porque tinham visão crítica e não conseguiam se calar.

A URSS levou a guerrilha comunista a muitos países, como Angola, Brasil, China e outros. Angola levou mais de dez anos sob guerrilha, com milhares de mortos, e a completa destruição econômica do país.

Cuba tornou-se também comunista em 1.961, depois do golpe de Fidel Castro em 1.959. O ditador está ainda no poder, e parece que morrerá governando.

Em Cuba hoje há cerca de 300 presos políticos, e no país não existe liberdade de imprensa. As duas emissoras de TV, as rádios, revistas e jornais são todos estatais, como pude ver quando lá estive em 2.002.

Na Coréia do Norte, desde a divisão da Coréia, o regime comunista tem sido duro e extremamente fechado. Hoje o mais fechado e retrógrado regime comunista do mundo.

Enquanto Cuba e China estão abrindo aos poucos sua economia, e também o Vietnã, a Coréia do Norte continua nos moldes mais radicais de controle da população e das idéias, sem a menor liberdade de expressão. Entraram no século XXI como estivessem na Idade Média cultural.

O século XX viu o crescimento absurdo do consumo de drogas.

As décadas de 1.960 e 1.970 transformaram o uso das drogas em coisa comum e parte integrante do lazer dos jovens. O movimento Hippie popularizou a maconha (marijuana), o LSD e a heroína. E nos anos seguintes surgiram a cocaína, em pó e líquida, o craque, o êxtase, e muitas outras drogas.

Jovens de idades cada vez menores entram no mundo das drogas. E não adianta somente o combate aos traficantes, enquanto as pessoas não deixarem de comprar e consumir drogas.

Os usuários de drogas são na prática sócios capitalistas dos produtores e vendedores das drogas. Assim, enquanto houver procura, haverá certamente oferta. Os traficantes sempre dão um jeito de chegar até os consumidores.

O século XX viu também a banalização do sexo. Na década de 1.960 nasceu o movimento de liberação da mulher, e com ele a liberação sexual, com o uso de preservativos e anticoncepcionais, tendo como objetivo não a proteção contra doenças, mas principalmente evitar a gravidez, para que as mulheres pudessem exercer livremente a sua sexualidade. Isso acabou levando à banalização do sexo.

Hoje em quase todo o mundo as pessoas fazem sexo como se fizessem um lanche. Prazer rápido e imediato, sem compromisso.

Como conseqüência, gravidez indesejada, doenças venéreas, AIDS, mães adolescentes, filhos sem pais conhecidos, famílias desajustadas, e tudo isso contribuindo para revolta, violência e desequilíbrio de toda sorte na sociedade.

O sexo chegou ao final do século XX bestializado. Na internet qualquer um pode entrar em sites de sexo, de pornografia de todo tipo, inclusive de zoofilia (sexo com animais). Cenas de cachorros, cabras e cavalos penetrando mulheres, e muito mais.

A violência em alguns locais do mundo, como no Brasil, por exemplo, se tornou também banal.

Nas favelas do Rio de Janeiro e em São Paulo organizações criminosas dominam, impedindo muitas vezes a entrada da polícia. Ateiam fogo em ônibus com pessoas dentro, ordenam o fechamento do comércio local, sem reação das pessoas, que ficam com medo das represálias. É o Estado paralelo, bandido, como dizem alguns jornalistas brasileiros.

Cenas de pessoas mortas nas ruas e nas portas de moradores das favelas do Rio se tornaram banais, e já não mais sensibilizam. Assaltos ousados a quartéis de polícia, desvio de armas das Forças Armadas, contrabando de armas sem controle, vendas de drogas nos morros, tudo quase liberado por muitos e muitos anos, e agora de difícil solução e extirpação.

Na Colômbia, os guerrilheiros comunistas se tornaram também traficantes, que seqüestram pessoas para pedirem resgates altos, para financiar a guerrilha. Os ideais de guerrilha ficaram em segundo plano. O dinheiro e a ambição passaram na frente.

Ao longo do século XX, as igrejas cristãs, que eram apenas quatro principais, a Católica, a Anglicana da Inglaterra, nascida por questões políticas, a Protestante, nascida no século XVI com a Reforma de Martinho Lutero, e a Ortodoxa, que possuíam alguma divergência real de culto, ou nasceram devido ao rompimento com o Vaticano, se multiplicaram às centenas.

Igrejas chamadas evangélicas nasceram tão rapidamente e de forma desordenada, visando ao que tudo indica meramente o enriquecimento de seus fundadores, que hoje talvez ninguém saiba exatamente quantas existem no mundo.

Nas cidades grandes brasileiras, muitas vezes há três ou quatro igrejas evangélicas diferentes em uma mesma rua.

Não há diferenças reais de dogma, muito menos de culto, entre as dezenas e dezenas de igrejas cristãs denominadas de evangélicas, denominação por demais vaga.

É por isso que hoje questionamos o seu surgimento e existência. Por que elas foram criadas? Com que finalidade? Será que Jesus, onde está, aprova tal disseminação de igrejinhas arrecadadoras do suado dinheiro dos fiéis?

Os jovens começam a ingerir bebidas alcoólicas cada vez mais cedo, devido às belas propagandas livremente transmitidas pelas emissoras de TV. Belas mulheres incentivam o consumo do álcool, e depois rapidamente uma curta frase diz: "Beba com moderação". É pura hipocrisia!

Em alguns países, como no Brasil, a propaganda do cigarro foi proibida na TV, nas revistas e out doors. Isso fez com que diminuísse o consumo do tabaco no Brasil. Esse hábito tão destrutivo e letal, que causa vários tipos de câncer.

A luta contra o tabagismo, no entanto, está ainda longe de ser vencida, porque a indústria de cigarros é muito forte, rica e poderosa.

O grande número de acidentes de trânsito ao redor do mundo, motivados principalmente pelo consumo de álcool, já justifica a adoção de igual medida em relação às bebidas alcoólicas, ou seja, a proibição de sua propaganda nos meios de comunicação, em todos eles. É uma guerra para o século XXI, pois será travada contra uma rede de indústrias ainda mais forte, unida e poderosa do que a do tabaco.

O século XX finalizou com um misto de avanço de informática, de engenharia genética, pesquisas espaciais, avanço na medicina e aberrações sexuais, libertinagem em alto grau, sem controle na internet, com violência urbana sem controle e sem limites, com corrupção mundial e banalização da violência e do sexo.

Além disso, o século XX terminou com uma população mundial de mais de 6 bilhões de habitantes, e um quadro preocupante de desmatamento, de destruição das florestas, de poluição de rios, mares e lagos, com secas e processo de desertificação em várias partes do globo, além de aquecimento global que está levando lentamente ao derretimento das calotas polares e também das geleiras das montanhas altas, como os Alpes na Europa e Andes na América do Sul.

A alimentação do tipo Fast Food, rápida, mas sem qualidade, está levando as pessoas a adoecerem mais. A poluição do ar está causando problemas respiratórios. A poluição dos rios está matando os peixes. O aquecimento dos oceanos está alterando o ciclo reprodutivo de alguns peixes.

A virada do século demonstrou um aumento da temperatura global, pela grande emissão de gases como o CO2; a destruição parcial da camada de ozônio, que serve para proteger o planeta das radiações solares danosas ao ser humano, deixando-nos mais expostos a essas radiações e mais propensos ao câncer de pele, o que exige um maior cuidado, e a utilização de filtros e protetores solares no dia a dia, principalmente as pessoas de pele mais clara.

A superpopulação concentrada nos grandes centros urbanos, chegando a viver dez milhõcs de pessoas em uma só cidade, levou a humanidade a um nível de estresse urbano jamais antes visto. Milhões de automóveis circulando nas ruas diariamente, causando congestionamentos longos e demorados, dificultando a ida para o trabalho e o retorno para casa. Marginalização das populações periféricas, principalmente nos países mais pobres, com a formação de imensas favelas, normal em grande parte da América Latina. Dificuldade na distribuição de água e energia elétrica para todas as residências, bem como de redes de esgoto.

O desafio do século XX em vencer todas essas dificuldade está longe de terminar. Trens urbanos e metrôs resolvem apenas em parte os problemas de transporte de massa em alguns países. Mas na maioria o problema parece ser mesmo insolúvel. O desafio da inclusão social dos pobres na economia produtiva, possibilitando que eles também se tornem consumidores é grande.

O problema da energia vai ficar cada vez mais evidente, à medida que a população mundial crescer ainda mais. O petróleo logo vai acabar. Se houver diminuição dos mananciais de água dos rios, as hidrelétricas já não servirão mais de solução para a questão da energia elétrica. Restará a energia nuclear, e a energia solar, ainda com tecnologia cara.

O século terminou com idéias inovadoras, como o biocombustível, na forma de álcool combustível, e outros tipos, desenvolvidos no Brasil.

A humanidade terá que encontrar formas alternativas de combustível, para substituir o petróleo e o carvão mineral. Esse desafio é para o novo século XXI.

Esse um quadro muito sintético do século XX.

No próximo capítulo, trataremos do Fim dos Tempos e do Juízo Final.

CAPÍTULO 10

O FIM DOS TEMPOS E O JUÍZO FINAL

Inicialmente, é importante frisar que o fim dos tempos não é a mesma coisa que juízo final, ou juízo universal. Trata-se de duas coisas diferentes.

Ainda há os sinais do fim dos tempos.

O juízo final, ou juízo universal, profetizado desde Isaías, Daniel, Miquéias, Zacarias e Jesus, e também revelado a João, e contido no livro Apocalipse, certamente acontecerá, como todas as profecias desses profetas já cumpridas em relação a fatos que para nós hoje já é passado.

As invasões das terras dos judeus no passado, com o cativeiro na Babilônia, profetizadas e cumpridas; o cerco e destruição de Jerusalém pelos romanos, profetizado em detalhes por Jesus, e já muito tempo antes por Moisés, e cumpridas no ano 70 d.C.; as guerras e rumores de guerras, os maremotos, os terremotos, as pestes, tudo demonstra o cumprimento das profecias antigas contidas nos livros da Bíblia.

Jesus falou em sinais do fim dos tempos, e entre eles mencionou a volta dos Judeus à sua terra, Israel, o que já foi cumprido em 1.948, quando da criação do novo Estado de Israel, bem como indicou também como sinal do fim dos tempos a pregação do evangelho por todo o mundo. E esses sinais indicados por Jesus diziam respeito à vinda do Senhor, ao Dia do Senhor, ao Dia do Juízo Universal, para usar diversas expressões antigas dos profetas, inclusive de Jesus.

Os sinais estão se cumprindo. E isso deve significar a proximidade do fim dos tempos das nações, de que falou Jesus. E a proximidade do Juízo Final, ou Juízo Universal.

Juízo, como utilizado na Bíblia, quer dizer julgamento. Também no moderno Direito utiliza-se a palavra juízo como sinônimo de julgamento. E até as pessoas comuns usam expressões como "juízo de valor" e "fazer um juízo", o que significa fazer um julgamento, emitir um julgamento.

Assim, *Juízo Universal* significa *julgamento universal*, ou seja, *julgamento de todos*. E *Juízo Final* significa *julgamento final*, não necessariamente destruição.

Desde cerca de setecentos anos antes de Jesus os profetas judeus já previram um julgamento último e coletivo, um juízo universal. E Jesus confirmou esse julgamento, que se daria com a sua volta. Também o Apocalipse, último livro da Bíblia, escrito no final do século I d.C. por João, apóstolo de Jesus, afirmou esse julgamento último e universal, e de toda a humanidade, não apenas dos judeus.

Para quem acredita na imortalidade da alma, como nós cristãos, e também os budistas e muçulmanos, bem como os judeus, não é idéia absurda a existência de um julgamento de almas em determinado momento da história humana.

Nem todos os judeus da época de Jesus acreditavam na imortalidade da alma, por incrível que possa parecer.

Os *saduceus*, por exemplo, na época de Jesus negavam a imortalidade da alma, tendo sido eles os principais responsáveis pela condenação de Jesus; os *fariseus*, puristas e nacionalistas, que esperavam do Messias a libertação do jugo romano, acreditavam na imortalidade da alma e na ressurreição do corpo.

Como se vê, os judeus na antiguidade tinham seitas com doutrinas divergentes, do mesmo jeito como hoje acontece, e do mesmo modo como existe entre os cristãos, muçulmanos e budistas.

É certa a efetivação do Juízo Universal, ou Juízo Final, de conformidade com as profecias dos antigos profetas judeus. E esse julgamento universal de almas se dará algum tempo depois do fim dos tempos, ou do tempo dado às nações, como disse Jesus.

Como vimos, tudo parece indicar mesmo que a contagem para o denominado fim dos tempos teve seu marco inicial com a volta dos judeus a Israel, à Palestina, à Canaã.

Quanto tempo vai levar para acontecerem as coisas previstas na Bíblia, de Isaías a Jesus e no Apocalipse?

O marco que demonstra o fim dos tempos das nações se deu em 1.948. Já se passaram 59 anos desde a criação de Israel, desde a volta dos judeus à Terra Santa, à Terra Prometida.

Os profetas antigos viam os acontecimentos futuros como se fossem acontecer logo. Mas o que vemos é que muitas vezes os acontecimentos levaram anos, séculos, e até mesmo milênios algumas vezes para se confirmarem.

Moisés, por exemplo, por volta do século XII a.C., descreveu o cerco romano a Jerusalém em detalhes, o que aconteceu mais de uma vez, sendo a primeira na época dos Babilônios, e depois no século I d.C., pelos romanos, no ano 70, cerca de mil e duzentos anos depois de sua morte.

Jesus anteviu a queda e destruição de Jerusalém que aconteceu no ano 70, pouco tempo antes de acontecer, uma vez que ele foi crucificado entre 32 e 34 d.C. Estando ele no templo, disse a seus discípulos que ali não ficaria pedra sobre pedra, o que de fato se cumpriu.

E Jesus descreveu acontecimentos que ainda não aconteceram, relacionados com o Juízo Universal, o Juízo Final, com o Fim dos Tempos das nações.

João Batista falava da chegada do Reino de Deus como se ele estivesse já muito próximo, mas ele ainda não chegou, 2 mil anos depois de sua morte.

Como se observa, muitas profecias bíblicas já se cumpriram, e outras ainda não.

Como vimos em capítulos anteriores, as duas grandes guerras do século XX, os terremotos, os maremotos, como o recente Tsunami, totalmente fora do padrão comum até então conhecido, e a volta dos judeus à Terra Santa são fortes indicativos de que está chegando o fim dos tempos das nações, ou seja, de que está chegando o momento do grande julgamento, do Juízo Final.

Intérpretes de Nostradamus fixaram uma grande destruição, mas atribuída a uma terceira grande guerra mundial, no ano 1.999, o que efetivamente não aconteceu, como já dito antes nesta obra. Todavia, os cálculos dos astrólogos e estudiosos de Nostradamus indicam a proximidade de uma grande destruição.

Documentos exibidos pela primeira vez em junho de 2.007 expõem o lado religioso pouco conhecido de um dos maiores cientistas da história. Isaac Newton, que morreu há 280 anos, é conhecido por seus trabalhos fundamentais da física moderna, astronomia e matemática.

Em um dos manuscritos, datado do começo do século XVIII, Newton, por meio dos textos bíblicos do Livro de Daniel, chegou à conclusão de que o mundo deve acabar por volta do ano de

2.060. Escreveu ele: "*Ele pode acabar além desta data, mas não há razão para acabar antes*", escreveu.

Em outro documento, o cientista interpreta as profecias bíblicas que contam sobre o retorno dos judeus à Terra Prometida antes do final do mundo. Segundo ele, se verá "*a ruína das nações más, o fim do choro e de todos os problemas, e o retorno dos judeus ao seu próspero reino*".

Uma das curadoras da exposição, Yemima Ben-Menahem, diz que os papéis de Newton vão de encontro à idéia de que a ciência é exatamente oposta à religião. "Estes documentos mostram um cientista guiado por um fervor religioso, por um desejo de ver as ações de Deus guiando o mundo", disse.

Os manuscritos de Newton, comprados da Inglaterra em 1.936, estão na Livraria Nacional de Israel desde 1.969.

Como se observa, o físico inglês que apresentou ao mundo a Lei da Gravitação Universal também era um estudioso e intérprete da Bíblia, e fazia cálculos a fim de tentar descobrir a época dos fatos descritos nas profecias, como as de Daniel e as do livro Apocalipse.

O ano 2.060 é por demais próximo, e em nosso século. Adiante analisaremos a lógica do cumprimento das profecias em época não muito distante, como também acreditava Nostradamus e acreditam alguns de seus intérpretes.

Como vimos também, Isaac Newton, há 280 anos atrás, fazendo cálculos, afirmou que os fatos descritos no Apocalipse aconteceriam a partir de 2.060, não antes desse ano.

A escritora A. Galloti, autora do livro que tem como título *Nostradamus – As Profecias do Futuro,* publicado em 1.999, calculou a grande destruição para o período compreendido entre 2.096 e 2.156, período em que passaria um cometa próximo da Terra, segundo a quadra II, 43, do livro de Nostradamus.

O povo Maia, da América Central, tinha um calendário, segundo alguns estudiosos, mais preciso, mais complexo e muito mais holístico que o nosso, e que teria previsto vários acontecimentos que de fato aconteceram, como, por exemplo, a chegada do homem branco na sua terra, o que se confirmou com a chegada dos espanhóis. Hernan Cortez chegou na América Central em 8 de Novembro de 1.519.

O calendário Maia previa que algo de muito grave se passaria no solstício de Inverno de 21 de Dezembro de 2.012. Tão grave seria o acontecimento que o mundo tal como o conhecemos desapareceria. Isto não quer dizer que o mundo acabaria, mas que um grande acontecimento transformaria o mundo.

Hoje se sabe que na data apontada no calendário maia, durante o solstício de 21 de dezembro de 2.012, a Terra estará alinhada com o Sol e com o centro da nossa galáxia, a Via Láctea. E se sabe também que no centro da Galáxia existe um buraco negro supermassivo.

Baseados em Einstein e em algumas informações astronômicas, há quem diga que o alinhamento com este buraco negro supermassivo levará a uma mudança do campo magnético terrestre, que acontece periodicamente, e que isso provocará Tsunamis, erupções vulcânicas, terremotos, etc.

Como podemos ver, intérpretes de Nostradamus, Newtom e também o calendário maia fixaram o século XXI, ou ao menos a partir dele, o início das catástrofes naturais previstas pelos profetas judeus antigos, inclusive Jesus, e também no Apocalipse.

É claro que as catástrofes ainda não aconteceram até este momento, 13 de julho de 2.007. Assim, quem arriscou palpite de que tudo aconteceria até o século XX errou. Só pode ser daqui para a frente. Mas quando?

Jesus também relacionou o aparecimento de falsos profetas e falsos cristos com a chegada do Dia do Juízo Final. Disse ele que naquele tempo se levantariam falsos cristos e falsos profetas, e que fariam prodígios que, se fosse possível, enganariam até mesmo aos eleitos.

O século XX foi demais rico em falsos profetas, e falsos cristos. Quantos cabeludos e barbudos ousaram afirmar serem o cristo. E quantos foram desmoralizados e desmascarados.

Os mais velhos devem ainda lembrar do pastor americano Jim Jones, evangélico, fundador de seita apocalíptica, o Templo do Povo, que se mudou dos Estados Unidos para a fronteira da Guiana, e que levou ao suicídio 914 seguidores em 11 de novembro de 1.978. Esse foi o maior massacre coletivo de seitas apocalípticas que se tem notícia até hoje. Quem não quis tomar o veneno foi morto a tiros. Homens, mulheres, crianças e até mesmo cães foram encontrados mortos na sede da seita (Foto 18).

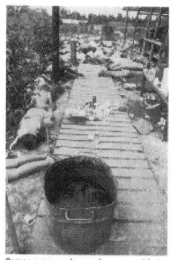

Corpos e copos de papel na comunidade de Jim Jones.

(Foto 18)

O século XX não foi a única época em que apareceram os falsos profetas, mas parece ter sido o período em que eles fizeram um maior estrago na sociedade, levando inúmeras pessoas ao suicídio coletivo para irem para o céu ou para escaparem da destruição do Juízo Final.

Pesquisando na internet, acerca de seitas apocalípticas e falsos profetas, encontrei o site de Roberto C. P. Júnior, mestre em ciências, escritor espiritualista e autor dos livros "Visão Restaurada das Escrituras" e "Jesus Ensina as Leis da Criação", muito bom, que apresenta um magnífico relato cronológico do aparecimento de seitas, falsos profetas e falsos cristos pelo mundo, desde a Idade Média. A seguir transcrevo grande parte do excelente material pesquisado e apresentado no site de Roberto C. P. Júnior.

"Em março de 1.993, pelo menos setenta seguidores da seita "Ramo Davidiano" morreram queimados num incêndio que teria sido provocado por eles mesmos. O dirigente da seita, David

127

Koresh, pregava palavras messiânicas misturando sexo, liberdade e resolução. Ele também dizia ser Deus.

Em outubro de 1.993, 53 habitantes de uma vila no interior do Vietnã cometeram suicídio coletivo. O responsável pelo desatino foi Cam Vam Lien, que recebeu vultosas somas em troca da promessa de um caminho rápido para o céu.

Em outubro de 1.994, 53 membros da "Ordem do Templo Solar" morreram num suicídio coletivo, incluindo o fundador da seita, o médico canadense Luc Jouret, que julgava ser um novo Cristo e pregava que o fim do mundo estava próximo. Os integrantes da seita acreditavam que, matando-se, viajariam para a estrela Sirius e lá teriam uma vida bem-aventurada. Em dezembro de 1.995, outros 16 membros da seita preparam por conta própria uma segunda excursão a Sirius; eles estavam ressentidos por não terem sido convidados para a primeira viagem. Dois integrantes do grupo preparam 14 homens, mulheres e crianças para essa segunda jornada, encapuzando-os com sacos plásticos e embebendo com gasolina seus corpos estendidos no chão, em formato de estrela. Atearam fogo a eles e depois se mataram com uma arma. Em março de 1.997, mais cinco membros da seita se "mudaram" para Sirius, ou seja, se suicidaram.

Em março de 1.995, membros da seita japonesa "Ensino da Verdade Suprema", provocaram um atentado com gás tóxico no metrô de Tóquio, matando dez pessoas e ferindo cerca de cinco mil. Fundada em 1.984, a seita tinha originalmente o nome de "Associação dos Eremitas Legendários com Poderes Miraculosos". O líder da seita, Shoko Asahara, que é cego e se considera a reencarnação de Buddha, dizia ser capaz de levitar e chamava Adolf Hitler de profeta. Ostentava os títulos de Sua Santidade, Venerando Mestre e Salvador do Século. Dizia que o mundo iria acabar em 1.997 e somente sobreviveria quem fosse membro do grupo. Os membros tinham de doar seus bens à seita e desembolsar até 10 mil dólares para ter o direito de beber o sangue do mestre. Já os menos abastados podiam, por 200 dólares apenas, tomar alguns goles da água suja do banho do guru. Os seguidores provocavam vômitos para expiar as culpas e 50 deles foram encontrados posteriormente em estado de coma, após um jejum de uma semana. Investigações policiais descobriram nos prédios da seita todos os ingredientes para a fabricação do gás sarin (utilizado no atentado de Tóquio), além de componentes de nitroglicerina, estoques de bactérias do botulismo, instalações para fabricação de armas de assalto e uma máquina de triturar ossos. Há indícios de que a seita planejava comprar blindados russos e ogivas nucleares. Em maio de 1.995 a seita de Asahara computava 10 mil seguidores no Japão e cerca de 20 mil em outros países.

Em maio de 1.996, o profeta chinês Wu Yangming foi executado com uma bala na nuca, depois de ter sido condenado por estupro. Wu, que se autoproclamava a reencarnação de Jesus Cristo e se intitulava futuro Imperador Sagrado, prometia o apocalipse a uma multidão de seguidores. Um relatório oficial do governo informava que, às mulheres (algumas de apenas 14 anos), Wu prometia a salvação em troca de sexo. Quando a polícia deu uma batida na aldeia onde ele se escondia, encontrou-o na cama com três de suas discípulas.

Em março de 1.997, 39 membros da seita americana "Portal do Céu" cometeram suicídio coletivo, na expectativa de que, se desvencilhando de seus corpos (chamados por eles de contêineres), embarcariam num disco voador que os aguardava escondido na cauda do cometa Hale Bopp. O líder da seita, Marshall Applewithe, que fora castrado para se purificar, acreditava ser um novo Cristo, com a missão de apresentar aos homens "um nível de evolução acima do humano". Em 1.993, ele havia publicado anúncios em vários jornais americanos e canadenses fazendo sua "última oferta" para quem quisesse se salvar. São dele também essas significativas palavras: *"Nossa missão é exatamente a mesma conferida a Jesus Cristo há dois mil anos. Eu estou para a sociedade de hoje na mesma posição em que estava a alma que habitava o corpo de Cristo. Estou aqui, portanto, para cumprir a última tarefa, prometida há dois mil anos. Como prometido, as chaves do Portal do Céu estão novamente no Ovni 2, como estavam em Jesus e seu Pai há dois mil anos."*

Em março de 1.998, uma multidão se aglomerou em frente ao número 3.513 da Ridgedale Drive, um subúrbio de Dallas, capital do Estado americano do Texas. Elas esperavam a chegada do Criador naquele endereço, anunciado com bastante antecedência pelo chinês Heng-Ming Cheng, líder da "Igreja da Salvação Divina". Duas semanas antes do evento, Chen afixou um cartaz na porta do referido endereço com os seguintes dizeres: ***"São todos bem-vindos para testemunhar a chegada de Deus, no próximo dia 31 de março, às 10 horas. (...) Qualquer um poderá fazer perguntas sobre religião, teologia e as sagradas escrituras diretamente a Deus"***. Para provar que seria Ele mesmo, o Criador atravessaria paredes e se multiplicaria em milhares de seres humanos, para cumprimentar cada um dos presentes e responder a perguntas em qualquer idioma.

Observando casos tão absurdos como esses, ficamos a pensar como foi possível haver pessoas que se deixassem seduzir por falsos profetas desse tipo, que têm esse título estampado nas testas. E não foram uma ou duas pessoas, mas dezenas e até centenas, milhares no caso da seita japonesa.

Os movimentos ditos "apocalípticos" provocam na verdade um dano muito maior do que o revelado quando de seus desmantelamentos. Em primeiro lugar, ao fazerem a pregação do "fim do mundo", "dos últimos tempos", do "Armagedon" e assuntos análogos, de forma tão absurdamente errada e ridícula, provocam nas pessoas sensatas uma compreensível repulsa por qualquer menção ao fim de uma era, e conseqüentemente também de um Julgamento Final.

Essas pessoas passam, assim, a tapar os olhos e ouvidos imediatamente diante de qualquer coisa que lhes pareça ter um ar religioso e relacionado com o Juízo Final ou o Apocalipse. Pondo tudo numa panela só, elas não poderão, evidentemente, verificar com imparcialidade se no meio de toda essa tolice existe algo que se coadune com a Verdade. As trevas obtêm dessa maneira a vitória que realmente lhes interessa: a de afastar os seres humanos de qualquer pensamento a respeito do Juízo Final, fazendo com que eles, em virtude dessa negligência (que não deixa de ser também indolência), acabem se perdendo.

E este processo já vem de longa data. Segue abaixo um relato cronológico das maiores sandices já divulgadas a respeito do "fim do mundo" e assuntos análogos:

No ano 960 da nossa era, um alemão de nome Bernard anunciou que o fim do mundo se daria quando a sexta-feira santa coincidisse com a anunciação da Virgem. Quando isso ocorreu, em 992, a cristandade, temerosa, acorreu em massa às igrejas para rezar.

Em 1.179, o astrólogo Juan de Toledo previu imensas catástrofes para o ano de 1.186, que poderiam levar ao fim do mundo e ao Juízo Final. O pânico se alastrou pela Europa e Oriente Médio. O arcebispo de Canterbury decretou uma semana nacional de penitência. O imperador de Constantinopla mandou murar todas as portas e janelas do seu palácio, enquanto uma grande parte da população cavava para si abrigos subterrâneos ou refugiava-se em cavernas e grutas.

Em 1.523, um astrólogo inglês anunciou que o fim do mundo fora marcado para o dia 21 de fevereiro de 1.524, e que começaria com a destruição de Londres por um dilúvio. O pânico foi tal que mais de 20 mil pessoas abandonaram a cidade para se refugiar nas colinas dos condados de Essex e Kent. O clero local construiu para si uma fortaleza na colina de Harrow, e lá se instalou com provisões para dois meses.

O anabatista alemão Melchior Hofman anunciou a volta de Cristo à Terra para 1.533, quando o mundo seria destruído pelo fogo, com exceção da cidade de Estrasburgo, que se tornaria então a Nova Jerusalém. Muitos adeptos se desfizeram de todos os bens terrenos para salvar suas almas.

Em 1.693, Jacob Zimmerman calculou que o fim do mundo teria lugar em outubro de 1.694, e fundou uma colônia na Pensilvânia para aguardar lá a chegada do Juízo Final. Seus discípulos construíram um tabernáculo de madeira com um telescópio no telhado, para poderem observar o céu e os astros no momento final.

Em 1.806, uma albergueira inglesa de nome Mary Bateman anunciou que uma de suas galinhas punha ovos sobre os quais se podia ler "Cristo está chegando". Ela havia tido uma revelação de que o mundo seria destruído pelo fogo, e que o Juízo Final viria quando a galinha agraciada tivesse botado 14 ovos com a inscrição sagrada.

Depois de estudar a Bíblia por dois anos, em particular o Livro de Daniel, William Miller se convenceu de que o mundo seria destruído pelo fogo no ano de 1.843. A partir de 1.840 o número de seus adeptos começou a crescer, até atingir centenas de milhares por toda a costa leste dos Estados Unidos. No início do ano fatídico ele construiu um tabernáculo em Boston, para cuja consagração acorreu uma multidão de quase 4 mil pessoas.

Em 1.844, uma vidente do Hawaí, chamada Hapu, anunciou que fazia parte da Santíssima Trindade juntamente com Jesus e Jeová, e ameaçou com os piores castigos divinos aqueles que se recusassem a crer em suas palavras. O sucesso com os havaianos foi imediato quando ela afirmou que não era mais necessário trabalhar, já que o fim do mundo estava próximo.

Em 1.895, um sacerdote protestante publicou um livro em Berlim em que anunciava o fim do mundo para 1.908. Havia lá a previsão de uma guerra européia para 1.897, o aparecimento de um novo Napoleão em 1.899, um enorme terremoto em 1.904, a ascensão ao céu dos 144 mil eleitos em 12 de março de 1.908 e outras coisas semelhantes.

No início do século XX, os adeptos da seita russa "Irmãos e Irmãs da Morte Vermelha" estavam certos de que o fim do mundo ocorreria no dia 13 de novembro de 1.900. Convencidos de que deveriam suicidar-se, 862 deles decidiram morrer na fogueira. Quando a polícia chegou, já havia uma centena de irmãos carbonizados.

Alguns anos depois da tragédia na Rússia, o arcanjo Gabriel apareceu à jovem americana Margaret Rowan, comunicando-lhe que o fim do mundo seria exatamente à meia-noite da sexta-feira, 13 de fevereiro de 1.925.

Em 1.938, um pastor protestante chamado Long teve a visão de uma misteriosa mão escrevendo numa espécie de quadro-negro a data "1.945", enquanto uma voz lhe comunicava que o fim do mundo teria lugar no dia 21 de setembro daquele ano, às 17h33min, momento em que tudo o que houvesse na face da Terra se vaporizaria e se desintegraria. Long angariou milhares de adeptos com sua história.

Na década de 1.950 a canadense Agnès Carlson fundou uma seita denominada "Os Filhos da Luz", com a promessa de que o fim do mundo aconteceria em 9 de janeiro de 1.953.

No dia 18 de maio de 1.954, os engenheiros da cidade de Roma encarregados de cuidar do Coliseu constataram o aparecimento de grandes fissuras no monumento, que ameaçavam fazê-lo desabar. Foi o que bastou para um profeta de plantão anunciar que aquilo era o sinal do começo do fim, e que o mundo seria completamente destruído no dia 24 de maio daquele ano, ou seja, seis dias depois. Em seu livro O Fim do Mundo, Maurice Chatelain narra o que aconteceu: *"Milhares de romanos se precipitaram para o Vaticano, a fim de pedir ao papa que os absolvesse de seus pecados. Mas o papa os mandou de volta sem absolvição, explicando-lhes que, se o fim do mundo estivesse para chegar, ele seria certamente o primeiro a saber. Interrogando-se então sobre a serventia de um papa que não era sequer capaz de absolvê-los de seus pecados, os romanos voltaram em massa para a Praça de São Pedro, na segunda-feira, 24 de maio, para lá aguardar o fim do mundo e o Juízo Final. Mas o fim do mundo não ocorreu, e alguns operários foram mandados para reparar as paredes do Coliseu"*.

Em 1.960, o médico italiano Elio Bianco fundou uma seita denominada "Comunidade do Monte Branco", com cerca de 40 discípulos. Segundo Bianco, o mundo seria destruído no dia 14 de julho de 1.960, às 01h45min, pela explosão de uma bomba americana ultra-secreta.

Ainda na década de 1.960, astrólogos hindus chegaram à conclusão de que o mundo acabaria em 4 de fevereiro de 1.962, por conta de uma conjunção do Sol, da Lua e mais 5 planetas. Segundo Maurice Chatelain, milhões de crentes caíram de joelhos, implorando à deusa Chandi Path que os poupasse e fazendo queimar quase duas toneladas de manteiga para apaziguar sua cólera. Como nada aconteceu na data estipulada, concluíram que a deusa atendera suas preces.

No dia 13 de maio de 1.980, 700 adeptos da seita brasileira Borboletas Azuis se reuniram para esperar o dilúvio, armazenando alimentos e água, mas o dilúvio até hoje não chegou. Em 1.997 a seita ainda contava com 15 persistentes fiéis.

Em outubro de 1.992, o profeta Lee Jang-Rim levou cem mil fiéis da Igreja Missionária Dami, na Coréia, a esperar pelo minuto final, previsto para a meia-noite. Uma chuva incandescente cairia sobre o planeta, nuvens carregadas de dragões desceriam à Terra e os seus seguidores ascenderiam ao céu. Jang-Rim acabou processado pelos fiéis, 46 dos quais pelo menos haviam doado a ele todos os seus bens.

Em novembro de 1.993, Marina Tsvygun, líder da Grande Irmandade Branca, ordenou a centenas de seguidores que se reunissem na capital da Ucrânia, Kiev, para aguardar o fim do mundo. Como nada ocorreu, os fiéis deram início a um quebra-quebra na cidade e cerca de 500 pessoas foram presas.

No ano de 1.666, um judeu chamado Shabetai Zevi declarou ser o messias, anunciou que a redenção estava próxima e escolheu doze discípulos para serem juízes das tribos de Israel. Foi entusiasticamente aceito por judeus em todo o mundo. Em 1.759, um tal Jacob Frank sugeriu que era Deus encarnado e angariou grande quantidade de adeptos. No início de 1.814, uma senhora inglesa de 64 anos, chamada Joanna Southcott, anunciou que estava grávida do Espírito Santo e daria à luz, no dia 19 de outubro de 1.814, uma criança divina de nome Shiloh, que seria o segundo messias. Esta data marcaria também o fim do mundo e o Juízo Final. Para convencer os incrédulos, Joana pediu para ser examinada por 21

134

médicos, dos quais 17 declararam que ela estava realmente grávida. Maurice Chatelain conta o desenrolar do drama: *"Então a exaltação religiosa não teve mais limites. Milhares de fanáticos instalaram-se diante da casa onda ela morava e começaram uma longa vigília de orações, na espera do nascimento da criança sagrada que os iria salvar das labaredas do inferno. Muitos deles caíram de cansaço e houve inclusive três que morreram no local. Finalmente veio o dia 19 de outubro, mas o messias não chegou. Chamaram então os médicos, que constataram que Joanna nunca estivera grávida, mas gravemente doente, tanto da cabeça como do corpo. Ela morreu, aliás, dez dias depois, e seus discípulos pensaram que a volta do messias, o fim do mundo e o Juízo Final haviam sido transferidos para mais tarde".*

No nosso século, vários messias já se auto-anunciaram em todo o mundo. No Brasil, há um que se paramenta com o tipo de indumentária que Jesus usava em sua época, afirmando simplesmente ser a reencarnação de Cristo, título que ele rivaliza com um seu colega coreano. Há um outro, morador da cidade de São José dos Campos, que se intitula "filho do homem" e fundou uma seita chamada 'litáurica' (aura da pedra).

Esse tipo de gente, instigados por forças tenebrosas e de forma totalmente inconsciente, procura desviar a atenção de pesquisadores sérios em relação à passagem do Filho do Homem pela Terra. Constituem eles a mais perigosa e dissimulada armadilha das trevas em seu embate final contra a Luz, na tentativa de arrastar com elas o maior número possível de almas na destruição completa que já vislumbram. Por isso é tão necessária a máxima vigilância de que um espírito humano é capaz. O desenrolar progressivo do Juízo está separando automaticamente o joio do trigo, o legítimo do ilegítimo. Quem estiver preso ao ilegítimo e não reconhecê-lo a tempo, será afastado conjuntamente.

Os casos mencionados acima a respeito dos falsos profetas são os mais escabrosos. A maioria deles, porém, não se mostra de forma assim tão clara. Atuam dissimuladamente, na maior parte das vezes sob a aura de benfeitores da humanidade. É o caso, por exemplo, dos grandes escritores de livros sobre ocultismo e coisas afins. Eles conseguem cumprir a sua missão com admirável eficiência, como atestam as listas dos livros mais vendidos, invariavelmente repletas de títulos esotéricos.

Outro grupo de falsos profetas bastante em voga é o dos "videntes". Só no Brasil há cerca de trezentos com a capacidade autodeclarada de ver Nossa Senhora. Pode-se imaginar o sucesso que fazem. Um deles, que tem seu campo de atuação próximo à cidade de Fortaleza, costuma pedir à multidão que o acompanha, quando está em comunicação com a Virgem Maria, para que olhem o Sol (!), onde se pode ver os sinais divinos. Cerca de dez mil pessoas fixam então os olhos no Sol, e dali a poucos segundos já tem gente vendo o trono de Nossa Senhora, fachos de luz coloridos, dois sóis, uma lua e até a própria imagem da santa. A comoção cresce até explodir em aplausos. Só alguns poucos mostram coragem bastante para confessar que não viram nada, além de manchas impressas na retina pela luz solar. Alguns ufólogos da região explicam que ET's haviam feito um cortejo em homenagem à Nossa Senhora.

Na cidade paulista de Araraquara, 80 pessoas seguiram as orientações de um vidente e também olharam para o Sol, na expectativa de ter uma visão de Nossa Senhora da Rosa Mística. Resultado: 16 incautos com lesões na retina com perda de até 40% da visão. Um outro vidente, que atua no Rio de Janeiro, informa para quem quiser saber que a voz da Virgem Maria é mais linda que a de Roberto Carlos. Um padre de Belo Horizonte, professor de Teologia, diz que Nossa Senhora criou uma ciência nova, chamada "mariologia política"; isso porque as mensagens da virgem têm "conotações políticas".

Poderiam ser descritos centenas, talvez milhares de casos semelhantes, sobre o atuar dos falsos profetas. Mas não é necessário. Cada qual poderá reconhecê-los, se apenas quiser realmente. Para isso cada um dispõe da sua intuição, que não falha porque é a voz do espírito. A intuição, porém, tem de estar livre das ponderações do intelecto, caso contrário o ser humano tomará decisões baseado no que imagina ser a sua intuição, quando na verdade o que ele percebeu foram as considerações do seu próprio raciocínio.

O ser humano tem de libertar-se de tudo quanto tenta desviá-lo do caminho certo. Agora, no Juízo Final, isso representa para ele vida ou morte! Significa poder permanecer nesta Criação, ou ter de sucumbir no Juízo!

Os falsos profetas e apaziguadores não são necessariamente servidores conscientes das trevas. Ao contrário. A quase totalidade deles se consideram imbuídos dos mais elevados propósitos, encarregados de uma missão divina, acreditando realmente estarem auxiliando a humanidade com suas atuações. Eles servem *inconscientemente* às trevas, e apresentam-se como lutadores em prol da Luz.

O que eles procuram aparentar não deve ser levado em consideração, mas sim o que transmitem. O que eles *oferecem* tem de ser analisado, e com toda a objetividade e firmeza que uma pessoa é capaz de reunir. Hoje, mais do que nunca, é preciso distinguir pedras de pão.

A maioria das pessoas já se desencantou completamente das promessas de políticos, pois suas mentiras são facilmente constatadas, já que não se efetivam em atos visíveis. Os políticos espirituais também mentem da mesma forma, porém suas mentiras dizem respeito ao âmago do ser humano, ao próprio espírito, e por isso só podem ser percebidas por aqueles que mantêm viva a voz de seus espíritos, a intuição.

O leitor deixe sempre a intuição falar quando se defrontar com algo que diga respeito à sua vida espiritual, pois a esse respeito não se pode ser negligente.

"

Aqui termina a transcrição do texto do escritor Roberto C. P. Júnior.

Hoje vive na Índia um guru com pouco mais de 70 anos de idade que, apesar de não afirmar ser Cristo, nem o Messias, nem o Salvador, pousa de Deus. Senta em trono que mais se parece com um trono divino. E seus seguidores afirmam que ele já realizou todos os milagres realizados por Jesus em sua vida, inclusive a sua própria ressurreição. E no "museu" em sua comunidade, verdadeira fortaleza, o que se vêem são unicamente quadros de Jesus e ao seu lado pôster do guru na mesma posição, em clara comparação. É tão óbvio! Mas parece que ninguém percebe, mesmo não havendo nada de sutil na comparação. Quando lá estive, em dezembro de 1.995, fiquei a me perguntar a razão de tal comparação. Por que tal necessidade? Com que objetivo? Hoje tudo está muito claro. Mais um falso profeta, mais um falso Cristo, oriental, não totalmente assumido, para enganar mais facilmente. E por trás dele há um ser invisível de muita força e poder, que o manipula, usando a brecha da imensa vaidade do guru, que alimenta em seus seguidores de forma absurda a idolatria à sua imagem, chegando a serem vendidas no comércio interno da própria comunidade pôsteres dos pés do guru, para as pessoas afixarem na parede de casa e beijarem os pés dele. Chega a ser cômico. São milhares de pessoas que lá chegam diariamente para adorar o guru indiano, que sequer abre a boca para falar qualquer coisa. Dizem que ele não tem mais o que pregar. É um guru meio aposentado, que só desfila entre seus fiéis, como se fora Deus.

Segue foto de um "cristo" brasileiro do século XX, sentado no seu trono (Foto 19).

Foto: CARLOS FENERICH

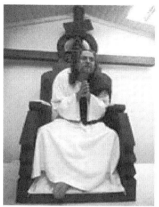

O ex-verdureiro Iuri Thais no seu templo, em Curitiba: "A Igreja Católica sucumbirá e eu levarei os eleitos à salvação"

A seguir, foto de fiéis de uma seita nordestina brasileira, na região seca, à espera do apocalipse (Foto 19).

Foto: ANDRÉ DUSEK

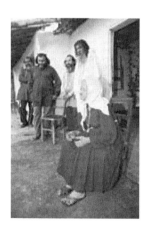

Os penitentes do Cariri: influência do "Padim Ciço" e espera do apocalipse   (Foto 20)

No Nordeste brasileiro, no sertão do Estado da Bahia, no final do século XIX, existiu também um homem que se apresentava com aparência de Cristo, de barbas e cabelos compridos, e uma túnica comprida, chamado Antonio Conselheiro, que com seu fanatismo e loucura levou o sertão brasileiro a uma guerra, que ficou conhecida como Guerra de Canudos, que teve fim trágico em 1.897. Seu arraial abrigava milhares de pessoas, e muitas morreram durante a guerra, sob o fogo das polícias e do Exército Brasileiro, pois Conselheiro era completamente insubmisso, e além de outras rebeldias não aceitava a República, recém proclamada no Brasil, em 1.889.

Antonio Conselheiro se dizia profeta, e profetizava que o sertão viraria mar, e o mar viraria sertão. Quem sabe um dia isso não se concretize? Mas a loucura e o fanatismo, junto com o messianismo de Conselheiro só causam desgraças para seus seguidores, que se armaram e enfrentaram de forma violenta e brutal as forças legais, até mesmo decepando cabeças de oficiais e as pendurando em estacas, liderados pelo próprio líder religioso. Como disse Jesus, "quem com ferro fere, com ferro será ferido!". E Antonio Conselheiro morreu de alguma doença desconhecida durante a guerra, e nem viu a derrota final de seu movimento messiânico, que foi totalmente aniquilado. Hoje as ruínas do Arraial de Canudos estão debaixo da água do Açude de Cocorobó.

Como disse Jesus de forma enfática, aquele dia e aquela hora nem ele nem os anjos no céu sabem, mas só Deus. Então, não adianta tentar calcular com base nos astros, etc. Se Nostradamus errou, ele que era um grande profeta, astrólogo e astrônomo amador, e também inúmeros astrólogos modernos que tentaram calcular o ano, e que indicaram o ano 1.999, não adianta calcular o dia e o ano da chegada do cometa e dos meteoros que causarão destruição no planeta.

Roberto C. P. Júnior pesquisou e demonstrou que durante mais de mil anos têm aparecido falsos cristos e falsos profetas, e não só no Ocidente, mas também no Oriente. E eles têm enganado a muitos. Mas todos os que têm indicado datas para o Juízo Final descrito no livro Apocalipse erraram, e sem uma só exceção.

Que a catástrofe descrita nos livros da Bíblia acontecerá, damos como certo, porque Jesus e os profetas judeus que o antecederam não mentiam e não erravam em suas profecias. Só não sabemos quando. Mas parece estar se aproximando esse dia.

A julgarmos cautelosamente por tudo que está escrito na Bíblia e também em Nostradamus, a vinda do Senhor, ou o Dia do Senhor, ou o Juízo Final, Juízo Universal, não representará de forma alguma o fim da humanidade e a completa destruição do Planeta Terra.

Pensar o contrário é ler de forma incompleta as escrituras bíblicas e também Nostradamus.

O próprio Jesus afirmou no Sermão da Montanha que os mansos herdariam a Terra. Ora, se a Terra fosse totalmente destruída, nada haveria mais para ser herdada. Isso seria ilógico e contraditório.

Se os mansos herdarão a Terra, como disse Jesus, é porque ela ainda continuará em condições de ser habitada, como no tempo do dilúvio bíblico que pegou muita gente desprevenida, mas que não acabou com a Terra.

E se os mansos herdarão a Terra, o que acontecerá com os que não forem considerados mansos?

Quem decidirá quem é ou não manso? E quando?

É exatamente isso o Juízo Final e universal!

Findo o tempo das nações, o fim dado aos povos e às pessoas para se transformarem, para deixarem de fazer guerra, de cometer crimes, de furtar, de matar, etc., e esse tempo já está terminado, ou terminando, virá logo o julgamento.

Para que seja separado o joio do trigo, os bons dos maus, os violentos dos pacíficos, os lobos dos cordeiros, será preciso haver mortes em grande escala, porque o julgamento será de almas. E essas mortes serão causadas exatamente pelas catástrofes anunciadas pelos profetas judeus antigos, por Jesus e pelo livro Apocalipse.

Casamentos entre pessoas do mesmo sexo, inclusive em algumas igrejas, crimes os mais hediondos possíveis em pleno século XX e na entrada do XXI, a volta das guerras de religião e do fanatismo, terrorismo matando pessoas inocentes, a banalização do sexo, o uso desenfreado de drogas alucinógenas entre adolescentes e jovens, e muitas outras coisas mostram que a humanidade parece ter chegado a um limite do suportável, e que precisa ser sacudida de alguma forma, como no tempo do dilúvio bíblico. A humanidade hoje parece estar muito pior do que no tempo de Noé.

A chegada de um cometa, acompanhado de grande quantidade de meteoróides, criará o quadro bíblico da duplicidade de sóis, da ausência de luz do sol, da lua e das estrelas. O cometa no céu, aproximando-se da Terra, será visto como um segundo sol. A sua queda por inteiro, ou de parte dele na Terra causará um impacto tão grande que levantará nuvens de poeira a cobrir grande parte do céu, subindo alto na atmosfera, encobrindo e impedindo por algum tempo que chegue até o solo a luz do sol, e também da lua durante a noite. Terremotos e maremotos também serão causados pelos impactos. Chuvas de meteoros de vários tamanhos cairão sobre a Terra, trazendo destruição e incêndios às cidades, e os que caírem no mar provocarão imensas ondas, que invadirão as regiões mais costeiras dos continentes, e as mais baixas principalmente.

O choque do cometa com o solo, a depender de seu tamanho e massa, e da localização geográfica do impacto, poderá provocar a alteração do eixo da Terra, a sua inclinação, provocando inundações em várias partes do planeta, e o surgimento de terras antes submersas nos mares. Quem sabe não apareça a Atlântida mitológica, como afirmou Edgar Cayce, famoso vidente, que afirmou que isso aconteceria antes do fim do século XX, e errou, como tantos outros profetas que indicaram datas para suas previsões antes e depois dele também erraram.

A queda de um cometa em Júpiter em 1.994 nos mostra que não estamos livres da mesma catástrofe. Lembremo-nos que o cometa causou uma mancha na atmosfera de Júpiter do tamanho da Terra, como vimos no primeiro capítulo. Se ele tivesse percorrido um espaço um pouco maior, e caído na Terra, agora o leitor não estaria vivo lendo estas palavras. Isso é uma ameaça real com a qual convivemos, devido à enorme quantidade de asteróides e cometas circulando em nosso sistema solar.

As visões do futuro não têm explicação científica. Como disse Nostradamus, elas *são a prova da existência de Deus*. Se a origem das visões do futuro não está na natureza nem nos homens, só pode estar em Deus. Mas na dimensão divina não existe tempo, nem datas. Assim, Deus não apresenta fatos e imagens com suas datas, mesmo porque cada povo tem seu próprio calendário. Os maias tinham um calendário no seu tempo que não coincidia com o calendário do tempo de Nostradamus, nem o dos judeus ou o dos romanos antigos, nem o dos antigos hebreus. Assim, impossível datar os acontecimentos vistos com a permissão de Deus. Tantos quantos se atrevam e se arvorem a indicar datas para fatos vistos na dimensão atemporal errarão sempre.

Como vimos no primeiro capítulo, ao tratarmos dos cometas, asteróides, meteoróides, meteoros e meteoritos, há cinturões de asteróides em nosso sistema solar com mais de 70 mil asteróides circulando ao redor de nosso sol, e muitos deles têm mais de mil quilômetros de comprimento. Além disso, a qualquer momento o choque entre dois asteróides pode deslocar um deles em nossa direção. E a depender do tamanho do asteróide, o impacto causaria sérios danos ao nosso planeta, e à humanidade que aqui vive.

De igual modo, vimos que há cometas conhecidos e de órbita razoavelmente conhecida e calculada, como o Cometa Harley. Mas há também inúmeros grandes cometas de órbita absolutamente desconhecida, que podem agora estar se dirigindo à Terra em um espaço longínquo, sem que possamos vê-lo e nos prevenir, porque os cometas são "invisíveis" até que se aproximem do sol, quando então passam a formar a cauda de gases, que se torna visível até mesmo a olho nu.

Assim, podemos estar com os dias contados, tendo mais um ano, dois, dez, cinqüenta, cem ou mais anos de existência física na Terra. Não temos como saber. Basta vermos as divergências de cálculos entre os estudiosos das profecias da Bíblia e de Nostradamus e também do calendário maia.

Ninguém sabe realmente quando um cometa nos atingirá, mas parece certo, se dermos crédito às profecias da Bíblia, especialmente ao livro Apocalipse, escrito pelo apóstolo João já em idade avançada. E freqüentemente são descobertos novos cometas, com trajetória (órbita) desconhecida.

Há alguns anos atrás foi descoberto um novo cometa, chamado de Cometa Lee, porque descoberto pelo astrônomo Steven Lee, o C/1999H1, que se encontrava atrás do sol e tem rota desconhecida. Em 2.038 provavelmente deve passar perto da Terra o cometa Westfal. Todos os meses são descobertos novos cometas, porque eles são muito numerosos. E as órbitas deles não são bem conhecidas.

O choque de um cometa com a Terra e uma chuva intensa de meteoros será a maior causa das mortes coletivas na Terra, provavelmente em tempo não muito distante, que pode acontecer ainda neste século XXI.

Após as mortes que se darão, as almas serão julgadas, pela sua consciência, pelos seus atos, pela sua vida, e somente os bons (mansos) permanecerão na Terra, como disse Jesus. Os maus, os perversos, os criminosos cruéis, os corruptos, os guerreiros conquistadores e todo tipo de gente sem escrúpulo serão colocados em outro lugar, que não será na Terra. Mas onde será?

A Bíblia não esclarece.

Hoje os maus ao morrerem estariam indo para o denominado "inferno", que seria uma região no mundo espiritual na própria Terra, uma outra dimensão, não material. Mas se os maus e violentos não ficarão mais aqui, mesmo no mundo espiritual, então temos que concluir logicamente que essas almas perversas e apegadas ao mal serão encaminhadas para alguma outra região no universo, provavelmente longe da Terra.

Somente isso levará à mudança da humanidade. Somente isso fará com que as nações não mais se adestrem para a guerra, e que o lobo se deite com o cordeiro, e animais diferentes, que antes eram caçador e caça, comam juntos e durmam juntos. Isso parece ser uma metáfora, que não pode ser levada ao pé da letra. Mas muito bela, a expressar e representar a nova ordem que reinará na Terra sem a presença das pessoas más e perversas, dos corruptos, dos guerreiros, dos assassinos.

Imaginem um mundo sem maldade, sem violência, sem guerra, sem fome, sem egoísmo, com boa distribuição das riquezas. É isso o que acontecerá no mundo futuro, mas somente depois da grande catástrofe, das mortes coletivas, do Juízo Final das almas humanas.

Até mesmo o Espiritismo, doutrina que também se considera cristã, pois adota também os evangelhos e venera a Jesus como seu mestre sustenta que um dia haverá uma grande catástrofe, como um dia teria já acontecido em outro planeta, na constelação de Capela, com o exílio daqueles espíritos perversos, que serão retirados da Terra e encaminhados para outro planeta em início de desenvolvimento humano.

Acreditemos ou não na versão espírita, no fundo, na essência, a idéia básica é a mesma, que é a separação do joio e do trigo, dos bons e dos maus, e apenas os bons ficariam na Terra, que deixaria de ser um planeta de expiação e provas para entrar na escala de planeta de regeneração.

É surpreendente a coincidência entre a idéia espírita e o Juízo Final e universal contido na Bíblia, pregado por vários profetas judeus e também por Jesus, bem como confirmado em sua essência por Nostradamus.

Após o Juízo Final as nações não mais investirão em armamentos como hoje. Assim, só o que os Estados Unidos gastam por ano com defesa, cerca de 1 trilhão de dólares, talvez já seja suficiente para acabar com a fome no mundo. Imaginem quanto se gasta no mundo todo em defesa, polícia, grades, cadeados, correntes, tudo por causa dos assaltos e violência criminosa. A economia com tudo isso geraria uma espetacular qualidade de vida material na Terra, e para todos os povos.

O Juízo Final, o Juízo Universal, está próximo, e depois dele, consertadas as coisas na Terra, viverá a humanidade dias de paz, nos quais das armas serão feitos arados, e os tanques de guerra serão derretidos e virarão tratores para a agricultura. Não haverá necessidade de gastos elevados com polícia, forças armadas, e as pessoas poderão andar pelas ruas sem susto e sem medo de serem assaltadas ou agredidas por jovens delinqüentes de classe média sem educação e de má formação de caráter, nem por pobres favelados tentando sobreviver.

Um mundo melhor por muito tempo...quase um paraíso.

No próximo capítulo falaremos da transformação humana e do futuro da humanidade.

CAPÍTULO 11

O Santo Sudário – Um sinal do Fim dos Tempos

No final do século XX, e no início do século XXI, e do novo milênio, um dos maiores mistérios e enigmas da humanidade se prende a um lençol de tecido existente na Catedral de Turim, na Itália. E isto porque, segundo se acredita, seria o lençol no qual José de Arimatéia e Nicodemos teriam envolvido o corpo de Jesus no sepulcro, após o terem retirado da cruz.

Até a década de 1.960, o Santo Sudário era apenas artigo de fé para os católicos. Contudo, após se iniciarem as investigações científicas sobre ele, passou a ser também objeto de estudos e pesquisas, com a utilização da tecnologia mais avançada, o que tornou o lençol ainda mais famoso, e mais misterioso.

No Evangelho de São João (cap.20), está escrito que o primeiro discípulo a ver o interior do sepulcro, e os lençóis no chão, foi ele mesmo, e depois Pedro, que chegou ao local após ele. Teria um deles pegado o lençol e guardado? Teria sido Maria Madalena quem guardou o lençol?

No Santo Sudário, um lençol que mede 4,36 metros de cumprimento por 1,10 metros de largura, vê-se manchas de sangue, marcas de queimaduras por fogo, manchas de água e outras manchas que vistas de certa distância mostram a aparência de um homem em pé. Seguem fotos do Sudário em positivo e em negativo, para comparação (Fotos 21, 22, 23 e 24).

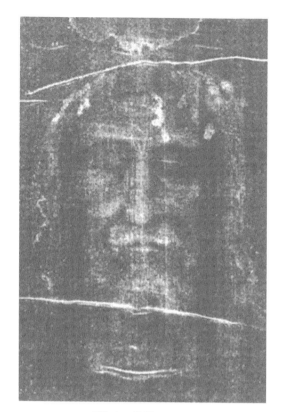

(Foto 21)

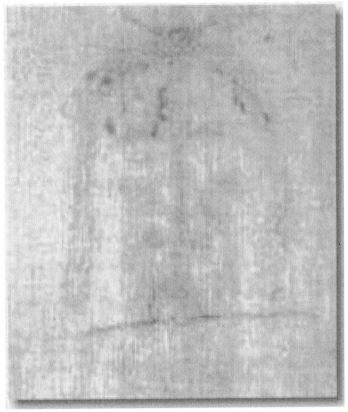

(Foto 22)

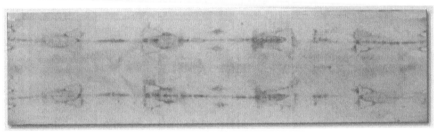

(Foto 23)

148

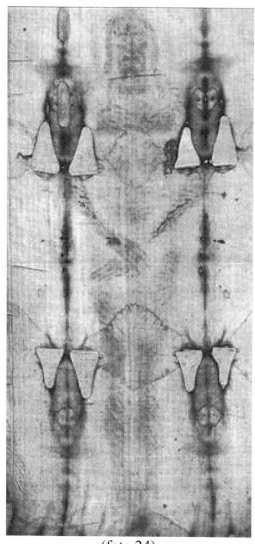

(foto 24)

As investigações sobre o Santo Sudário se iniciaram com as primeiras fotografias tiradas dele por Segundo Pia, um advogado nascido em Turim em 1.898.

Ao revelar as fotos, ele percebeu que os negativos são magníficos positivos, demonstrando com isso que a imagem do Santo Sudário é um perfeito negativo fotográfico. Como se teria formado a imagem em negativo em época muito anterior à invenção da fotografia?

A segunda série de fotografias foi feita em 1.931 por José Enrie, e levando-se em consideração a época, elas são muito boas, e inclusive são as mesmas até hoje usadas para a divulgação do Santo Sudário pelo mundo.

Sobre essas fotos de 1.931 começaram a trabalhar os primeiros cientistas interessados no apaixonante enigma do Santo Sudário.

O tecido do Santo Sudário é de uma textura chamada "espinha de peixe" ou "espiga", um tipo de sarja. Ele foi tecido à mão, em um tear, segundo os pesquisadores, e com linho também fiado à mão, e apresenta alguns fios de algodão junto com os de linho. Ele é compacto, opaco e de cor cru, estando bem conservado. É suave e leve.

Em 1.973, Gilbert Raes, do Instituto de Tecnologia Têxtil de Gant, fez estudos sobre pequenos fios que retirou do sudário, e concluiu que a textura do tecido correspondia àquela dos tecidos da época de Jesus. E foi ele quem encontrou fios de algodão entre os de linho, levando-o a acreditar que o tecido foi feito em um tear no qual também se fiava algodão. Mas no início da era cristã não se fiava algodão na Europa, e sim no Oriente Próximo. Assim, segundo Raes, o Sudário podia perfeitamente bem ter sido tecido na Judéia no início do século I d.C, século no qual Jesus foi morto.

A imagem vista no Sudário é o que mais interessa a todos, e ela mostra um homem que sofreu uma morte semelhante à que, segundo os evangelhos, sofreu Jesus de Nazaré.

Segundo Stevenson, um engenheiro de uma equipe que investigou o Sudário de Turim, olhando-se diretamente para o sudário, a olho nu, é difícil distinguir os detalhes da imagem, por ser ela tênue, quase fantasmagórica. Ela vai se desvanecendo até se converter em uma mancha imprecisa à medida que vamos nos aproximando do lençol, de tal forma que, se chegarmos a alguns centímetros dele, somente distinguimos as áreas com imagem e as áreas sem imagem. Porém, quando se olha o lençol estando a quatro ou cinco metros dele podemos perceber todos os seus detalhes perfeitamente. Afirmou Stevenson que esse fenômeno ótico curioso se deve à falta de limites definidos entre as zonas com e sem imagens no tecido. Não há perfis nítidos, e as bordas da imagem estão desfiadas.

A figura que se vê no Santo Sudário possui características muito interessantes. Ela é superficial. O que significa isso? Um fio de linho é formado por cem a duzentas fibrilas, e a imagem do Sudário só afeta em profundidade as duas ou três primeiras fibras. E o que se vê a olho nu é a descoloração amarelada das fibras de linho mais próximas da superfície do tecido.

A imagem é extremamente detalhada, pois mostra diminutos arranhões que dilaceraram a pele nas proximidades dos sinais dos açoites.

A imagem resiste ao calor, pois mesmo o incêndio de Chambery não a afetou. Há, assim, estabilidade térmica.

A imagem resiste também à água, pois, quando houve o incêndio acima citado, a água usada para apagá-lo, fervendo dentro da urna onde se encontrava o Sudário, não afetou a imagem.

A imagem é resistente a todos os reagentes químicos conhecidos, que não a descoloram nem a dissolvem.

Não há vestígios de pigmentos na imagem, o que demonstra que ela não foi pintada.

Não há indicativo de direção na imagem, como sempre fica claro nas pinturas, de qualquer tipo, seja a pintura a óleo ou de outro tipo qualquer. O artista sempre pinta de uma direção para outra com o pincel.

A imagem é um negativo fotográfico, ou seja, só é perfeitamente entendida quando fotografada e visto o seu negativo.

A intensidade da imagem varia em função da distância entre o lençol e o corpo.

O professor Judica-Cordiglia, que estudou profundamente as imagens do Sudário, em seu livro "L'Uomo della Sindone", escreveu: "Se considerarmos o conceito unitário do organismo e o significado biológico do psiquismo, e aceitarmos a correlação que vários autores sustentam existir entre as características psíquicas e somáticas, temos de enxergar neste Homem um indivíduo psiquicamente perfeito". E continua: "O Homem do Santo Sudário media 1,81m, pesava cerca de oitenta quilos e tinha medidas antropométricas que nos permitem considerá-lo o protótipo do Homem perfeito, estando além e acima de qualquer tipo étnico". Isso nos lembra a hipótese de a genética de Jesus não ser realmente a de seus pais terrenos, e daí ele não ser exatamente como os judeus de seu tempo, do ponto de vista físico.

A primeira equipe de cientistas teve acesso ao Santo Sudário em 1.969, mesmo ano em que o homem pousou na lua, e somente depois de duas décadas uma outra equipe com equipamentos mais sofisticados e modernos teve acesso a ele e realizou estudos mais profundos, em 1.978.

Os estudos revelaram também que a coroa de espinhos do homem do Sudário era como um capacete, que lhe encobria toda a cabeça, até a nuca, o que deve ter provocado sofrimentos enormes; que o homem recebeu um golpe, provavelmente de vara, no lado direito do rosto, que se apresenta afetado; que o homem foi flagelado (açoitado) pelo método romano, que era em si já um castigo, dado somente aos que não fossem ser crucificados, pois o prisioneiro era açoitado até perder a consciência. Os réus que seriam crucificados eram açoitados pelo método judeu, que era composto de trinta e nove golpes, recebidos no corpo desnudo, pelo menos a metade superior do corpo, o que servia para debilitar o réu e apressar a sua morte na cruz. A flagelação do homem do Sudário foi praticada por dois verdugos experientes, que não golpearam a zona do pericárdio para não provocar a morte do réu. Foram dados mais de cento e vinte golpes, deixando marcas por todo o corpo, com exceção da região do coração.

Os estudos demonstraram ainda que o homem foi amarrado pela perna direita, e deve ter levado muitas quedas, o que teria acontecido no caminho para o calvário, a julgar pelos hematomas nos joelhos. Como não há lacerações da pele na região dos joelhos, concluiu-se que ele estava vestido durante o trajeto, e provavelmente vestindo uma túnica longa, até os pés, comum na época.

O homem do Sudário foi pregado na cruz com cravos, não amarrado. E os cravos foram enfiados nos pulsos, não nas palmas das mãos, como sempre se pensou. Estudos realizados com cadáveres demonstraram que um homem crucificado pelas palmas das mãos não poderia ser mantido na cruz, pois as palmas das mãos se fenderiam, por não conseguirem suportar o peso do corpo. O cravo foi colocado no que se conhece por "espaço de Destot", ou pela articulação rádio-cubital inferior, como defende o Dr. Antonio Hermosilla em seu estudo "La Pasión de Cristo vista por un médico".

Em 1.968, durante escavações feitas em Jerusalém para construção de casas, encontraram um esqueleto de um homem, que foi identificado pelos arqueólogos como sendo Yohanan, pois encontraram o seu nome escrito no local. Ele havia sido crucificado depois da Grande Revolta do ano 70 d.C., e tinha sido pregado na cruz com cravos que lhe foram colocados no punho, entre os ossos rádio e cúbito, segundo o patologista israelense Dr. Nicu Haas, da Universidade Hebraica de Jerusalém. Verificou ainda o patologista que Yohanan teve os ossos das duas pernas, tíbia e perônio, fraturados, pelo que parece por um golpe único e devastador de um porrete. Com isso, os estudiosos do Sudário tiveram mais um elemento de estudo e comparação, tendo concluído que o homem do Sudário foi crucificado pelo método romano vigente à época, e que confirma os relatos dos evangelistas.

O homem do Sudário teve os dois pés pregados com um só cravo, tendo o pé esquerdo sido colocado sobre o direito.

O homem do sudário recebeu um golpe de lança nas costas, do lado direito do peito, entre a quinta e a sexta costelas, correspondendo exatamente à forma do ferro de uma lança romana, chamada em latim de "lancia". Esse golpe de lança tinha por objetivo garantir a morte do réu, impedindo que ele fingisse estar morto. Se Jesus estivesse vivo, no momento do golpe de lança ele se moveria, e morreria depois, pois o golpe atingia o coração.

O homem do Sudário não teve as pernas fraturadas, coincidindo com os relatos dos evangelistas sobre Jesus, mas recebeu o golpe de lança no lado direito do peito, lado do coração, e dele saíram água e sangue, segundo os evangelhos.

Os especialistas sustentam que a ponta da lança deve ter atingido a pleura e depois o pulmão direito, e a posição do golpe justifica o líquido que escorreu, e também o sangue.

O Sudário não mostra sinais de decomposição cadavérica, o que, em casos normais de um morto há mais de vinte e quatro horas deveria mostrar.

O Dr. Max Frei, palinólogo e criminalista, professor da Universidade de Zurique, Suíça, e fundador e diretor do laboratório científico da polícia suíça em Neuchatel, e da polícia alemã de Hiltrup, teve acesso ao Santo Sudário, e em uma simples tira de papel adesivo, que aplicou ao tecido, recolheu amostras do "pó" existente na beira do lençol. Comparando os vários tipos de pólen encontrados no sudário com aqueles encontrados nas diversas camadas geológicas, concluiu que o sudário não poderia ser uma falsificação feita na Europa na Idade Média, porque nele há vários tipos de polens iguais aos encontrados na Terra Santa, e alguns de plantas que somente crescem na Terra Santa. O Dr. Max encontrou no Sudário polens iguais aos encontrados no fundo do Mar da Galiléia e do Mar Morto, em camadas geológicas que são da época de Jesus. A Europa carece de vários tipos de pólen somente encontrados na flora oriental. E foram encontrados polens de plantas das regiões por onde a tradição conta que passou o Santo Sudário.

Feitas ampliações do tecido do Sudário até 5.000 vezes, não se encontrou qualquer sinal de pintura. E a pintura afetaria não só as fibras superficiais, mas também as fibras mais profundas. E nenhuma pintura pode ser realizada sob a forma de negativo tridimensional. Assim, para os cientistas que estudaram o Sudário, está totalmente afastada a possibilidade de ter sido pintada a imagem do homem do Sudário. Então, como se formou a imagem?

O Dr. Cordiglia, cirurgião italiano que fez experiências com mais de dois mil cadáveres, para tentar chegar a algo semelhante à imagem do Sudário, concluiu que fracassou, e que é humanamente impossível conseguir isso. Disse ainda que não há explicação adequada para a formação dos sinais no Santo Sudário.

Alguns cientistas da NASA integraram o grupo denominado de STURP (Shround of Turim Research Project), o Projeto de Investigação do Sudário de Turim. Ao STURP se deve a maior parte dos descobrimentos científicos, tendo se formado em 1.977. Foram eles que descobriram a existência de uma relação matemática entre a distância do corpo e a luminosidade, e a partir daí puderam estabelecer uma imagem tridimensional do homem do sudário.

Descobriu-se que nos olhos do homem do sudário havia duas moedas, uma em cada olho, e já se descobriu a mesma coisa em uma caveira em um cemitério judeu do século I. É importante lembrar que isso era um hábito dos gregos antigos, e que os gregos dominaram a Palestina por bom tempo, na época de Alexandre, o Grande, e após a sua morte, o que pode ter contribuído para a instalação desse hábito de colocar moedas nos olhos dos mortos entre os judeus, ao menos nos mais ricos, e mais influenciados pelos costumes gregos. As moedas, segundo os gregos, eram para o barqueiro que faria a travessia do rio que levava à terra dos mortos. Vemos esse costume grego no filme Tróia, e em muitos outros.

Os cientistas da NASA descartaram a possibilidade da formação da imagem do Sudário por contato, tanto químico como bacteriológico. Pouco a pouco foi se firmando a hipótese que eles chamaram de "chamuscadura".

Em 1.981, O Dr. Baima Ballone, italiano, professor de medicina legal, encontrou sangue nas manchas do sudário, mas fora da imagem, e conseguiu reconhecer o grupo AB.

Os cientistas do STURP analisaram os negativos do Sudário com o Ordenador VP-8, o mesmo aparelho que analisou as imagens recebidas do planeta Marte, e descobriram que as imagens que o Ordenador VP-8 lhes devolvia eram tridimensionais, enquanto toda fotografia convencional é plana. O que dava a tridimensionalidade era exatamente a correlação da distância do corpo e da luminosidade da imagem. E a maior surpresa foi obtida quando se observou a parte dorsal da imagem. Os músculos dorsais e deltóides apareciam abaulados, e não planos, como deveriam aparecer na espalda de um morto cujo corpo se apóia em uma pedra sepulcral. E os cientistas concluíram: *"Parecia que o cadáver se vaporizara, emitindo uma estranha radiação que teria sido a responsável pela formação dos sinais do Santo Sudário. Quando se produziu a imagem deve ter havido uma radiação, desconhecida para a ciência, que foi igual em todos os pontos do corpo. Só assim poderiam ser impressas partes tão diferentes e distantes como a nuca e os pés com a mesma intensidade luminosa. Essa energia só pode ter saído do interior do corpo. De outra forma não se poderia explicar que a espalda e o peito tivessem irradiado com igual intensidade. É muito provável que no momento em que se produziu a radiação o corpo estivesse leve, em levitação, e por isso os músculos dorsais não ficaram aplanados. Não sabemos como a imagem se formou. Não é pintura, não foi por contato, não é uma impressão por calor. Não sabemos o que é. Mas podemos afirmar que não se trata de uma fraude. A alteração física do corpo no momento da ressurreição (a palavra não é minha) pode ter provocado uma liberação breve e violenta de alguma radiação diferente do calor - que pode ou não ser identificável pela ciência - e que abrasou o tecido. Neste caso, o Sudário é uma quase fotografia de Cristo no momento de retornar à vida, produzida por uma radiação ou incandescência de efeitos parcialmente análogos àqueles do calor...Concluindo, aceitar que a imagem do Santo Sudário seja uma imagem por 'abrasamento' - seja qual for a forma exata em que isso aconteceu - justifica o seguinte enunciado: o Santo Sudário só é explicável se serviu alguma vez para envolver um corpo humano ao qual aconteceu algo extraordinário. Não pode ter sido de outra maneira".*

Segundo os cientistas Stevenson e Habernas, depois de todas as conclusões dos estudos realizados no Santo Sudário, a probabilidade de o homem cuja imagem aparece no Sudário não ser Jesus de Nazaré é de um contra oitenta e dois milhões novecentos e quarenta e quatro mil.

Em 1.988, foi realizado o teste do carbono 14 para que se pudesse aferir a idade do tecido, e ele concluiu com a datação seguinte: entre 1.260 e 1.390.

Conforme se verifica nas informações até aqui lançadas, apenas o teste do carbono 14 destoou do restante das conclusões de todos os cientistas que já estudaram o Santo Sudário. E hoje já se contesta os resultados do teste realizado, porque não se levou em consideração o que todos sabiam, que nas fibras do tecido se encontram incrustados cera, pólen, microorganismos e também colônias de bactérias que continuam vivas, e que isso poderia influir na datação do tecido. Matéria orgânica mais recente pode ter contribuído para "rejuvenescer" o tecido, ou seja, indicar antiguidade menor do que a real. A errônea datação pelo carbono 14 não teria decorrido do método empregado, mas pela contaminação do lençol pelo estudo, que não pôde ser isolado de sua longa e complexa história de conteúdo de carbono.

Além do questionamento atual sobre as condições em que foram realizados os testes, há ainda suspeitas sobre a lisura dos laboratórios que os realizaram, e há até mesmo um livro que sustenta que houve uma conspiração para induzir o resultado (A Conspiração Jesus), que relata de forma investigativa toda a trama.

O Dr. Rinauld afirmou que a imagem do Sudário parecia ter sido produzida por uma radiação muitíssimo bem dosada. Se tivesse havido muita radiação, a imagem teria ficado excessivamente escura. E diz ainda ele: "... é exatamente como se 'alguém' tivesse tido a intenção precisa de invocar a imagem".

O Dr. Dimitri A. Kouznetsov, cientista russo e professor dos Laboratórios de Métodos de Investigação, em Moscou, e Prêmio Lenin, usando um dos laboratórios que realizaram a datação do Sudário, provou seu erro de datação, em não considerar a história de carbono 14 do tecido e os efeitos de incêndios (calor) também sobre o tecido, alterando sua datação.

Conforme informação contida na revista brasileira SUPER INTERESSANTE, ano 13, n.9, de setembro de 1.999, o Santo Sudário voltou à baila no XVI Congresso Internacional de Botânica, nos Estados Unidos. Foram feitas análises em grãos de pólen encontrados no Santo Sudário, e os resultados indicaram que o manto foi tecido antes do século VIII. Isto coloca ainda mais em dúvida os resultados do teste de carbono 14, colocando-o sob suspeita, ao menos. E abre maior perspectiva de certeza quanto aos resultados dos outros exames feitos por cientistas no Santo Sudário.

Mais de trezentos testes foram realizados no Santo Sudário, e nenhum concluiu que ele era fraudulento.

Acaso tivesse de fato o tecido do Santo Sudário sido confeccionado na Idade Média, no período que o teste do carbono 14 indicou, há muitas perguntas que ficariam sem respostas, e constatações sem explicação, como por exemplo:

1 - A imagem do Santo Sudário é um negativo fotográfico, e a fotografia só foi inventada no século XIX;

2 - O tecido do Sudário é uma sarja de linho, e este tipo de tecido só foi fabricado na Europa quase em meados do século XIV. Assim, teria o falsificador ido ao oriente expressamente para buscar o tecido?

3 - O Sudário contém polens iguais aos que se encontram nas camadas sedimentares de dois mil anos atrás no Lago de Genezaré e de outras zonas da Terra por onde se pôde demonstrar que o Santo Sudário passou. Conheceria o falsificador tanto assim os polens que os foi buscar expressamente para colocá-los no tecido, a fim de serem descobertos sete séculos depois? Sequer existia microscópio na época em que o teste do carbono 14 indicou como sendo da fabricação do tecido.

4 - Existem no Sudário fios de sangue que se conseguiu demonstrar corresponderem a sangue venoso e arterial. Como teria conseguido o falsário colocar no tecido tipos diferentes de sangue

quando ainda não se conhecia a circulação do sangue venoso e arterial?

5 - As imagens do Sudário são anatomicamente corretas. Suas características patológicas e fisiológicas são claras e revelam alguns conhecimentos médicos ignorados até cento e cinqüenta anos atrás;

6 - Qual teria sido a técnica do falsário que ele levou para o túmulo sem repetir em outra obra?

7 - Como o falsário colocou no tecido sangue pré-mortal e pós-mortal, nele existente? E como pintou com albumina do soro as bordas das marcas dos açoites?

Os cientistas do STURP, após fazerem ampliações das fotos, acabaram descobrindo moedas nos olhos do homem do sudário, e depois se identificou o que nelas está escrito em grego, que em português corresponde a DE TIBERIO CESAR, mesma inscrição que se encontra nas moedas chamadas léptons, cunhadas por Pôncio Pilatos entre o ano 29 e o ano 32 da nossa era, com bronze da Judéia. Isso é quase um certificado de Pilatos de que o Santo Sudário data daquele tempo.

A única conclusão a que podemos chegar, após conhecer as conclusões dos cientistas que estudarem a fundo o Santo Sudário, principalmente os integrantes do grupo STURP, é que realmente o lençol com as imagens não é fraudulento, mas sim autêntico. E que ele de fato envolveu o corpo de Jesus depois de morto e retirado da cruz.

Além dessa conclusão anterior, somos forçados a concluir também que Jesus efetivamente morreu na cruz, afastando aquela hipótese de ter sido ele retirado vivo da cruz e que depois teria vivido na Índia. E ainda, a concluir que Jesus realmente retornou à vida no mesmo corpo que havia sido crucificado, ou seja, ressuscitou, como prometeu muitas vezes que faria, e como estava predito pelos profetas antigos de Israel.

As conclusões dos cientistas corroboram os relatos dos evangelistas, em nada contradizendo essencialmente o que sobre a morte de Jesus foi escrito. Confirmam a lapidação (açoite); a perfuração do peito no lado direito, por lança romana, depois de já estar morto; a colocação de uma coroa de espinhos na cabeça; o fato de não ter tido as pernas quebradas, ao contrário do costume romano, o que comprova que Jesus já estava morto quando lhe foram quebrar as pernas; as quedas no caminho para o Calvário.

O Santo Sudário é a prova material de que Jesus existiu, morreu na cruz e depois saiu novamente vivo do sepulcro. Ou seja, é a prova que só no final do século XX a ciência reconheceu que Jesus realmente ressuscitou, produzindo o prodígio que ele comparou ao do profeta Jonas. E a sua imagem no Santo Sudário foi produzida por ele intencionalmente, de forma controlada, e em negativo, por irradiação de alguma forma de energia ainda para nós desconhecida, irradiada de dentro de seu corpo, estando este em levitação acima da pedra do sepulcro, para somente ser visto de forma clara e estudada no final de século XX, quando teríamos tecnologia e conhecimentos suficientes para realizar os estudos que foram feitos pelo STURP. Foi tudo deliberado e premeditado. Só no século XIX a fotografia foi inventada. Assim, antes disso não se podia investigar o Santo Sudário, como passou a ser feito após ser ele fotografado. Só no século XX passamos a conhecer a radiação, e muitas outras coisas, inventamos o microscópio eletrônico, conseguimos ampliar fotos milhares de vezes, etc. Equipamentos usados pela NASA para estudar fotos de Marte mostraram a tridimensionalidade da imagem, ao contrário dos negativos das fotos comuns. Só então poderíamos atestar a autenticidade do Santo Sudário, e tudo indica que Jesus sabia já desse fato, e previu tudo. Esse foi um de seus muitos milagres, mas o único com prova material para nós, e para a ciência, mesmo para os cientistas materialistas, que não conseguem explicar como a imagem se formou no tecido do Sudário de Turim. Não existe atualmente tecnologia para fazer outro igual. Não é fraude. Então só pode ser mesmo uma "fotografia" que Jesus tirou de si mesmo quando ressuscitou, para a posteridade, para nós, que nascemos no século XX, ou no XXI.

Jesus não foi um homem igual aos outros que habitaram ou habitam este planeta. Era um homem dotado de faculdades paranormais variadas, e em grau elevado. Tinha imenso potencial de cura, captava os pensamentos das pessoas presentes, via o passado individual das pessoas, materializava seres vivos e objetos inanimados, influenciava as forças da natureza, trazia mortos de volta à vida e muitas outras coisas.

Jesus não era um louco, um lunático, nem era fanático ou radical. Muito pelo contrário. Os textos dos evangelhos demonstram que ele era um homem inteligente e extremamente habilidoso no trato com as pessoas, inclusive com aqueles que o queriam derrubar e prender. Sempre se saía bem das armadilhas que preparavam para ele envolvendo as leis vigentes, notadamente as leis de Moisés, como no caso do trabalho ou realização de qualquer atividade no sábado.

Jesus pregou e fez milagres durante cerca de nove a onze anos, e foi muito famoso ainda em vida. Quando saía da Palestina, indo para terras vizinhas, como as cidades de Sídon e Tiro, na Fenícia, era reconhecido e procurado, tendo que se esconder muitas vezes, o que comprova sua fama mesmo fora de sua terra.

Raramente alguém contesta os milagres de Jesus alegando que a Igreja Católica pode ter acrescentado seus relatos aos evangelhos. Mas, a esse argumento ou alegação apresentamos o seguinte: os livros sagrados dos judeus não relatam milagres como os efetuados por Jesus em relação a nenhum outro profeta ou líder político.

Ninguém antes de Jesus, em Israel ou em outro país, como Grécia, Índia, Egito e China curava como Jesus. Não há indicativos históricos de curadores com o seu potencial, ou de alguém que tenha ressuscitado mortos como Jesus.

Poderia alguém sustentar que é tradição no Oriente as fábulas, lendas e contos fantásticos envolvendo poderes fantásticos de certos homens. Isto é em parte real. Contudo, na tradição judaica, somente Moisés teria feito coisas fantásticas, como abrir o Mar Vermelho e lançar pragas sobre o Egito. Nenhum outro profeta judeu teve poderes fantásticos, segundo se lê em seus livros, que compõem a Bíblia. Assim, não era comum atribuir aos profetas poderes como os que tinha Jesus. Isto reforça a crença de que os textos dos evangelistas traduzem a verdade e a realidade do que eles presenciaram ou ouviram ou dos relatos ouvidos de quem presenciou os fatos.

Jesus não era um homem infeliz com tendências ao suicídio. Não era um depressivo. Era trabalhador, tendo exercido o ofício de carpinteiro até os trinta anos, quando assumiu a condição de Messias. A partir dessa idade, passou a pregar e curar de forma incessante e habitual, tendo produzido muitos fenômenos paranormais. E apesar de perseguido desde muito cedo, soube se esquivar dos inimigos até quando decidiu se deixar prender e matar, porque isto fazia parte de seus planos, e dos planos de Deus, conforme as escrituras sagradas. Jesus não se matou, mas se deixou matar, para que pudesse ressurgir três dias depois, como previsto pelos antigos profetas, e como previamente afirmado por ele mesmo. Sua prisão não foi uma surpresa para ele. De certo modo ele a provocou, principalmente quando expulsou os vendedores do Templo de Salomão, pois os vendedores estavam lá com autorização dos sacerdotes do templo, sendo muitos deles criadores dos animais que eram vendidos no local para o sacrifício. O comércio de animais e outras coisas era controlado pelos próprios sacerdotes, e Jesus feriu seus interesses materiais. Além disso, o ciúme, a inveja e o despeito já haviam incendiado a cabeça dos sacerdotes do Sinédrio, principalmente ao verem Jesus entrar em Jerusalém como um rei, aclamado pela população da cidade, que estava cheia de judeus de todas as partes, porque era a época da maior festa judaica, a Páscoa.

Jesus não tinha bens pessoais durante seu tempo de pregação como Messias. E até as doações que recebia eram partilhadas com os pobres. Não tinha ambições materiais. E se tivesse, poderia ter ficado muito rico cobrando pelas curas que produzia em pessoas ricas.

Jesus não teria morrido como morreu se não tivesse incomodado tanto os poderosos do Sinédrio, sede do poder religioso em Israel. E isto demonstra que era independente, e que não se vendia nem se dobrava aos governantes. Não se corrompia, nem se desviava um passo de sua missão, sendo, no entanto, astuto bastante para se livrar das armadilhas que considerava precoce. Não podia morrer antes do tempo certo.

Tudo que foi registrado a respeito de Jesus nos leva a crer que ele era mesmo um homem incomum, extraordinário em todos os sentidos. Inteligente, astuto, pacífico, bondoso, duro nas horas certas, manso e suave na medida correta. Sua vida tinha um propósito, que ele bem soube cumprir. Cabe-nos agora entender bem as razões de sua vinda à Terra, a razão de sua morte na forma descrita pelos evangelistas, e o que ele queria deixar para a posteridade.

Como vimos, o Santo Sudário é um "retrato" feito de Jesus por ele mesmo, através de radiação emanada dele. E ele sabia que só no século XX poderíamos ter essa certeza, pois só nesse século a ciência teria condições de analisar o tecido do Sudário da forma como foi feita. O que será que há de tão especial neste momento da humanidade para ter Jesus planejado que seu retrato só agora fosse conhecido? Não estaremos nos aproximando realmente do que ele chamou de Fim dos Tempos, ou do Dia do Juízo? Os Sinais dos

Tempos não estarão se tornando presentes já nesses momentos, desde o século XX, com os terremotos, inundações, guerras e rumores de guerra, falsos profetas e falsos Cristos às dezenas em todo o mundo?

No século XX o evangelho já estava divulgado em todo o mundo; os judeus retornaram à Terra Prometida, Israel, em 1.948; e o Santo Sudário finalmente revelou a imagem de Cristo e aspectos de sua morte como descritos nos evangelhos, confirmando-os.

Com esta obra, nosso maior propósito é fazer as pessoas despertarem ao menos a curiosidade em relação a Jesus, suas profecias, e as revelações que ele fez a seu apóstolo João, e contidas no livro Apocalipse, passando a ler com maior atenção os evangelhos, e principalmente dando maior importância ao que ele disse e fez. Ele não era um homem comum como nós, e por isso deve ser analisado com maior atenção, lido nas entrelinhas, sem preconceitos e condicionamentos religiosos, políticos ou ideológicos.

Jesus foi um homem extraordinário, fantástico, sem nenhum comparativo com outra pessoa. Disse que estaria conosco até o fim dos tempos. E se ressuscitou dos mortos, demonstrou com isso seu poder sobre a morte corporal. Com suas pregações e sua morte deixou claro que há vida além da morte, e que seu reino não era deste mundo. Assim, nos deu a certeza de que continuaremos vivos mesmo depois de nossa morte física, o que é um grande consolo e esperança, independentemente de a nova vida, a vida futura, ser em outra dimensão ou na Terra física.

Jesus continua muito vivo na mente das pessoas, e vivo, também, em algum lugar em outro mundo, em outra dimensão, trabalhando por nós, e a nos esperar. Sigamos seus passos e sua luz, pois foi para ser a luz do mundo que ele viveu, sofreu e morreu.

No século XX se iniciou uma verdadeira, mas sutil, campanha para tentar desmoralizar Jesus e retirar a sua força no mundo, o que só pode ser atribuído às forças das trevas.

Autores espertos, e às vezes sem escrúpulos lançaram idéias mirabolantes acerca de um suposto relacionamento amoroso entre Jesus e Maria Madalena, sem qualquer respaldo e amparo em documentos históricos.

Criaram uma farsa acerca de uma linhagem real dos Merovíngios na França, e sobre a criação do Priorado de Sião, que de fato somente foi criado no século XX, ao que parece em 1.956.

Pesquisas históricas e investigações já concluíram ser falsa a suposta linhagem Merovíngia, bem como a data antes apontada para a criação do Priorado de Sião. Com isso, toda a base da estória (não história) do livro O Código Da Vince caiu por terra.

O History Channel, em recente documentário, em julho de 2.007, mostrou a investigação feita, e a farsa derrubada. O homem que havia apresentado a linhagem Merovíngia na França confessou, sob juramento, que havia forjado a lista da suposta linhagem.

O único objetivo era mesmo a desmoralização de Jesus. Talvez nem mesmo os escritores tenham se dado conta disso. A manipulação das trevas é por demais sutil.

Não há absolutamente nenhum respaldo em documentos antigos acerca de suposto envolvimento amoroso entre Jesus e sua seguidora Maria de Magdala, ou Maria Madalena.

O documentário do History Channel mostrou o pedaço do papiro encontrado no Egito, de suposto evangelho, considerado apócrifo, e não aceito pela Igreja Católica, e que menciona que Jesus beijou Maria Madalena. Alguns escritores sustentam que o manuscrito afirma que Jesus beijou Maria Madalena na boca. Todavia, na verdade o papiro contém um furo logo em seguido à palavra beijo, não se podendo saber se de fato o texto fala em beijo na boca, mas apenas beijo. Até isso é inventado, para tentar desmoralizar Jesus e retirar a sua força.

Jesus optou por não se casar, como todos os profetas antes dele, porque isso era o comum, como no caso de João Batista, seu contemporâneo.

Veja-se que nenhum escritor escreve sobre caso amoroso de João Batista, de Daniel, Elias, Isaías ou outro profeta judeu anterior, e isso porque o objetivo é desmoralizar apenas Jesus, o mais importante profeta, e mais que um simples profeta, o Filho do Homem previsto nas escrituras antigas de Israel. O Messias.

As trevas só querem desmoralizar e retirar a força de Jesus. E os ambiciosos embarcam nessa onda, nessa idéia, vendo nisso uma oportunidade de ganhar rios de dinheiro, o que de fato acontece.

A humanidade adora escândalos. E quanto mais famoso o difamado, melhor.

Temos visto muita gente ler o livro O Código Da Vince e terminar convencido de que Jesus de fato se casou com Maria Madalena e que ela teve um filho seu, vivendo até hoje a sua

163

descendência. As pessoas nem questionam. E não pesquisam para ver a base real e concreta da teoria. Tomam como verdade absoluta.

Os ingênuos acreditam em tudo.

É preciso criar uma couraça contra esse tipo de difamação de figuras históricas ilustres, e não acreditarmos em toda teoria mirabolante que aparecer.

CAPÍTULO 12

A Transformação e o Futuro da Humanidade

Se considerarmos a evolução da humanidade apenas a partir do surgimento da chamada civilização, há cerca de 6 mil anos, até nossos dias, veremos que fizemos grandes progressos, mas que também ainda estamos deixando a desejar em muitos aspectos.

As guerras e lutas diminuíram muito; a expectativa de vida aumentou espetacularmente; os meios de transporte e comunicação avançaram incrivelmente; os medicamentos, as técnicas cirúrgicas e os equipamentos dos hospitais mudaram por completo, salvando muito mais vidas; a educação nas escolas se aperfeiçoou em muito; a diplomacia alcançou níveis nunca antes imaginados, evitando conflitos armados entre as nações; a produção de alimentos, de roupas, de remédios e de bens de consumo em geral atingiu níveis incríveis, e hoje só não consome quem não tiver dinheiro. Mas ainda há crimes hediondos e bárbaros no mundo; o fanatismo religioso se recusa a desaparecer do mundo; as aberrações sexuais, a banalização do sexo e da violência, e insensibilidade com a dor alheia ainda deixam muito a desejar.

No Brasil, por exemplo, nos últimos anos, um repórter da emissora de TV Rede Globo teve a cabeça decepada por traficantes de droga em um dos vários morros da cidade do Rio de Janeiro, quando estava investigando para elaborar matéria jornalística. E por uma espada de samurai. Em pleno século XXI. E um garoto de 6 anos foi arrastado por um carro, preso pelo cinto de segurança, por quatro bairros também do Rio de Janeiro, por jovens assaltantes que tomaram o veículo da mãe dele em assalto e não deixaram que ela antes tirasse a criança do veículo, tendo o garotinho ficado preso pelo cinto de segurança. O menino teve a cabeça arrancada do corpo, depois de ser arrastado por vários quilômetros, em cena bárbara, desumana, chocante, e que nos faz pensar que ainda vivemos numa certa barbárie em alguns lugares do mundo.

Traficantes vendem drogas a jovens e crianças sem pensar no seu futuro, sem a menor dor de consciência; policiais de vários países se misturam aos bandidos e a eles se igualam para ganharem um pouco mais de dinheiro; políticos de quase todos os países se corrompem, para enriquecerem rápida e facilmente, sem a menor preocupação com as necessidades das pessoas que votaram neles; líderes políticos se apegam ao cargo e ao poder e não mais querem largá-lo, buscando sempre a reeleição para continuar mandando, e desmandando; cientistas usam conhecimentos para fabricar armas cada vez mais potentes e letais, apenas por dinheiro, sem pensar nas mortes diárias ao redor do planeta com as suas armas.

Há hoje no mundo um misto mesmo de civilização e barbárie, lembrando o livro de igual nome, de autoria de vários pensadores modernos.

Enquanto construímos no espaço uma nova estação espacial, importante para o futuro e talvez até para a própria sobrevivência da humanidade, aqui embaixo palestinos matam palestinos dentro de Israel; muçulmanos matam muçulmanos no Iraque, numa guerra civil não declara entre Xiitas e Sunitas, facções da mesma religião. Muçulmanos fanáticos matam também cristãos no Iraque, só porque eles são ocidentais, mesmo depois de viverem todos no mesmo país durante tantos e tantos séculos sem qualquer problema. Só o fanatismo e a intolerância religiosa geram isso.

Na Índia, logo depois da declaração de independência, em 1.947, com Gandhi ainda vivo, hindus e muçulmanos que antes eram amigos e vizinhos começaram a matar uns aos outros, a incendiarem as casas uns dos outros, e acabaram tendo que dividir o país, nascendo assim o Paquistão, deslocando milhões de muçulmanos para o norte e hindus para o sul, coisa estúpida e odiosa, que ainda guarda ressentimento. Até hoje há tensão e trocas de tiros na fronteira entre os dois países, e não está totalmente descartada uma luta mais feroz entre eles.

Na Irlanda, durante muito tempo, católicos e protestantes brigavam ferozmente, e finalmente o IRA (Exército Republicano Irlandês) depôs as suas armas e a luta terminou.

Na Itália, a Máfia durante muito tempo aterrorizou a população e os governantes, que por fim decidiram fazer um combate duro e inteligente a essa organização ultrapassada, e venceu a guerra, sobretudo por causa da garra do juiz Falconni, que foi morto pelos mafiosos em um terrível atentado.

Ainda há no mundo alguns regimes comunistas cruéis, como o da Coréia do Norte, principalmente, totalmente fechado, sem direito de manifestação e crítica ao governo, sem imprensa livre, e tudo o mais que de ruim pode ter um regime comunista, inclusive a incapacidade de alimentar a população.

A China somente começou a melhorar as condições de vida de seu povo quando começou a adotar métodos capitalistas de produção, e abrir seu país às empresas estrangeiras. Hoje a China é o país que mais cresce, exatamente porque é o que mais empresas atrai, gerando emprego e renda para sua população. O comunismo implantado na China desde 1.949 não foi capaz de gerar uma sociedade próspera, do ponto de vista material, nem feliz, porque não tinham os chineses direitos e liberdade. Lembrem-se do massacre da Praça da Paz Celestial!

Em Cuba, Fidel Castro reina absoluto desde 1.959. Derrubou o governo que ele chamava de ditador (Fulgêncio Batista), prometendo implantar uma democracia, e terminou logo se apegando ao poder, que segura ferozmente até os dias atuais. Cuba é hoje um país extremamente pobre, os idosos não recebem remédio de graça, as policlínicas de bairro não têm estrutura, todos ganham baixos salários, levando ao surgimento e aumento de prostituição das mulheres cubanas em larga escala, inclusive estudantes universitárias e gente formada como nunca antes existiu em Cuba. Desde o fim da União Soviética, que sustentava Cuba, o país começou a afundar, pois nada produzia além de açúcar e tabaco. Somente recentemente, com o início da abertura da economia a algumas empresas estrangeiras, sobretudo da rede hoteleira, Cuba começou a melhorar, e a dar os primeiros passos para sair da pobreza. O governo finalmente saiu de seu estado letárgico ultrapassado e começou a investir no ensino de línguas estrangeiras e em informática, para o trabalho no turismo, única chance de salvação econômica de Cuba. Estive lá em 2.002, quando constatei tudo o que aqui narro, e muito mais.

Enquanto países como o Canadá e a Noruega possuem níveis elevados de desenvolvimento humano (IDH), outros ao redor do mundo vivem em grande atraso, com pessoas vivendo em palafitas, cabanas de palha, de papelão, de madeira, de barro, etc.

Em Nova Deli, capital da Índia, onde estive em 1.995, famílias inteiras viviam em minúsculas cabanas de pano velho e papelão nas calçadas no centro da cidade, em cumpridas avenidas. E havia na Índia naquela época mais de 400 milhões de miseráveis, numa população de 1 bilhão de pessoas.

Em países como o Brasil, vemos nos centros das grandes cidades edifícios luxuosos e condomínios de mansões, e quando nos afastamos para a periferia vamos nos deparando com casebres, barracos, cabanas de madeira...é um contraste triste de se ver, quando ainda se tem alguma sensibilidade.

O mundo está cheio de obesos, e gente passando fome.

Nos Estados Unidos 70% da população é considerada obesa, o que já é considerado epidemia. E 25% dos alimentos comprados nos restaurantes e lanchonetes vão para o lixo, porque os pratos e sanduíches são extremamente grandes, e nem todos conseguem comer tudo. E pesquisa indicou que esses 25% de alimentos jogados no lixo dariam para alimentar 80 milhões de pessoas, que é muito mais do que a quantidade de miseráveis que existe no Brasil, só para exemplificar.

O mundo produz muito mais alimentos do que seria preciso para alimentar toda a população do planeta. Mas esses alimentos não chegam às mesas dos pobres.

A globalização aumentou o volume de dinheiro circulante no mundo, como já dito antes, mas aumentou a desigualdade entre pobres e ricos. Há menos ricos no mundo, porém eles têm mais dinheiro; e há mais desempregados, sem renda, sem salário.

Há muito a ser modificado no mundo.

O século XX produziu a erotização da sociedade, principalmente a ocidental, a partir do movimento de liberação feminina.

Hoje os adolescentes cada vez mais cedo querem ter vida sexual ativa, mesmo sem qualquer preparo emocional para isso. E a gravidez indesejada e não planejada é apenas uma das muitas conseqüências danosas desse hábito "moderno". E os milhões de abortos anuais no mundo são também conseqüência do sexo desvairado, da liberação excessiva do sexo, do amor livre, e da falta de equilíbrio e maturidade para a vida sexual.

Na primeira metade do século XX, os adolescentes de 13 a 15 anos dificilmente tinham relações sexuais. Hoje, meninas de

13 a 15 anos estão cada vez mais buscando iniciar sua vida sexual. E poucas, no Ocidente, chegam aos 18 anos virgem.

O sexo foi totalmente desvinculado do casamento. É a busca do prazer pelo prazer, e só. Sem compromisso.

Namoro está ficando cada vez mais raro. Os jovens agora chamam de "ficar". Simplesmente ficam uns com os outros por uma noite, numa festa, ou depois da balada em bares, e nunca mais se falam, muitas vezes. O sexo está se tornando cada vez mais animal e banal.

As relações estão ficando cada vez mais superficiais. E isso já atinge os casamentos também.

Pessoas se casam imaturas, e meses ou poucos anos depois já estão se separando. E os filhos ficam à deriva, de uma casa para outra, conhecendo e convivendo com vários namorados de suas mães e namoradas de seus pais. Os filhos de pais separados têm duas casas.

O que tem de filho rebelde porque seus pais se separaram enquanto eles ainda eram crianças não é brincadeira.

É preciso ter mais maturidade emocional antes de se partir para um casamento, porque esse passo importante na vida das pessoas afetará muitas outras, sobretudo os filhos.

A sociedade se tornou tão erótica que hoje em grande parte das propagandas, para vender qualquer coisa, é colocada imagem de mulheres com roupas provocantes, sensuais, quando não quase nuas, para chamar a atenção dos homens, que se tornaram presas fáceis da indústria da propaganda erótica, devido ao seu apego ao sexo e à forma das belas mulheres usadas nas propagandas.

De um aparelho de telefone celular a um carro, de um fogão a um guarda-roupa, tudo requer uma bela mulher na propaganda. E isso levou ao incremento da profissão de modelo. Meninas cada vez mais novas deixam de estudar e se aventuram no mundo das passarelas, com o sonho, muitas vezes realizado, por um único desfile.

A propaganda do sexo na televisão, em telenovelas no final da tarde, incentiva cada vez mais o sexo entre os adolescentes.

A sociedade também se prendeu a uma escravidão da forma. As modelos e artistas belas fazem com que as mulheres que trabalham e criam filhos nunca consigam competir com elas, e fiquem em eterna frustração. Além disso, os maridos vendo na televisão, out doors e no cinema belas mulheres malhadas sentem cada vez mais desejo de se envolver com as belas e jovens mulheres "mecânicas" e artificiais da telinha, e também ficam frustrados, e sentem o seu desejo diminuído pelas esposas que não têm tempo para as academias e não são como as modelos da televisão. A competição é absurda, descabida, e despropositada.

Deu-se na sociedade do século XX uma grande inversão de valores.

Enquanto jogadores de futebol, modelos, artistas e esportistas ganham salários milionários, o resto da população, que trabalha nas diversas profissões, ganha salários baixos. É a inversão da estória infantil da formiga e da cigarra. Hoje, quem passa o verão cantando enquanto o outro está trabalhando para juntar alimento para o inverno terá mais dinheiro e mais conforto do que aquele que passou o verão trabalhando, como as formigas, quando o inverno chegar. A cigarra hoje é a certa, e não a formiga, em nossa sociedade de valores invertidos.

Hoje garotos deixam de ir à escola para ir jogar bola. E quem pode dizer que futebol não dá futuro a ninguém? Olhem os salários milionários dos grandes jogadores hoje. Basquete, vôlei e outros esportes hoje dão muito dinheiro em vários países.

Ser delegado de polícia, médico do Estado, professor de escola pública está em completa desvantagem em relação a quem segue uma carreira esportiva de sucesso, ou a de modelo, desde que a garota seja realmente bela e tenha talento.

No século XXI teremos que rever essas distorções todas, para que as profissões mais importantes para a sociedade voltem a ter o seu devido valor, como os professores e médicos, bem como os cientistas das várias áreas.

Há ainda outras inversões de valores. Hoje alguns bandidos passaram a ser considerados como heróis, como no caso do famoso bandido brasileiro Lampião. Era apenas um líder de quadrilha, que só crimes cometia. Nunca pretendeu fazer revolução para ajudar as pessoas. E hoje muita gente adora e venera lampião. Já se pretendeu até colocar estátua em sua homenagem. E parentes de ex-cangaceiros chegam a dizer na televisão que se orgulham do que seus antepassados fizeram. Se orgulham de seus pais ou avós terem sido criminosos comuns?

Hoje a pessoa comete um crime bárbaro e logo depois do julgamento um escritor ou produtor de cinema logo o procura na prisão para comprar a sua estória e produzir um livro ou um filme que venderá mesmo, e faturará milhões de dólares.

O louco do Antônio Conselheiro, fanático religioso que causou uma guerra no sertão nordestino brasileiro, a famosa Guerra de Canudos, no final do século XIX, causando milhares de mortos e aleijados, órfãos, viúvas e viúvos, já tem estátua no interior da Bahia.

Isso é uma grande inversão de valores.

Ser esperto hoje é sinônimo de inteligente. Mas a esperteza desonesta que toma conta de alguns países como o Brasil é uma tremenda inversão de valores. Políticos desviam dinheiro público e recebem propina com tanta naturalidade, como se isso não fosse errado, que até nos deixa perplexos. Isso se tornou o comum, o normal para muita gente. E não podemos nos esquecer que somos nós, o povo, que colocamos os políticos nos cargos públicos.

Ao escolhermos políticos desonestos, isso pode ser um indicativo de que também nós somos iguais a eles, e que não achamos nada demais eles fazerem o que fazem. E o futuro de nossos filhos? No que eles acreditarão? Em quem eles votarão?

O sistema de transporte individual chegou a níveis absurdos, com milhões de veículos circulando nas grandes cidades, gerando grande poluição, estresse nos congestionamentos, perda de tempo nos deslocamentos e diminuição da qualidade de vida das pessoas.

Uma cidade como São Paulo, uma das maiores do mundo, para onde vou com freqüência, vive uma permanente crise de trânsito. Rodízio entre os veículos, de acordo com o número da placa do carro. Trânsito sempre lento, congestionamentos diários e certos, com grande demora para ir a qualquer lugar. E isso não é exclusividade de São Paulo. Uma cidade como Salvador, capital do Estado da Bahia, no Brasil, onde moro, já vive em certas horas e locais congestionamentos que lembram São Paulo. E há muitas e muitas cidades ao redor do mundo com o mesmo problema. E parece não ter solução.

O individualismo levou a humanidade a optar pelo transporte individual. Há famílias com dois ou até três carros na garagem. Mas as cidades não têm como alargar suas ruas e avenidas, que vão ficando cada vez mais estreitas diante do volume crescente de veículos.

A cada dia milhares de novos carros ganham as ruas nas cidades do mundo, gerando mais congestionamentos, mais poluição, mais aquecimento global e mais estresse. E a qualidade de vida das pessoas cai cada vez mais, e a qualidade do ar também.

A poluição dos rios, lagoas, lagos e mares colocam em risco o manancial de água potável da humanidade. E as calotas polares e também as geleiras das montanhas estão derretendo ligeiramente. Já existe uma grande preocupação com a falta de água no futuro, o que é matéria de freqüentes matérias jornalísticas em todo o mundo.

A população mundial cresce ainda, sobretudo nos países mais pobres, onde não há instrução, meios contraceptivos, e onde as religiões impedem qualquer forma de controle de natalidade. Assim, breve seremos 7 bilhões de habitantes no planeta, e depois 8 bilhões...e por aí vai.

Com a diminuição das guerras, com o maior controle e cura das doenças, e maior previsão de catástrofes naturais, livrando mais pessoas, os reguladores populacionais humanos naturais estão deixando de conter o crescimento populacional.

Na antiguidade, as guerras freqüentes, as doenças várias e as pestes matavam muita gente, e isso era um regulador populacional. Hoje a população já não tem o mesmo tipo de freio. O homem era o predador do próprio homem, e isso diminuiu muito.

A humanidade precisa mudar.

É preciso haver mais solidariedade ainda entre os povos. É preciso investir na educação e no controle de natalidade dos pobres, para conter a multiplicação da miséria. É impensável uma família ter de quatro a oito filhos e esperar que o Estado sustente a todos. O Estado somos todos nós. E não é justo que aqueles que planejam suas famílias tenham que sustentar os filhos dos que não planejam.

A ciência está se desenvolvendo cada vez mais, e ela acabará encontrando soluções para muitos problemas humanos, como as doenças congênitas, os vírus e bactérias novos e super-resistentes, o problema da poluição e dos combustíveis, o problema da água, etc.

A moral humana, no entanto, não tem acompanhado a contento a velocidade das mudanças científicas e tecnológicas. A moral humana não evoluiu muito, em seu conjunto, na mesma velocidade do avanço da ciência.

Hoje temos ainda pessoas que se comportam de modo muito semelhante aos humanos de dois mil anos atrás, como os romanos, os gregos, os persas, os "bárbaros".

Pessoas "civilizadas" ainda saem de suas casas para um jantar levando arma de fogo. E matam por motivos muitas vezes fúteis. Uma simples discussão no trânsito, que poderia tranqüilamente terminar em uma delegacia de polícia ou num tribunal pequeno muitas vezes termina no cemitério.

Há uma música brasileira, da banda Titãs, que diz "polícia para quem precisa, polícia para quem precisa de polícia". Isso bem demonstra que há pessoas que ainda precisam de polícia, para vigiarem seus atos, nem sempre corretos e honestos. E há pessoas que não mais precisam de polícia.

Quanto mais polícia nas ruas, mais pessoas violentas, desonestas e violadoras de direitos há na cidade. É claro que isso não é regra absoluta, pois existem países com muita violência urbana, como no Brasil, sem a correspondente quantidade de polícia nas ruas, mas neste caso é por falta de condições da administração pública, o que é diferente.

Precisamos nos tornar mais honestos, respeitando as coisas públicas, e também o direito dos outros de possuírem seus bens. Precisamos respeitar as regras de trânsito, os sinais de trânsito, mesmo sem a presença do policial. Respeitar as filas, a ordem de preferência, etc.

Grande parte da Europa já atingiu esse nível de educação, e também o Japão. Mas muitos países mais pobres estão longe dessa realidade.

Precisamos nos tornar menos agressivos, menos violentos, tanto no falar quanto no agir no dia a dia. Isso vai fazer das cidades lugares mais calmos e menos estressantes para se viver.

Precisamos cuidar mais de nossas crianças e jovens, retirando-os das ruas e dando-lhes educação, esporte, lazer, comida e profissão. A maior violência começa nas ruas, com os menores pedindo nos semáforos, e muitas vezes roubando, ameaçando com cacos de vidro, pregos, canivetes, facas, quando não com revólveres mesmo. Essa ainda é uma realidade em muitas cidades brasileiras.

Acredito que para a humanidade tenha sido fixado um tempo para o seu desenvolvimento moral, não apenas para o desenvolvimento científico e tecnológico.

O desenvolvimento científico e tecnológico já chegou a níveis muito bons, neste início de século XXI. Todavia, o ser humano ainda dá mostras diárias da bestialidade, do desajuste, do desequilíbrio, da agressividade animal, às vezes pior do que os animais.

Acho mesmo que esse tempo dado para a evolução moral da humanidade está se esgotando. As "crianças" humanas já passaram do tempo de amadurecer. Resistem a crescer. E por isso virão as catástrofes descritas no Apocalipse, em complementação a tudo quanto antes já havia falado Jesus e outros profetas judeus antes dele.

Os sinais do fim dos tempos estão aí, quase todos, como vimos ao longo desta obra. E outros se mostrarão no devido tempo, que pode ser amanhã, no ano que vem, daqui a dez ou cinqüenta anos, ou mais. Ninguém sabe, nem mesmo Jesus, como por ele mesmo afirmado.

Ele nos recomendou a oração e a vigilância, para tentarmos evitar o sofrimento que virá. Mas nos deu a certeza de que as coisas por ele previstas aconteceriam. Assim, não se trata de possibilidade de se concretizarem as profecias sobre o Juízo Final, mas de certeza.

A vinda de um cometa acompanhado de inúmeros meteoros e sua queda na Terra é uma certeza, afirmada por Jesus, sobretudo. E ele fez revelações mais detalhadas a João, seu apóstolo mais novo, que estão contidas no livro Apocalipse.

Decifrando o Apocalipse, depois de anos de estudos, e só agora tomando coragem para escrever a respeito, porque somente aos 48 anos me sinto mais maduro, e depois de mais de 18 anos trabalhando como Juiz do Trabalho, com uma grande prática na análise e interpretação de textos e sua comparação, bem como a análise comparativa de depoimentos às vezes divergentes de testemunhas.

Minha profissão me deu grande ferramenta para a leitura e interpretação sistemática dos textos bíblicos. Além disso, estudo religião, filosofia, misticismo e muitas outras coisas desde os 17 anos, o que me deu uma visão mais larga e profunda dos escritos bíblicos.

Devemos nos preparar para o que vier. Se não acontecerem os fatos neste século, poderá ser no próximo, mas o fim dos tempos das nações está se concretizando, e o Dia do Juízo Final está mesmo próximo.

Não pretendo fazer nenhuma forma de terrorismo, como alguns poderão pensar. Não sou fanático de forma alguma.

Apenas meus estudos e tudo o que venho acompanhando no mundo pela TV, jornais, revistas, livros, internet, nas ruas, etc., têm me mostrado que estamos chegando ao limite de nosso estilo de vida e civilização, e que precisamos mudar mesmo.

O modelo de cidades gigantes, com transporte individual não pode mais subsistir. A pobreza tem que acabar. O egoísmo do capitalismo tem que ceder lugar a um capitalismo mais humanista. O socialismo sem direito de manifestação e liberdade de expressão tem que desaparecer. As pessoas têm que sair de casa sabendo que a ela retornarão, sem medo de serem mortas nas sinaleiras por um adolescente que quer um relógio, um colar, uma bolsa ou uma carteira de dinheiro.

A destruição daquele dia, do Dia do Juízo Universal, reduzirá enormemente a população da Terra, e aqui somente ficarão os mansos, como disse Jesus, aqueles que não são lobos do seu irmão, que são incapazes de fabricar armas para ameaçar e ferir o seu próximo, que são incapazes de levar uma nação à guerra, incapazes de assaltar e roubar os pertences de seu irmão humano, incapazes de ferir os animais apenas para o seu deleite nas caçadas estúpidas, incapazes de poluir as águas dos rios e dos mares apenas para verem suas empresas prosperarem, incapazes de mentir para serem eleitos a cargos públicos, incapazes de desviar dinheiro público para suas contas em outros países.

Como se vê, muita gente precisa mesmo ser expulsa da Terra para que ela mude de nível, para que ela se renove, e dê um grande passo qualitativo.

A humanidade do futuro será uma humanidade pacífica, sem armas de forma alguma, próspera do ponto de vista econômico, e com uma conduta ética e moral muito melhor do que a da humanidade de hoje.

Pode parecer crueldade divina a destruição que virá. Mas ela, mesmo sendo uma catástrofe natural, que muitos podem inclusive atribuir ao mero acaso, ou a forças cegas da natureza, na forma da vinda de um cometa em nossa direção, sem que ninguém tenha planejado isso, provocará a renovação da Terra, seja no seu aspecto físico, seja no moral dos homens.

Os dinossauros foram extintos para que a humanidade pudesse surgir, pois com eles os humanos não sobreviveriam. Os dinossauros também eram seres vivos. Mas a sua era passou. Novas espécies teriam que surgir. E eles eram um empecilho para as novas espécies menores, como os mamíferos, e depois os símios, até a chegada do homem, na visão da ciência.

A natureza muitas vezes destrói coisas velhas para criar coisas novas. É a renovação. Até estrelas e planeta são destruídos pelo universo afora.

O Homem de Neandertal, já humano, provavelmente foi destruído e extinto pelo homem moderno, a nossa espécie. Homem acabando como homem, por serem um pouco diferentes fisicamente. Deve ter havido o genocídio do Homem de Neandertal pelo Homem moderno.

Assim, também, a velha humanidade será em parte destruída, para dar nascimento a uma nova humanidade.

Terrenos já cansados serão submersos, e renovados com o tempo; e terras submersas virão para a superfície do planeta, novas e férteis.

A poluição sofrerá um freio brusco, com a destruição de grande parte dos agentes poluentes: veículos, embarcações, fábricas, etc.

Uma verdadeira parada para balanço. Um fechamento para balanço.

Depois desses dias, muitas coisas mudarão. A humanidade nunca mais será a mesma. Nem o globo terrestre, que sofrerá uma certa inclinação em seu eixo, ao que indicam as profecias. O clima no planeta sofrerá mudanças.

Ninguém, no entanto, deve ter medo. A alma é imortal!

Mas as almas dos maus, dos que resistirem à mudança, que se comprazem no mal, não mais ficarão aqui na Terra. Irão para o Inferno, que poderá ser em um lugar no mundo espiritual, não na Terra, ou irão para planeta mais atrasado e em início de desenvolvimento, conforme a crença de cada um.

Uma coisa é certa, os maus serão retirados da Terra. Portanto, quem quiser continuar aqui que trate de se adequar às novas condições da futura humanidade.

Egoísmo extremo, agressividade, violência, desonestidade, inveja que leva a tomar o que é dos outros, corrupção, ambição desmedida. Nada disso terá espaço na nova humanidade, na Terra futura, depois daqueles dias previstos no Apocalipse.

Assim, quem quiser permanecer aqui, que comece a mudar já, porque não sabemos nem poderemos prever exatamente quando chegará o Dia do Juízo Final, o dia do último julgamento das almas que vivem na Terra.

Apocalipse é Revelação. E tudo está revelado!

Ouça quem tiver ouvidos para ouvir!

Veja quem tiver olhos de ver!

Acredite se quiser!

Mas ele virá!

E breve!

Que Deus nos dê sabedoria e forças para mudar, e para nos prepararmos para o dia do Juízo Final que se aproxima.

E que assim seja!

REFERÊNCIAS BIBLIOGRÁFICAS:

BÍBLIA SAGRADA, Edição Barsa de 1.969;
ENCYCLOPAEDIA BRITANNICA DO BRASIL PUBLICAÇÕES LTDA (BARSA), livros e CD-ROOM, Edição de 1.997;
NOSTRADAMUS – AS PROFECIAS DO FUTURO, de A. Galloti, Editora Nova Era, 2ª Edição;
OS MILAGRES DE JESUS CRISTO, Luiz Roberto Mattos, edição particular;
O SANTO SUDÁRIO: MILAGROSA FALSIFICAÇÃO?, de Julio Marvizón Preny, Editora Mercúrio, 1.998;
REVISTA SUPER INTERESSANTE: Ano 12, nº 6 (junho de 1.998);
REVISTA GLOBO CIÊNCIA, Ano 7, nº 77;
REVISTA TERRA, maio de 2.003, Ano 12.

Printed in Great Britain
by Amazon

47051002R00106